A Guide for Health and Beauty Therapists

A GUIDE FOR
Health and Beauty Therapists

Volume 1: Face, Hands and Feet

SECOND EDITION

Gaynor Winyard

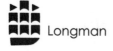 Longman

Addison Wesley Longman Limited
Edinburgh Gate, Harlow
Essex CM20 2JE, England
and Associated Companies throughout the world

© Longman Group UK Limited 1990
© Addison Wesley Longman Limited 1996

First published 1990
Fourth impression 1994
Second edition 1996

British Library Cataloguing in Publication Data
A catalogue entry for this title is available from the British Library

ISBN 0-582-24790-X

Set by 3 in $9\frac{1}{2}$/11pt Palatino
Produced by Longman Singapore Publishers (Pte) Ltd
Printed in Singapore

Contents

Contra-indications   Dry hands   Moist and clammy hands
Enlarged knuckles   Warts   Self assessment

Foreword

There are books, and books, on beauty – and there will no doubt be more to come. But, while many make pleasant reading, few treat the subject with such clinical accuracy as this guide by Gaynor Winyard.

To call it a guide is almost too modest, for the author tackles her subject – or more accurately we should say subjects (plural) – by going into detail at the outset on the structure of the human cell and the tissues and systems of the body.

This, surely, is the right approach, for unless the beauty therapist seriously addresses the deeper physiological aspects, she will never appreciate that beauty is very much more than skin-deep. For it is, in the final analysis, a matter of *health*.

Quite properly, Gaynor Winyard provides us with chapters on skin types, lesions, diseases and tumours and pigmentary disorders. And many a lay person would be grateful for the chapters that cover care of the hands, and in particular the nails which always either make or mar a hand's appearance.

The technical side of therapy is also treated in some depth, with a chapter on electrophysics, and invaluable guidance on high-frequency currents and heat treatments.

This responsible and thoroughgoing attitude to the subject of beauty will surprise no one who knows Gaynor Winyard. Her remarkable grasp of her subject comes from a very wide experience of all facets of beauty therapy, and we should not forget that she is an innovator as well as 'a guru'.

As Director of the flourishing Stobo Castle Health Spa in the Scottish Borders, she continues to put her knowledge to excellent use, guiding and still teaching her bright young team.

Students in the many schools and colleges nationwide where beauty therapy is taught will find this the textbook *par excellence* as – one fancies – will their peers who lead the courses, and who will surely give *A Guide for Health and Beauty Therapists* the warm welcome it deserves.

MG
October 1990

Acknowledgements

The author and publishers are grateful to the following for permission to reproduce copyright material:

Churchill Livingstone for our Figs 3.1–2, 4.2–3, 4.4(b)–(d), 4.5(a) & (b), 4.6, 5.1–2, 5.3(a), 5.4, 6.3–5, 6.8–9, 20.2, 26.1–2, 26.4, 26.9 and 32.6–8 from *Anatomy and physiology in health and illness* by J.S. Ross & K.J.W. Wilson; our Figs 4.4(a), 4.7, 20.1 from *Physiology for health care* by J. Hubbard & D. Meehan; our Fig. 5.5 from *Anatomy & physiology* by Cambridge Communication Ltd.

Addison Wesley Longman Limited for our Figs 6.1–2, 7.6, 22.6 and 22.7(b) from *Advanced hairdressing science* by F. Openshaw; our Figs 7.1–4, 7.7–9, 14.1–10, 16.1, 16.3, 26.3, 26.7–8, 27.1, 28.2–3, 28.6–7, 28.9, 28.12 and 31.1 from *Cosmetic make-up and manicure* by A. Eaton & F. Openshaw; our Figs 22.7(a), 22.14, 36.2 and 36.6 from *Beauty therapy science* by R. Bembridge.

Thanks are also due to John Woodruff, Cosmetic Chemist, for his technical and professional contributions, and to Mike Devlin who took the photographs.

Acknowledgements

1 The salon

Beauty therapists usually commence their careers as an employee, or by renting space in a hairdressing salon or leisure club to gain invaluable experience. Later, renting or taking a lease or purchase of premises for a salon, may be considered. The location of the salon is paramount, it should be easy to find, convenient for clients travelling by public transport and, ideally, have car parking space. If possible try to find ground-floor premises, it is always easier for clients to walk straight into the salon, rather than having to climb stairs.

Layout of the salon

This is very important and should be given very careful thought and possibly engaging the services of an expert. Even though you may only start your salon for the face, hands and feet, you must adhere to certain standards to comply with the laws of any country to commence trading. There must be adequate lighting, power sockets, ventilation, heating, hot and cold water supply, fire extinguishers, toilet facilities for clients and staff, a rest area for staff and adequate working space in the salon. When planning the layout of the salon consideration should be given to a reception area, treatment cubicles and a laundry area. The decor of the salon is a personal choice but it is wise to adapt the colour scheme to the type of client you are hoping to attract.

Equipment for the salon

The amount of equipment purchased will depend on the amount you can afford, your specialist skills and the space available. For the face, hands and feet, one multipurpose treatment couch will suffice. The following is a list of suggested items:

- trolley/s to hold equipment with drawers for treatment materials for the face, hands and feet, and small instruments
- adjustable stool/s
- magnifying light or Wood's light (this can be supplied with a bracket which is clamped to the trolley, so saving space)
- sterilising unit
- facial steamer
- galvanic machine
- high-frequency unit
- vacuum-suction machine
- brush-massage machine

- cosmetic stand (this is often provided by the manufacturer or supplier)
- electrolysis machine.

Some stock and other miscellaneous items are also required and these have been listed under 'preparation' for each treatment in following chapters.

Health and safety in the salon

There are health and safety laws in every country, some are more strict than others but all insist that health and safety procedures are carried out in the salon to protect staff and clients. Most countries, including the UK, send inspectors to salons periodically to check the standards. They will send the manager/owner of the salon a report on their findings. Any areas that the inspectors find contravening health and safety requirements should be corrected as soon as possible. If on their return the measures suggested have not been carried out it could jeopardise the business, i.e. by being fined or prosecuted, which would result in bad publicity, possibly loss of trade and staff and could end in the closure of the business.

Responsibility of employer

Laws in every country vary but they all state that the employer must maintain a safe and healthy working environment; ensuring that all employees are trained in safety procedures for electricity, gas, chemicals, storage and disposal of waste and hazardous materials and security. Salon and personal hygiene should be continually supervised.

The employer of the salon must ensure that electrical equipment is checked and certified, at least annually, by a qualified electrician; that the fire extinguishers are of the recommended type, checked periodically and a written record kept by the salon. Emergency or fire exits must be clearly marked and all entrances and exits kept completely clear. The salon should also be well ventilated and lighting must be adequate.

A first-aid box should be easily identified, containing the following:

- a guidance card
- sterile bandages of different sizes
- assorted waterproof plasters
- sterile and unsterile dressings
- an eye bath and sterile eye pads
- surgical adhesive tape
- bandages (including crêpe and a triangular bandage)
- an antiseptic solution
- medical wipes, cotton wool, scissors, tweezers, safety pins and disposable gloves.

At least one member of staff should be trained in first-aid and know how to deal with minor accidents and what to do in an emergency.

Symptoms and conditions together with immediate first-aid suggestions are covered in Chapter 16, Volume 2.

A list of the safety procedures should be displayed in the staff area
for anyone to read and should include telephone numbers for emer-
gencies (e.g. electrician, electricity board, gas fitter, gas supply emergency service (if the salon has a gas supply), plumber, the local doctor,
hospital, fire station and police station.

Responsibility of employee

An employee, on the other hand, should make sure that the safety procedures are understood, make every effort to avoid injury to clients/
staff and report to the employer any potential hazards immediately
(e.g. light bulbs failing, fuses blowing, wires fraying, defective furniture or equipment and blocked sinks or drains). Salons should have an
'action' book to record any defects and this should be brought to the
attention of the employer on a daily basis. Remember, the spoken
word can be forgotten but the written word can hardly be ignored!

Salon safety

Electricity

It is very important that leads/flexes are maintained in pristine condition (no fraying wires exposed) and all broken plugs are replaced
immediately. You should ensure that the correct fuse is used for all
equipment (see Chapter 21 on Electro-physics) and that electrical circuits are not overloaded. All electrical equipment (including wall
heaters) must be disconnected from the sockets at the end of the day.
You should always ensure the mains are switched off before repairing
fuses or switches. Always switch off the light switch before replacing a
lamp and disconnect electrical equipment prior to cleaning. Remember,
electricity and water rarely mix, so never have wet hands or stand on a
wet floor when handling live electrical equipment.

Gas

There are salons with a *gas* supply, be it for heating the premises and/or
water. If you should smell gas, speak to someone in authority, check
any gas appliances to see if they are switched on without a flame and
check the pilot light. If there are, turn them off immediately and open
windows to get rid of the gas. Should you not find an appliance which
has been left on then you may have a leak and the gas should be turned
off at the mains. You will find the mains tap near your gas meter. It is
wise then to explain the situation to the clients in the salon and to take
them to a safe area. Whatever happens do not allow anyone to smoke
or use a naked flame. Do not turn electrical switches either on or off as
a small spark inside the switch may ignite the gas. Seek immediate
assistance by either telephoning the gas fitter or the gas emergency
service.

Chemicals

In most countries there are laws which govern the use of chemicals especially those of a hazardous nature. In the UK COSHH (Control of Substances Hazardous to Health) Act is applicable and it is necessary to carry out certain safety precautions. To help you, manufacturers will produce a Product Safety Data Sheet for all their products which will state whether any item is hazardous, toxic or flammable and how they should be stored; the method of mopping up spillage and any first-aid procedures to be taken if ingested, inhaled or if an irritant to the skin or eyes.

As a general guide:

Flammable products in a salon include items such as acetone, aerosols, liquids containing alcohol, nail polish thinners and removers, some equipment cleaners and sterilising agents. These should be kept in closed containers, clearly labelled, away from heat and sunlight and separated from oxidisers, e.g. hydrogen peroxide. Large quantities must be stored in a fire resistant area. If a fire should occur the extinguisher should be foam, powder, carbon dioxide or water fog, water should not be used in a jet and always advise the firemen of their presence. In the unlikely event of ingestion give plenty of milk or water and obtain immediate medical advice. Excessive exposure to inhalation may cause dizziness and fresh air is advised. Prolonged contact with the skin should be avoided and if eyes are affected, irrigate them well with water and if irritation persists medical help should be sought. All spillages should be cleaned up with a detergent and water.

Skin irritants or sensitisers include such items as hydrogen peroxide, eyelash tints, skin bleach, most nail technology products and some equipment cleaners or sterilising agents. These should be re-sealed after use or kept in closed containers and stored in a cool, dry place. Hydrogen peroxide, because it can give off oxygen when heated, can be a fire risk if stored near flammable products. In a beauty salon the bottles are usually very small and the risk is minimal but play safe and keep them apart. Contact with the skin should be avoided where possible, gloves can be worn when using cleaners or sterilising products. There are exceptions (see Chapter 16 on eyelash tinting) when a patch test is performed to check for any allergies. Should a client have an adverse reaction to a product remove it immediately and wash well with plenty of warm water and blot dry. For accidental ingestion, inhalation or contact with the eyes follow the same first-aid procedure as for flammable products.

Fine powders e.g. loose powder in cosmetics, talcum powder or powder used for certain types of masks can cause irritation by inhaling the very fine particles. Care should be taken when using these to avoid inhalation and lids must be replaced immediately after use. If you are dispensing large quantities of powder, a face mask should be worn and these can be obtained from any pharmacy. For accidental inhalation wash the skin and eyes well and move to the fresh air.

Disposal of waste products

This will vary from Council to Council in the UK and from country to country abroad. As we become more and more environmentally minded waste is becoming classified, inasmuch as it is divided into areas, e.g. paper, bottles, cans, hazardous materials etc.

Presently, it is possible in most areas to put used paper, i.e. from couches, tissues, disposable head caps, make-up capes etc., together with used disposable brushes, cotton wool, wooden spatulas, gauze, etc., in a plastic bag and tied.

Bottles and cans should be separately bagged and it may be necessary to take these to a bottle bank and cans to a special area.

Hazardous materials include needles and glass phials and these must be put into a metal box with a lid and labelled (e.g. a Sharps box); aerosol cans (which should never be punctured) and any flammable product. You should seek advice from your local environmental department for the disposal of waste. In the UK the new Environmental Protection Act, Duty of Care, became effective in April 1992 and it applies to everyone who has to dispose of waste. At the moment it seems more applicable to large businesses but inevitably smaller businesses will soon be involved. Many countries in Europe have very strict laws pertaining to waste. At the end of the day, all waste must be secured/contained and removed from the salon.

Fire

Materials such as towels, blankets, sheets etc., should not be put over gas or electric heaters, as this prevents the circulation of air whereby the heater could over-heat or the materials could dry, burn and catch fire.

Cigarettes can often be the cause of a fire when they are not extinguished properly and thrown into a bin. If you *do* allow clients or staff to smoke, and this is not recommended, make sure there are ashtrays available. A little water can be added to the ashtray before the contents are thrown away.

Although a fire in the salon is unlikely, you must familiarise yourself with the fire extinguishers and/or blanket, where they are situated and the exits to be used. You should also know how to deal with a fire, e.g. if a person's clothes catch fire smother them with damp towels or if a bin ignites, close the lid to starve the fire of oxygen. In the case of other fires, if possible, close windows and doors and use the appropriate fire extinguisher or blanket without risk to yourself. Should you be unable to contain the fire, make sure clients (and any other personnel) have left the premises, then telephone the fire brigade or dial 999 giving the name of the salon and the address, then leave the building.

Accidents

Accidents can be prevented by being alert at all times. Ensure that:

- there are no trailing leads/flexes to trip over

- spillages (water or products) are mopped up immediately
- electricity, gas and chemicals are handled safely
- accidents are written into an 'accident' book, giving name, date, time and cause, together with action taken immediately and any follow-up information recorded.

Salon security

The security of the salon is usually the responsibility of the salon owner, i.e. to provide locks/bolts to doors and windows, double locks to external doors and usually installing a burglar alarm, to ensure adequate protection for both the premises and contents. There is always a greater risk of burglary when the salon is closed and during the hours of darkness. Liaison with the police is very helpful as they have personnel to advise on security, they may suggest leaving a light on outside or inside the salon, checking security for the rear of the building, holding a key to the premises, perhaps linking the burglar alarm to the police station or even an answer-phone system for the front door.

The employer or a senior member of staff will be responsible for the keys and for locking up the salon and that includes ensuring that stock cupboards are locked, doors and windows checked, the external doors double locked and for switching on the alarm (if installed). Very little money, perhaps a small float, should be left in the till. Banking should be done during the day but if it has to be deposited in the night safe, it is wise to be accompanied. The external doors to the salon should be locked from the inside during the time that you are preparing to open or close the salon, especially if you are on your own.

The reception area is vulnerable during business hours with clients arriving and leaving, telephone enquiries etc., and at the same time ensuring that retail stock on display is not handled or stolen. It is safer to have stock in a locked glass cabinet, or shelves in front of the reception desk with lockable glass doors. You can always arrange an eye-catching display of dummy products in the reception area or, if you have a window, on the window sill. The police should be advised if theft occurs and it will be helpful to them if you write a report giving any relevant information. No person, other than staff and clients should enter the salon without producing identification, e.g. inspectors, readers of the gas or electricity meters or Council employees etc.

Money is the greatest temptation of all! Larger salons will have a full-time receptionist but smaller salons may not have this luxury. It is preferable to have an electronic till with only one or two people having keys for access but if this is not possible, always take out the larger bank notes and put them in a safe place out of sight.

Stock is money and it should be safeguarded in a similar way. Retail stock should be kept separately from salon stock, i.e. consumables, and a good system for recording both should exist. It is better if the manager/owner or one member of staff has a key to storage areas, and is responsible for the issuing of stock and keeping records, i.e. the date, the item taken out, checking the quantity left, re-ordering levels and recording orders received. Dependent on the size of the salon and the procedures adopted, all stock should be physically checked at least once a month.

Personal property, whether belonging to clients or staff should be kept in a safe area. Staff handbags etc., should be kept preferably in a locker or locked cupboard/area, or at least out of sight. The therapist should ensure that clients' property, i.e. handbags or jewellery is kept safe and is visible to the client.

Salon hygiene

Hygiene practices in the salon are paramount to prevent cross-infection and, to reassure clients, must be apparent by the obvious use of disposable materials, the sterilisation of equipment and a high standard of cleanliness throughout the salon.

Blood infections

With the advent of the deadly virus condition known as *AIDS* (Acquired Immune Deficiency Syndrome) people have undoubtedly become very sensitive and conscious of hygiene standards particularly in beauty salons and health and leisure areas. The virus responsible is HIV (Human Immunodeficiency Virus) and has been found in human blood, semen and saliva, but fortunately it does not live long outside the body. It attacks the body's natural immune system and makes the system more vulnerable to other infections and it is the build-up of these other infections that eventually result in death. A blood test is the only way to verify whether a person has the AIDS virus. If the result is HIV positive, it will mean that the person has been exposed to the virus but may not develop AIDS. However, that person is a 'carrier' of the disease and is capable of passing on the virus to someone else through infected blood or tissue fluid. You are only at risk if the infected blood, from an HIV positive person, enters a break in your skin, be it a cut, an abrasion or eczema.

Prevention, by covering broken skin, is the most important aspect until more is known about the disease and immunisation is possible.

Other infectious blood diseases include hepatitis, both A and B. Hepatitis is the inflammation of the liver which may be secondary to other disorders, e.g. amoebic dysentery, cirrhosis; it may be drug induced or it may be a viral infection. *HAV* is the virus hepatitis A, and is found in infected faeces and is caused by infected food or drink. *HBV* is the virus hepatitis B, which is transmitted in blood and tissue fluids and is highly infectious. Unlike the AIDS virus, HBV can survive outside the body for a very long time. However, for this disease, immunisation is now possible.

Strict hygiene practices are paramount in the salon as a tiny drop of blood or even dried blood is infectious. You will now appreciate how important it is to cover broken skin with a plaster. If blood is spilt in the salon, disposable gloves must be worn and it should be wiped up immediately with household bleach. Extreme caution should be exercised if there is a need to handle used sanitary towels or tampons. There are companies, e.g. Rentokil who provide a service, but they are expensive.

The use of the autoclave (see below) will sterilise implements as heat will destroy the viruses as will most disinfectants if used correctly.

Sterilisation

Sterilisation is the destruction of bacteria (which are described in Chapter 9), and in the salon it can be carried out in several ways.

The most effective method for small implements is the use of an autoclave (see Fig. 1.1.) which acts on the same principle as a pressure cooker. It has two compartments, the upper area has a tray for implements and the lower area is for the water, which is contained under pressure at 121 °C (282 °F) for fifteen minutes. Most autoclaves used for beauty therapy have an automatic timer and pressure gauge, a steam release valve to allow steam to escape and a safety valve (in case the valve becomes blocked). Word of caution, *never* attempt to open the lid of the autoclave until all the steam has escaped, otherwise scalding may result.

Another method most commonly used is the ultra-violet cabinet (see Fig. 1.2.) which can accommodate larger implements, including brushes, glass electrodes and ventouses. However, UV radiation will only sterilise the surfaces the rays touch, so it will be necessary to turn

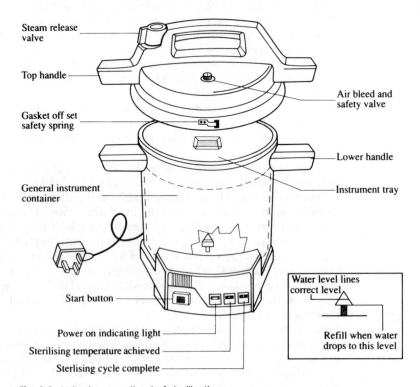

Fig. 1.1 Autoclave method of sterilisation

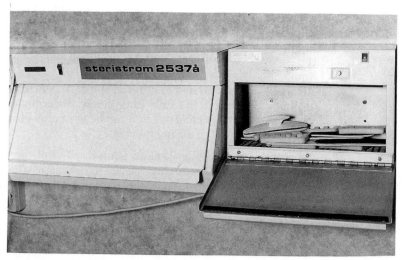

Fig. 1.2 Ultra-violet cabinet

the implements after fifteen minutes. However, if for any reason, blood has come into contact with the implement UV radiation may not destroy all bacteria, it must be placed in a disinfectant first. The cabinet itself must be cleaned regularly, especially the tubes to ensure their efficiency.

For very small items, a glass-bead steriliser can be used. There are several types and the temperatures reached can vary between 190–300 °C (374–572 °F). Read the manufacturer's instructions as you may need to turn on the steriliser for quite some time before use. Instruments like scissors, cuticle knives etc., should be put well down into the beads for the required time. Because of its limited use in the salon this steriliser is rarely used.

Disinfectants

These can be used as they also work against bacteria and fungi if used long enough and the solution is strong enough, e.g.,

1. Coal tar derivatives – e.g. Dettol, which includes phenol and cresols, is diluted according to the manufacturer's instructions. Salon surfaces can be cleaned and it can also be used in a container to immerse implements.
2. Hypochlorites – e.g. Milton or Domestos, which are a form of chlorine bleach, are very effective against all germs including viruses and spores. However, hypochlorites can corrode metal so are not recommended for manicure tools and the ends of electrodes.
3. Quats – (quaternary ammonium compounds) e.g. Savlon or Cetrimide, will prevent bacteria from spreading. However, they are not compatible with anionic detergents, i.e. soaps or shampoos as their effectiveness is cancelled out.
4. Glutaraldehyde – e.g. Cidex, a 2 per cent solution will remain

effective for 14–18 days, after which time it must be thrown away. Implements including metal instruments should be immersed in the liquid for about ten minutes. It is advisable to wear thin surgical-type gloves (which are commercially available) when using the liquid.

5. Alcohol – e.g. methylated or surgical spirit, 70 per cent isopropopyl alcohol can be used, but only once before discarding and it has a very effective bactericidal effect. It can be used on tools and the skin and has the benefit of drying quickly.

Whatever method of sterilisation is used, all implements, brushes, sponges etc., must be thoroughly washed in hot soapy water and dried prior to the use of a disinfectant (wet implements, sponges etc., dilute the solution) before being placed in an ultra-violet cabinet or autoclave.

General hygiene in the salon should include the following:

- flooring and walls should be easy to clean, curtains and blinds should be washed regularly
- keeping the salon spotlessly clean, including all fittings, windows, ledges, equipment, trolleys, washhand basins and toilets
- regularly laundering a blanket (if used for facials)
- using fresh couch paper for each client
- providing each client with clean towels
- washing your own hands prior to, and sometimes during, a treatment
- using implements that have been cleaned and sterilised
- ensuring surface areas are wiped daily with a disinfectant, including, at least once a week, couches, legs of trolleys and chairs
- making sure equipment and implements are sterilised immediately after use and are kept in a hygienic area, i.e. an ultra-violet cabinet or in surgical spirit, e.g. cuticle knives and nippers etc.
- using the correct method of waste disposal after each treatment
- disposable gloves are removed from wrists and turned inside out.

Salon plumbing

Washbasins and toilets are connected to the main drainage and if allowed to become blocked, will not only cause unpleasant smells but increase bacterial growth in the stale water. Where basins are concerned, before calling out the plumber, try to dislodge the blockage with a plunger and if this does not work have a look at the waste trap which can be found beneath the sink. Usually there is a screw plug on the S bend which can be opened. Place a bucket under the bend, unscrew the plug and let the waste water flow out and you can see if the blockage is between the basin and the S bend. Another means to clear a blockage is to pour a solution of sodium hydroxide (caustic soda) into the waste pipe. Great care should be taken when handling this substance, gloves must be worn as it is corrosive to skin and eyes. Once the blockage has been removed, replace the screw plug, flush the basin clear with running water and dispose of the contents of the bucket.

If these means fail, call out the plumber as it is obvious that the obstruction is beyond the waste trap.

Burst pipes often happen in extremes of cold weather and you should find out where the relevant stop-cocks are situated so that they can be turned off in an emergency.

Toilets must be cleaned regularly followed by the use of a household bleach. A covered bin should be supplied in the ladies' toilet for sanitary towels. Blockages in the toilet are often caused by insoluble towels or tampons. Any problems with toilets must be reported immediately to the employer or senior member of staff for a plumber to attend.

Salon ventilation

Ventilation is the process where stale air is replaced by fresh air and this can be achieved by the use of extractor fans and/or opening windows above head height. If the salon is warm and humid, there is a build-up of carbon dioxide in the air, oxygen levels are reduced, smells produced by certain products linger through lack of circulation and all provide ideal conditions for bacteria and infection to spread. The ideal temperature in the salon should range from 16–24 °C (60 to 75 °F), which can be maintained by a thermostatically controlled heating system or by air conditioning. It is important to keep the salon fresh and comfortable for clients and to provide you with ideal working conditions. Find out how to regulate the ventilation and heating systems in your salon.

Salon lighting

Lighting in the salon should be adequate, not be so bright as to cause a glare, but adequate enough to prevent accidents in the salon or cause eye-strain. Natural daylight is ideal but often has to be augmented with artificial light. Some areas may require increased lighting, e.g. passageways and staircases, in other areas, diffused lighting will make the light softer. Warm white fluorescent tubes imitate daylight and are useful when applying colours for make-up or using nail polish. For close work, special lighting is needed, e.g. a magnifying light. You should ensure that the lighting is sufficient and report any faulty bulbs or flickering tubes to the employer, or write it in the action book so that these can be replaced.

Personal hygiene and appearance

Personal hygiene and appearance are paramount. The salon will be judged on the appearance of the receptionist and therapists. In our particular industry image is all important, therefore, you should ensure *that*:

1. Intimate personal hygiene is carried out to prevent body odours, e.g.

at least daily showers/baths; the use of deodorants/anti-perspirants; bad breath is avoided by regular dental hygiene and when necessary the use of a breath freshener.
2. You do not smoke, the smell will not only come from your breath, but also from your hair and clothes.
3. You always wear a clean, pressed overall and make sure it is loose enough to allow movement.
4. Jewellery is not worn, with perhaps the exception of a wedding ring and/or discreet ear-rings.
5. Hair is clean and kept well off the face.
6. Shoes are clean and comfortable, preferably with closed toes and rubber soles.
7. If tights/stockings are worn, make sure these are fresh and not laddered.
8. Light make-up is worn and refreshed during break times.
9. Your nails are short and clean and devoid of nail polish.

In other words you are 'squeaky' clean and immaculate!

Self assessment

In order to commence trading you must adhere to certain standards, name at least six of these.

- as a manager/owner of the salon, what training are you responsible for?
- name at least nine items which should be included in the first-aid box
- as an employee, how would you ensure that defects are reported?
- what would you do if you could smell gas?
- what steps would you take to safeguard money, stock and personal property in the salon?
- what is AIDS? and state the main difference between AIDS and Hepatitis B
- describe three ways to sterilise implements
- name at least three disinfectants that work against bacteria
- what measures would you take to ensure general hygiene in the salon?
- why is good ventilation so important?
- how would you dispose of hazardous materials?
- how would you achieve strict personal hygiene and an immaculate appearance?

2 Reception and initial consultation

Reception

The following is primarily for beauty therapists working in a beauty salon rather than a hairdressing salon, or a health and leisure club, where the reception desk for appointments is shared. With public awareness now-a-days of the treatments available, clients expect friendly and efficient service by trained staff, value for money and excellent facilities.

Reception area

The reception area creates the first impression of your salon, so it should be pleasant in decor and spotlessly clean. The furniture should be comfortable and literature and magazines up-to-date. If you have room for a display unit ensure that the products are attractively presented, clearly priced and regularly rearranged when cleaning. A price list for treatments should be clear and easy to read and placed in a prominent position. If beverages are supplied make sure empty cups and saucers are removed immediately and the table wiped.

The reception desk itself should look uncluttered, with only the appointment book, telephone, holder for pens and pencils etc., and a jotting pad. If the desk is large enough, an electronic till could sit on top, a price list for treatments and/or products could be displayed and, perhaps, a small arrangement of flowers (these should *look fresh* daily!). Underneath keep telephone books, box for client's cards (in the absence of a computer), possibly the till and other miscellaneous items you may require, e.g. small bags for products and leaflets etc.

The receptionist

The receptionist should present an immaculate appearance, have an attentive and caring attitude to clients which in turn will represent the professional image of the salon. Communication skills are very important, whether talking to a client in person or over the telephone. The information should be given in a clear and confident manner. If the receptionist is not a beauty therapist the salon owner or manager should explain the treatments, or better still, treatments are given to the receptionist so that accurate knowledge can be imparted to the client.

The responsibilities of the receptionist

Responsibility covers the following:

- enquiries
- recording an appointment
- keeping client record cards
- processing payments
- cashing up payments at the end of the day
- selling retail products
- handling complaints
- retail stock control
- ordering stock.

Enquiries usually start over the telephone and you should answer with a greeting, name of salon and your own name, e.g. Good morning, West End Beauty Clinic, Sarah speaking. A multitude of questions may be asked by clients from, where are you? Is there parking for a car? What is the number of the bus or nearest station? What hours do you open? Do you have a late night?, to, do you do 'such-and-such' treatment? How much does it cost? The response should be business-like but friendly, you may be talking to a prospective client. If the person seems apprehensive it may be appropriate to suggest that he/she just comes in for a consultation and explain that there is no charge and no obligation to take the treatments suggested.

Recording an appointment must be made accurately (the date, the time, the treatment requested) using the client's surname and where possible a telephone number. The appointment book will vary from salon to salon, larger salons will have a heading for each therapist whereas smaller salons will put the therapist's initials against the client's name. If you are not a therapist keep a list handy of the length of time required for each treatment to avoid over-lapping appointments. Remember, clients will demand efficiency from you but not from themselves, they can arrive late, they can cancel at the last minute or not arrive at all! Whatever happens, courtesy prevails, you are giving a service and you need to maximise your salon's clientele. Clients may often arrive without a booking to see if they can be 'fitted in' immediately! Occasionally this is possible or they may have to wait for a few minutes, this is where your expertise in handling clients comes in useful, providing a beverage and magazines and very general conversation, perhaps talking about the various treatments given in the salon or retail products available. Never 'hard sell' as this will inevitably irritate the client.

Keeping client records accurately, i.e. in alphabetical order, is very important. The card should give the name and address of the client (telephone number if available) and a list of appointments taken (if applicable). When an appointment is made the date, time and treatment, should be entered on the card and given to the therapist on the due date. After the treatment liaise with the therapist concerned and talk to the client to arrange a further booking. Enter this on the card, the appointment book and then file. The client's card will have other information entered by the therapist and is therefore confidential and should not be left around for others to view.

Figure 2.1 is a sample record card with the client's name, address,

West End Beauty Clinic

Mr/Mrs/Ms ....   Address ....

Surname ....

Forenames ....   Postcode ....

Tel. No. Day ....   Tel. No. Eve ....

Medical history ....   Date of birth ....

....   No. children/ages ....

Medication ....

....   Dr Name ....

Allergies ....   Dr Tel. No ....

Contra-indications: ....

Reverse side of card

Date	Treatment given	Retail sales	Initials
....	....	....	....
....	....	....	....
....	....	....	....
....	....	....	....
....	....	....	....
....	....	....	....
....	....	....	....
	Comments		
....	....	....	
....	....	....	

Fig 2.1 Suggested record card for client

telephone number etc. and the reverse side of the card shows the dates, treatments given and retail products purchased.

With computerised systems, and these are on the increase, client information can be fed into the computer for future reference.

Processing payments takes various forms such as cash, cheques and credit cards. Most salons have an electronic till which produces a receipt and, as there are many versions, you should familiarise yourself with the different codes used and how it operates. In the event of a fault with the machine or an electric power cut, it is advisable to have a duplicate receipt book beneath the desk.

If payment is made by cash, give the change (if any) and the receipt to the client before putting the money into or closing the till.

To process a cheque, ensure that it is filled in correctly, i.e. check that it is made out to the salon correctly, the date, the amount, both in words and figures and that it is signed. Request to see the client's cheque card, verify the signature and write the card number (and your initials) on the back of the cheque before returning the card and receipt. Any discrepancies appearing on the cheque, must be initialled or signed by the client. The cheque is kept safely in the till or locked drawer.

Larger salons may have facilities for processing credit and debit cards. Credit cards are issued by Banks (e.g. Access, Visa, Mastercard) or by UK Building Societies (e.g. Abbey National, Halifax). Charge cards are a type of credit card issued by companies (e.g. American Express or Diners Club). Debit cards (e.g. Connect, Switch) enable monies to be transferred from the client's bank account. The salon would need a special terminal which is connected through to a central computer to enable the card to be 'swiped' through and this gives automatic authorisation; or the salon may have a credit card printer using special carboned vouchers (in triplicate) where the details are written in and an imprint is made. The top copy is given to the client and the salon keeps the duplicates in a safe place. Both systems require the client to sign the receipt and this should be verified by checking the signature on the reverse side of the card. All card companies take a commission and this varies from 1.5 per cent to 5 per cent.

Taxes are levied on the sale of goods or services and these vary from 10 per cent to 25 per cent according to each country or, as in the USA, from State to State. These appear as service tax or sales tax and in the UK as value added tax (VAT) which is payable to Customs & Excise quarterly. VAT is levied when the turnover on sales and services exceed the annual figure determined by the Government. Some salons may not have to pay VAT as their turnover is too small, but larger salons will apply VAT either within their price structure or add it on to the total bill. The manager/owner will be responsible for the payment of VAT but you will need to know how it should be applied (if applicable).

Records are kept for all receipts and payments and most salons have a cash book. You may be required to enter these as they are made. The manager/owner of the salon will also record payments made into the bank and reconcile the totals in the cash book against bank statements.

Cashing-up payments at the end of the day confirms the day's takings. When you open for business in the morning the till will contain a float, which is merely an amount of money to provide clients with change. It can also be used for petty cash for small items (i.e. tea, coffee, milk) or money may be kept in a separate cash box, but whatever method is used, receipts for these must be kept and entered into the cash book. At the end of the day, put aside the day's float and add up *all* the receipts (some electronic tills will give the final total of payments received for treatments and products). Count all the money, cheques and vouchers for credit cards received and the two should equate. The manager/owner of the salon usually assumes responsibility of the day's takings, including making out a summary sheet for the vouchers received, for payment into the bank. A new float may be put into the till for the next day.

Selling retail products is an important aspect for the salon. The therapist carrying out the treatment will have advised using certain products and written these on the client's card but may not have the time to follow through and sell, or no advice has been given during the treatment, e.g. if the client comes in for electrolysis, skin care or cosmetic products may not have been discussed. To be able to sell with confidence, you, as the receptionist, should have a sound knowledge of the products and how and when they should be used and also the treatments offered by the salon. Talking and listening to the client is paramount, ask questions, be they closed (i.e. the reply may be a simple yes or no) or open, whereby the receptionist invites conversation. Explain how the product should be used or how the treatment will benefit the client and do not hesitate to mention the price. It is possible to use link selling, e.g. if a client purchases a lipstick you could suggest a matching nail polish. Many salons offer a commission for retail sales and this may cloud judgment in selling. Never 'hard' sell, i.e. push a sale, it sometimes has the opposite effect, the client feels pressurised into buying and you lose the sale, or worse, the client may not come back to the salon. It is important that you listen, keep eye contact all the time, keep quiet until the client has made a decision. Any purchase made by the client should be entered on the record card and this will help for future sales.

Handling complaints is initially the responsibility of the receptionist. When a client returns a faulty product ensure that it is truly defective, that it has not been misused by the client and has been sold by the salon. In the UK laws are in place to safeguard the sale of goods and the retailer is responsible for the sale. If you feel the complaint is genuine offer a refund of money or replace the product. Any uncertainty should be referred to the manager/owner of the salon. The complaint should be dealt with sympathetically and an apology will go a long way! The product can always be returned to the supplier for a replacement or refund of money. The manufacturer of a product will carry a product liability insurance which provides the necessary cover.

If complaints concern a treatment or a reaction to a certain treatment, this should be referred to the therapist or manager/owner of the salon. The business will have a public liability insurance which covers injuries or reactions to treatments if caused by negligence on the part of the staff or salon. The client should be shown to a quiet area for discussion where the complaint can be listened to without interruption. Details of this type of complaint should be recorded just in case the client decides to seek compensation from the salon. This, however, is usually the responsibility of the manager/owner of the salon.

Retail stock control should be carefully monitored. On receipt of stock from a supplier, products should be checked off against the order and delivery note. The supplier should be advised if stock arrives damaged or if there is any discrepancy.

The control of stock can be carried out very simply by using stock sheets, cards or a stock book and, in larger salons, by a computer. The manager/owner will advise you on the salon's stock control system and you should familiarise yourself with the procedures being used. New stock should be coded, entered into the control system, priced, placed in a locked cupboard or stock room and gradually transferred to the display area and placed behind existing stock, effecting a first in, first out method. Remember, unseen stock cannot be sold and stock is money tied up. Although it is important not to run out of certain products, you should be careful not to over-stock. Stock which has exceeded its 'shelf life' will either have to be sold off cheaply or thrown away and the salon loses money. On the other hand, panic buying from a supplier will involve the salon in extra costs for packing and postage. It will be seen from the sales records which are the fast or slow moving items and re-ordering should equate with these. Stock checks should be carried out weekly and the stock held, and that which has been sold should balance out. Mistakes can happen, pilfering can occur and, if you are responsible for the retail stock, the manager/owner should be advised of any discrepancies – however small.

Ordering stock may combine both retail and salon stock (i.e. consumables used for giving treatments). Use a salon order form and when filling it in for the retail side, check with the therapists to see if salon sizes are also required from the same supplier. Make the order out clearly and always retain a copy on file to tie up with deliveries. Orders are posted or 'faxed' (i.e. both the salon and the supplier must have fax machines), if the latter, the original order can be the copy retained on file. Suppliers often send out literature on 'special offers' for a set period of time, or a bulk-buying offer for seasonal products, check to see if any are applicable. Also find out if there is any discount offered by a supplier, sometimes it is offered if orders exceed a certain amount of money. You will have to calculate whether it is worth ordering an item or two more to obtain the discount. Usually there is a minimum and maximum figure for each item of stock to assist in re-ordering. No doubt the manager/owner will have negotiated prices and terms with suppliers and possibly free delivery, so when the order is complete, it should be authorised.

Note: Finally, small salons may not be able to afford the luxury of a receptionist and the therapists will have to share the duties between them and this involves organising their time very efficiently between treatments, to ensure paper work is completed, including stock control (both salon and retail) banking and keeping client record cards up-to-date. The telephone still has to be answered and appointments booked, clients welcomed into the salon etc., but careful planning will always leave someone free to attend to these areas.

Initial consultation

The receptionist (or therapist in a small salon) initiates a consultation for new clients and when an appointment is made time should be allowed for this, either on its own or when it is associated with a treatment. The name, address and telephone number should be entered on the card.

The consultation should take place in a quiet area, devoid of distraction, where the client can be at ease and appreciate confidentiality by the therapist. Initially find out what the client wants, listen carefully and establish a good rapport. Discuss the various treatments you can offer which are suitable for the client before going on to suggest what is actually needed. Remember some clients are not always familiar with all the treatments available, e.g. hair removal may not always require depilatory waxing, electrolysis may be more appropriate.

For facial treatments a skin analysis is essential (see Chapter 11) and a time factor for this should be allowed. Give reasons for your choice of treatment, impart your technical knowledge simply and you will find the client will have confidence in you and the salon and return on a regular basis. Always advise the price of the treatment or treatment plan and the cost of the retail products for home care. You may decide to charge less for a course of treatments instead of charging these on an individual basis. Suggest a general maintenance routine, be it skin care, diet or exercise etc. Never guarantee 100 per cent success for any treatment, so much depends on the client, whether she heeds your advice or whether home-care products are used regularly. Wait for the client to make a decision, then you can sell or proceed with the treatment/s, sell the retail products or give appropriate skin-care samples and/or make a future appointment.

During or immediately after the consultation a record should be made of the advice, treatment suggested and products or samples given. This should be written on the reverse of the client's record card. The information can be transferred into a computer for future reference, i.e. if the salon has a computer, the necessary soft-ware and ideally a printer to print out the client's record on return visits.

If a treatment plan is agreed, suggest appointment times and ensure these are entered on the card and in the appointment book (the date, time and initials of the therapist). Clients will often request the same therapist for their treatments and the receptionist should ensure that the particular therapist is free at the time requested.

Self assessment

- what does a client look for when entering a salon?
- how would you record an appointment?
- how would you keep client record cards?
- what would you look for when processing a cheque?
- how would you account for petty cash?
- how would you close a retail sale?
- how would you deal with a complaint?
- give reasons why stock control is so important
- what do you look for when re-ordering stock?
- what results do you expect to achieve after a consultation?

3 Structure of the human cell

The cell is the fundamental unit of all living matter. Although cells may be widely differentiated and very specialised in their function, they have the same basic structure.

The cell is a minute mass of protoplasm which is a slightly opaque, colourless, jelly-like substance, held together by a cell membrane (see Fig. 3.1). A cell generally consists of 70–80 per cent water; 15 per cent proteins, which are divided into three types – amino acids, simple proteins and polypeptides; 1 per cent carbohydrates; 3 per cent lipids (fatty substances) and 1 per cent nucleic acids and minerals (i.e. sodium chloride, potassium chloride and magnesium).

The cell membrane acts as a selective sieve, through which certain substances are absorbed and others rejected. Therefore, it is semipermeable and composed of protein threads and lipids. Between the threads and lipids are spaces (or pores) which allow minute molecules to pass into the protoplasm. Even larger molecules of nutrient material can be dissolved in the lipids of the cell membrane. Also other nutrients can be transported across the cell membrane by chemical substances, generally known as 'carriers'.

Therefore, three methods are involved in supplying the cell nutrient:

1. by diffusion through the 'pores';
2. by dissolving in the lipids;
3. by 'carriers'.

The chemical structure of the protoplasm varies according to the activity and condition of the cell.

In the middle of the cell is a globular mass known as the nucleus which is surrounded by its own membrane, the nuclear membrane. This is the control centre of the cell and it plays an important role in influencing growth and reproduction. The nucleus has a network of filament or fibres and these are known as chromatin. It is this part of the cell that contains deoxyribonucleic acids (DNA), which are the genetically inherited information required for the maintenance of cells and their reproduction. When the cell is reproducing, the network of chromatin filaments assumes the form of a twisted skein which divides into a number of V-shaped loops known as chromosomes. Each cell of the human body has 46 chromosomes arranged in 23 pairs.

Note: Genes are segments of the DNA molecule and each gene carries a specific hereditary trait. These traits are physical, biochemical and physiological. Therefore, genes affect not only the physical appearance of an individual but also physiological make-up, the tendency to de-

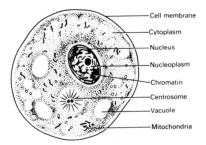

Fig. 3.1 Basic simple cell

velop certain diseases and the daily activities of all the cells of the body. A child, in receiving a set of genes from its parents will develop characteristics which reflect those of the parents, grandparents and other ancestors, but the child is also affected in various ways by, for example, environmental influences such as diet, training and education.

Between the nucleus and cell membranes the protoplasm is known as cytoplasm. This contains small granules called ribosomes which are the site of protein synthesis. Genetic information is passed from DNA in the nucleus to the ribosomes by means of ribonucleic acid (RNA) so enabling protein synthesis to take place. The cytoplasm also has small rod-like structures called mitochondria. These are involved in oxidative reactions which take place in the cell and also act as a storehouse for nutrient materials which are needed to replace worn-out cytoplasm. Within the cytoplasm there are clear circular spaces called vacuoles and these are the recipients of the waste material or secretion which the cytoplasm has formed.

In the cytoplasm, near to the nucleus, a small spherical body is seen called the centrosome which is surrounded by a radiating thread-like structure. The centrosome has two barrel-like cylinders called centrioles. These are believed to produce the asters and spindles upon which the chromosomes travel during cell division.

Cell division

The cells of the human body reproduce or divide in a complicated manner which is known as mitosis. This can best be described as occurring in several stages or phases (see Fig. 3.2).

Prophase

The centrosome divides into two (each centrosome contains a centriole). The two centrosomes move to opposite poles of the cell but remain attached by thread-like spindles.

Metaphase

The chromatin becomes more concentrated and more definite in shape and forms dark rod-shaped structures. The nuclear membrane disap-

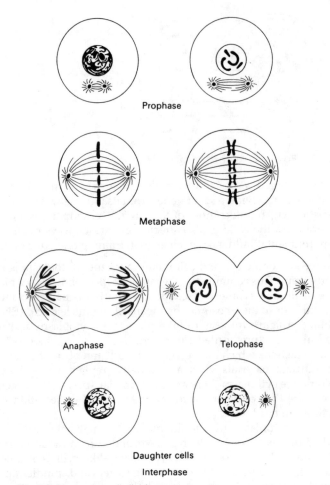

Prophase

Metaphase

Anaphase   Telophase

Daughter cells

Interphase

Fig. 3.2 Stages in cell division

pears and the chromosomes arrange themselves around the centre of the cell and appear to be attached to the spindles of the centrosomes which are now at either pole of the cell.

Anaphase

The chromosomes begin to divide longitudinally into two equal parts. The two groups of chromosomes begin to move away from each other to the opposite poles of the cell and arrange themselves around the centrosomes. At this stage the spindles break.

Telophase

A constriction appears around the centre of the cell body. The nuclear membrane reappears and the spindles disappear entirely. To complete the cycle the constriction of the cytoplasm increases until the cell is divided, the chromosomes disappear and the filament-like structure chromatin is re-formed. The cell has now completed its division and the two cells formed are known as the 'daughter' cells, which in turn will grow and reproduce by mitosis.

Cell activities

The activities of the cell are as follows:

Metabolism is, generally speaking, the physical and chemical process taking place in the cell. The cell receives its nourishment from the bloodstream through its semi-permeable membrane. Because of this nourishment heat and energy are produced, worn-out protoplasm is built up and repaired and secretions or enzymes are also generated.

Respiration and excretion   As oxygen is required for metabolism, it is absorbed through the semi-permeable membrane. Cellular respiration takes place, that is, oxidation of nutrient material providing heat and energy and forming waste products, such as carbon dioxide and water which are expelled through the semi-permeable membrane.

Growth and reproduction   Cells, of course, grow until they are mature and ready to reproduce (mitosis).

Movement and irritability   This means that a cell can respond to a stimulus be it physical, chemical or thermal.

Self assessment

- the cell consists of 70–80 per cent water, how is the balance made up?
- describe the methods involved in supplying the cell with nutrients
- what is meant by DNA and what is its function?
- explain the phases of mitosis
- describe the activities of the cell.

4 Tissues of the body

The body is composed of millions of cells and they are arranged in patterns, thus forming the tissues of the body. The tissues then form into patterns and become organs; likewise the organs become systems. Each pattern is really a highly specialised group, but no group can operate on its own: they are wholly dependent upon one another. The main fundamental tissues are:

1. epithelial tissue (or epithelium);
2. connective tissue;
3. muscle tissue;
4. nervous tissue.

Epithelial tissue

Epithelial tissue consists of cells closely packed together, supported by a basement membrane; the matrix or intercellular substance is reduced to a minimum. The membrane supplies the cells with their nourishment. Epithelial tissue has two main structures, simple and compound. Membranes are a modification of simple epithelium.

Simple epithelial tissue

This consists of a single layer of cells. There are four types, renamed according to their shape and the functions they perform.

Squamous epithelium (often known as 'pavement')

These cells fit closely together, rather like a pavement, producing a very smooth surface. They provide the inactive lining of the alveoli of the lungs, the heart, blood vessels and lymphatic vessels. Because they are so flat they allow substances to pass through them easily (see Fig. 4.1(a)).

Cubical or cuboidal epithelium

As the name would imply this consists of cube-shaped cells fitting closely together. Its function is secretory; it absorbs substances – for example, the tissue forming the tubules of the kidneys and some of the glands (see Fig. 4.1(b)).

Columnar epithelium

These cells are of much greater height than width and consist of a single layer of cells of cylindrical shape, which produce a secretion or are

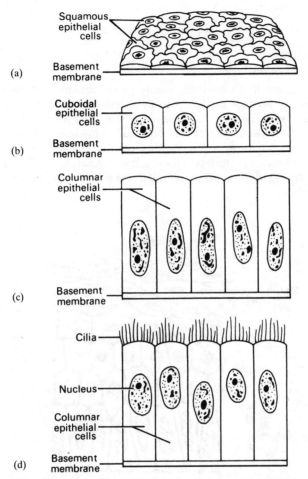

(a)
Squamous
epithelial
cells

Basement
membrane

(b)
Cuboidal
epithelial
cells

Basement
membrane

(c)
Columnar
epithelial
cells

Basement
membrane

(d)
Cilia

Nucleus

Columnar
epithelial
cells

Basement
membrane

Fig. 4.1 Simple epithelial tissue – (a) Squamous (b) Cuboidal (c) Columnar (d) Cilated columnar

capable of absorption. It forms the lining for the small and large intestines, the stomach, gall bladder and bile ducts (see Fig. 4.1(c)).

Cilated epithelium

This is also formed by cylindrical-shaped cells, the only difference being that on the free edges of the cells are minute hairlike processes known as cilia. These have the effect of performing a sweeping movement in one direction, dependent on the area of the tissue. This epithelium forms the lining of the bronchi, trachea, larynx and nose and moves particles of dust etc., upward from the lungs. It is also found lining the uterine tubes and helps to move the ovum towards the uterus (see Fig. 4.1(d)).

Compound epithelium

This contains two or more layers of cells and may be divided into several types.

Stratified epithelium

The deepest layer consists mainly of columnar epithelium and the superficial layer is made up of flattened cells (squamous). You may hear of non-keratinised and keratinised stratified epithelium. The former will be found on wet surfaces, that is, the lining of the mouth, the conjunctiva of the eyes, the pharynx and the oesophagus. The latter will be found on a dry surface, where a layer of keratin will prevent injury to or drying of the underlying cells, that is, the skin, hair and nails (see Fig. 4.2(a)).

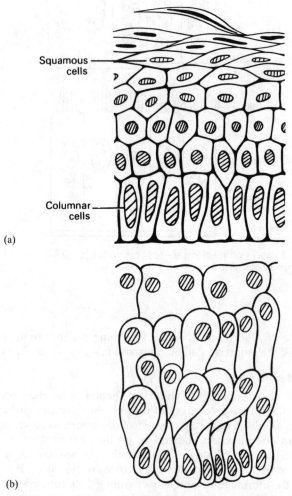

Squamous cells

Columnar cells

(a)

(b)

Fig. 4.2 (a) Stratified epithelium (b) Transitional epithelium

Transitional epithelium

This is composed of several layers of pear-shaped cells. It is so called because it is believed that the cells represent a transition between stratified squamous and columnar epithelium. They are usually found in the linings of hollow organs as they are subject to change through contraction and distention, i.e. kidneys, ureters and bladder (see Fig. 4.2(b)).

Membranes

These consist of thin layers of epithelial tissue that cover a surface or divide an organ and are designed to secrete lubricating fluids. The most important membranes are mucous, serous and synovial.

Mucous membrane

This is covered with epithelium, lining canals and cavities which communicate with the exterior of the body, i.e. digestive, respiratory and genito-urinary tracts. The cells forming the membrane produce a slimy fluid called mucus which contains a protein, mucin. The secretion is formed within the cytoplasm of the cells and as it accumulates the cells become distended and finally rupture, so discharging the mucus. The organs which are lined have a slippery moist surface. As the cells fill up with mucus they look like a goblet and this is what they are called, i.e. goblet cells (see Fig. 4.3).

Serous membranes

These line the cavities which have no communication with the exterior of the body. The membrane has a double layer of squamous or pavement epithelial tissue, visceral and parietal. The visceral layer surrounds the organ and the parietal lines the cavity in which the organ lies. Between the two layers the membrane exudes serous fluid. These membranes are found in the thoracic cavity, the pleura around the lungs, the pericardium of the heart and in the abdominal cavity. The purpose of the serous fluid is to ensure that organs move without damage or friction to one another, e.g. when the heart beats it changes shape and size, but friction damage is prevented by the pericardium (the fibroserous sac enclosing the heart) and its serous fluid.

Synovial membrane

This is the inner layer of specialised epithelial cells in the articular capsule of a synovial joint. They exude a clear, sticky yet oily fluid which acts as a lubricant to joints, helping to maintain their stability and activity as a nutrient to the articular cartilage. Synovial cells remove damaging material from within the joint cavity.

Connective tissue

As already said, tissues consist of specialised cells. Basically, connective tissue is a fibrous type of tissue which supports the various structures of the body. The cells are more widely separated than in epithelial tis-

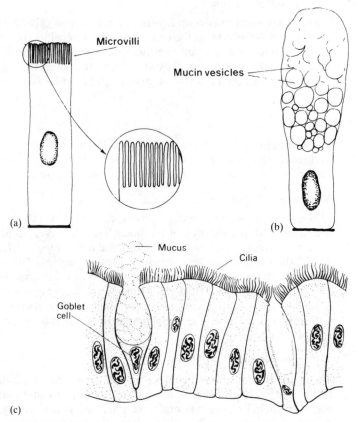

Fig. 4.3 Ciliated columnar epithelium with goblet cells (a–c)

sue and so the intercellular substance is increased. The matrix may be either a semi-jelly-like substance or dense and rigid. The cells are some-times referred to as 'stellate cells' which simply means star-shaped and polyhedral – having many sides or surfaces, from which fine processes branch out to form bundles of minute fibrils. It is the density of these fibres together with the absence or presence of certain chemicals which make connective tissue soft and rubbery or hard and rigid.

Areolar tissue

This is a loose connective tissue with a viscous matrix into which are woven an irregular arrangement of fibres and a variety of cells.

These cells include fibroblasts which secrete the collagen and elastic fibres, macrophages and plasma cells, which absorb bacteria and de-fend the body against foreign matter and fat cells which store fat.

These fine fibres may be white and wavy or yellow, straight and taut. The former run through the matrix, forming a network and consisting of collagen held together by mucin. Collagen has structural and pro-tective properties and therefore helps to repair or replace cell damage.

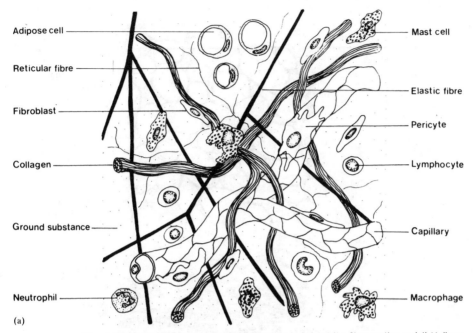

Adipose cell

Reticular fibre

Fibroblast

Collagen

Ground substance

Neutrophil

(a)

Mast cell

Elastic fibre

Pericyte

Lymphocyte

Capillary

Macrophage

Fig. 4.4 (a) Areolar tissue (b) Adipose tissue (c) White fibrous tissue (d) Yellow elastic tissue (e) Lymphoid tissue

Fine yellow fibres, composed of elastin, are essential for suppleness and elasticity.

This tissue is found in every part of the body. It lies between the muscles; supports blood vessels and nerves; provides a lining for the digestive tract; helps to bind the inner organs to their main structure; and also lies under the skin for pliability (see Fig. 4.4(a)).

Adipose

This is a fatty tissue deposited in most parts of the body and it consists of small vesicles (fat cells) lodged in the meshes of areolar tissue. These vary in size, are specially adapted for storing droplets of fat (a type of lipid) and are embedded in a vascular areolar tissue. Adipose tissue is present in all subcutaneous tissue with the exception of the eyelids, the penis and inside the cranial cavity. It helps to support the organs of the body, i.e. the kidneys. This tissue not only forms a protective covering for the body but gives it shape. It also constitutes a storage depot for excess food (see Fig. 4.4(b)).

Adipose tissue is a metabolically active tissue in as much as it releases fat in response to nervous and hormonal activity. In this way it provides a source of heat and energy for use in the body.

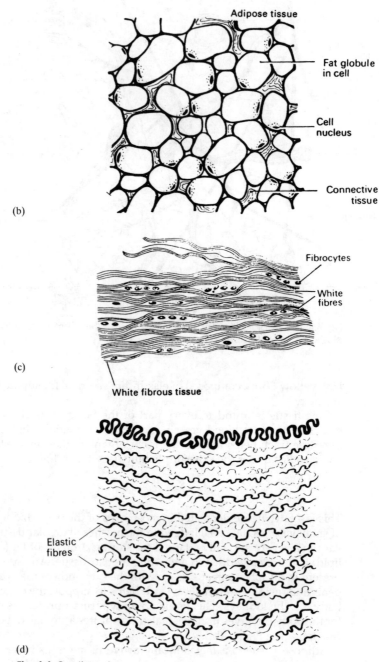

(b)

(c)

(d)

Fig. 4.4 Continued

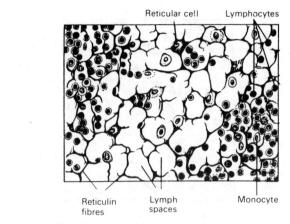

(e)

Fig. 4.4 Continued

White fibrous tissue

There is very little matrix and very few cells in this very strong connective tissue and what cells there are lie in rows between bundles of white fibres. This tissue is found in many areas for many purposes; that is to say, it forms an outer specialised covering for bones and is then known as periosteum; it forms the ligaments, thereby binding bones together; it forms muscle fascia (which is muscle sheath); it forms tendons which bind muscle to bone and to help to support the bones at the joints, e.g. ankle and wrist – for example, an aponeurosis, where one muscle connects with another ending in a flat expanding tendon or fibrous sheet, i.e. between the frontalis and occipitalis muscles of the skull. It also provides a protective covering for some of the internal organs (the brain, kidneys, lymphatic nodes and blood vessels) (see Fig. 4.4(c)).

Yellow elastic tissue

Again this contains very few cells and the matrix itself consists mainly of masses of yellow elastic fibres. Because of its elasticity it is capable of considerable extension and retraction. Some ligaments consist entirely of yellow elastic fibres. It is found in organs where alteration of shape is required, e.g. large arteries, the trachea, bronchi and lungs (see Fig. 4.4(d)).

Lymphoid tissue

This is a connective tissue with meshes that lodge lymphoid cells, lymphocytes. Its matrix is semi-solid with very fine branch fibres. The tissue is found in the lymphatic nodes, the spleen, tonsils, adenoids, appendix and in the solitary glands of the intestines (see Fig. 4.4(e)).

Cartilage

This is a specialised fibrous connective tissue and, as the matrix is quite

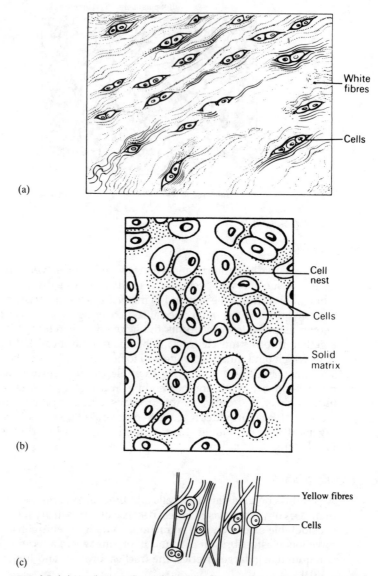

(a)

White fibres

Cells

(b)

Cell nest

Cells

Solid matrix

(c)

Yellow fibres

Cells

Fig. 4.5 (a) Hyaline cartilage (b) White fibrocartilage (c) Yellow elastic cartilage

solid, it is much firmer than any other connective tissue. It is similar to bone but without its mineral content. It cushions the bones at the joints and therefore prevents jarring between bones. It also gives shape to external features, for example, the nose and ears.

Hyaline cartilage

This has a blue–white appearance and its matrix is smooth and solid. The cells are arranged in groups of two or more and when they come into contact with each other their edges appear straight. This cartilage is found on the articular surfaces of bones; it forms the costal cartilages which attach the ribs to the sternum; it also forms part of the larynx and supports the trachea and bronchi so that they do not collapse when swallowing (see Fig. 4.5(a)).

White fibro cartilage

Like the tissue, with dense masses of white fibres with few cells in a solid matrix and therefore tough and slightly flexible, this type of cartilage is found as pads, known as the intervertebral discs, between the vertebrae; also as semi-lunar cartilages which lie between the articulating surfaces of the bones of the knee joint. It is also present around the rims of the bony sockets of the hip and shoulder joints (see Fig. 4.5(b)).

Yellow or elastic cartilage

This type of cartilage contains yellow or elastic fibres (as shown in Fig. 4.5(c)) which run through the solid matrix, the cells lying between the fibres, and is found in the pinna (the external ear) and the epiglottis.

Muscle tissue

Composition of muscle tissue is 20 per cent protein, 75 per cent water and 5 per cent mineral salts, glycogen and fat. The muscle is generally a bundle of long slender cells or fibres that have the power to contract. Muscles are responsible for locomotion and play an important part in performing vital body functions. They also protect the contents of the abdomen against injury and help support the body.

Muscle fibres vary in length from less than a millimetre to several centimetres. They also vary in shape and in colour from white to deep red. Each muscle fibre receives its own nerve impulses so that fine and varied motions are possible. Each has its small stored supply of glycogen which it uses as fuel for energy. Muscles, especially the heart, also use free fatty acids as fuel. At the signal of an impulse travelling down the nerve, the muscle fibre changes chemical energy into mechanical energy and the result is muscle contraction.

Some muscles are attached to bones by tendons. Others are attached to other muscles and to the skin, producing a smile, a wink or other facial expressions. All or part of the walls of the hollow internal organs, such as the heart, stomach, intestines and blood vessels, are composed of muscle. The last stages of swallowing and of peristalsis are actually a series of contractions by the muscles in the walls of the organs concerned. There are three types of muscular tissue.

Voluntary (striped)

These muscles are controlled by the conscious part of the brain. They are skeletal muscles that enable the body to move and there are more than six hundred in the human body. We say they have 'striated' fibres, and this is because the contractile fibrils that form them are connected

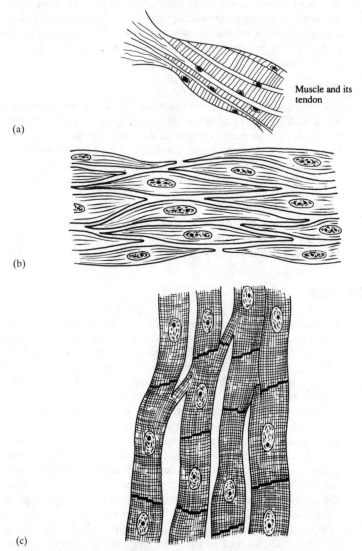

Muscle and its
tendon

(a)

(b)

(c)

Fig. 4.6 (a) Voluntary striped (b) Smooth muscle fibres (c) Cardiac muscle
fibres

in such a way that they appear to be striped. The nuclei are always on
the outer edges. The fibres are grouped together in a sheath of muscle
cells. Bundles of fibres are enclosed in a delicate web called the perimysium and these bundles are also separated from one another by a
connective tissue derived from perimysium, termed endomysium,
which serves to support blood vessels and nerves running between
them. Finally the entire muscle is surrounded by a sheath of areolar tissue known as epimysium.

Unlike the involuntary muscles, which can remain in a state of contraction for long periods without tiring and are capable of sustained rhythmic contractions, the voluntary muscles are readily subject to fatigue. They also differ from the involuntary muscles in their need for regular and proper exercise (see Fig. 4.6(a)).

Involuntary (smooth)

These muscles are not under the control of the conscious part of the brain and they respond to the nerve impulses of the autonomic nervous system. They are countless short-fibred, or smooth, muscles of the internal organs. They form part of the walls of the arteries, veins, some lymphatic vessels, the organs of the digestive, respiratory and uro-genital tracts. They are also found in the skin in the arrector muscles of the hair (arrectores pilorum) and the sweat glands. The muscle fibres are shaped like spindles and each has a single rod-shaped nucleus. Smooth muscle does not contract very quickly or powerfully but it never fatigues (see Fig. 4.6(b)).

Note: Control of smooth muscle can be learned, for instance, control of the bladder sphincter.

Cardiac

As the name implies, these are muscles of the heart. They are involun-tary and consist of striated fibres but are quite different from the fibres of the voluntary muscle. Unless the muscle is injured in some way, it contracts and relaxes at a rhythmic pace. The rate of contraction can change and is controlled by the nervous system (see Fig. 4.6(c)).

Nervous tissue

Some knowledge of the nervous system is required as it is important in your work to know how the nerve operates in dealing with the skin and muscles.

Nervous tissue consists mainly of two different structures: grey matter which forms the nerve cells and white matter which forms the nerve fibres. Nervous impressions and impulses originate in the grey matter and are conducted by the white matter.

The nerve cell, which is called a neuron, is the fundamental unit of the nervous system. A neuron is a specialised cell capable of being stimulated and able to conduct impulses. Surrounding the nucleus of the neuron is cytoplasm from which nerve fibres extend. These fibres carry messages in the form of electrical charges and chemical changes. A nerve cell may have one slender fibre or it may have two or more which are called unipolar, bipolar and multipolar respectively. Most neurons are multipolar which have a single fibre called an axon and several branches off, called dendrites. The latter are stimulated by other nerves or from a receptor organ such as the skin. Rather like a two-way radio, the dendrites receive messages and the axon and its nerve end-ings transmit messages. The point at which an impulse is transmitted from one nerve cell to another is called a synapse (see Fig. 4.7).

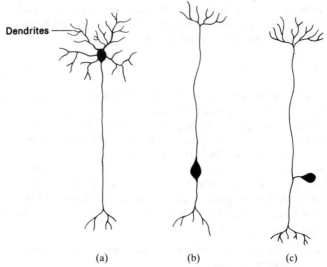

Fig. 4.7 (a) Multipolar neurons (b) Bipolar neurons (c) Unipolar neurons

Nerve fibres come together from the extremities of the body joining into cables running to and from the brain via the spinal cord. They promote sensation and motion. Nerves are nourished through the blood and lymph vessels surrounding them.

Types of nerves, put very simply are as follows.

Sensory (or afferent) nerves

These are also known as ascending nerves, because they carry impulses from all parts of the body and the sense organs to the brain. The nerve endings are located near the surface of the skin; therefore sensations of heat, cold or pain are conveyed by these nerves.

Motor (or efferent) nerves

These are also known as descending nerves because they carry impulses from the brain and spinal cord to the muscles and to glands.

Mixed nerves

These contain both sensory and motor fibres carrying impulses to and from the brain.

Self assessment

- describe the two main structures of epithelial tissue
- name the most important membranes
- which membrane secretes mucin?
- where would you find synovial fluid?
- in which connective tissue would you find collagen and elastin fibres?
- what is adipose tissue and where is it present?

- which tissue forms ligaments and muscle fascia?
- where would you find hyaline cartilage?
- what is the difference between voluntary and involuntary muscles and how does each respond?
- name the two different structures of nervous tissue and state how they perform
- what is a neuron?
- what is a synapse?
- explain the difference between afferent and efferent nerves.

5 Systems of the body

The human body can be divided into 9 systems:

skeletal
muscular
circulatory
lymphatic
nervous
digestive
respiratory
genito-urinary
glandular

In this volume only parts of the first five systems, which relate to the face, hands and feet are described. The remainder and the last four systems are included in the second volume pertaining to the rest of the body.

Skeletal

Bones, all 205 of them in the human body, form the skeletal systems.

Structure of bones

Despite their hard, rigid appearance, bones are living organs subject to growth. When fully formed they are composed of 25 per cent water, 30 per cent organic matter and 45 per cent inorganic salts. Bone tissue is made up of both compact and cancellous (spongy) substances which receive nourishment through the blood vessels (capillaries) which make their way through the periosteum into the cancellous substance.

Compact bone

This would appear to be a solid structure containing no empty spaces but its composition is fibrous rather than solid, giving the bones resiliency. It forms the hard bone found in shafts of long or flat bones, i.e. humerus (bone of the upper arm) and scapula (the shoulder blade). Throughout the compact bone runs the Haversian system which contains the following.

A central hole which is called the Haversian canal and this runs longitudinally. It contains two blood vessels with some delicate connective tissue and some nerve fibres. Around the canal there are layers of bone tissue known as **lamellae**.

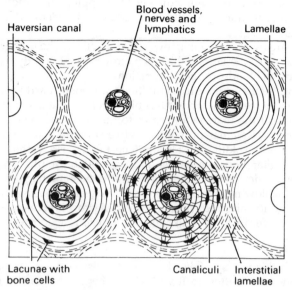

Haversian canal

Blood vessels, nerves and lymphatics

Lamellae

Lacunae with bone cells

Canaliculi

Interstitial lamellae

Fig. 5.1 Cross-section of bone

Between the lamellae, there are spaces known as **lacunae** which contain lymph and bone cells.

Between the lacunae and the canal are fine channels called **canaliculi** which carry nourishment to the bone cells.

Lastly, between the Haversian systems there are other lamellae with their own lacunae and canaliculi running in various directions called the **interstitial lamellae** (see Fig. 5.1).

Cancellous bone

Encased within the layers of the compact bone is the tissue that makes up most of the volume of bone called cancellous or spongy bone because it contains little hollows, like those of a sponge. It does not have a Haversian system but consists of a web-like arrangement of red-marrow-filled spaces separated by trabeculae (thin processes of bone). Blood vessels run through every layer of bone conveying nutritive elements and oxygen. Bone tissue contains a large number of nerves and the basic chemical in bone is calcium phosphate which gives strength and hardness.

Marrow

The innermost portion of the bone is a hollow cavity containing bone marrow. It is a network of blood vessels and special connective tissue fibres that hold together a composite of fat- and blood-producing cells.

The chief function of marrow is to manufacture erythrocytes, leucocytes and platelets (red and white blood cells – see pp. 46–7). These blood cells normally do not enter the bloodstream until they are fully developed, so that the marrow contains cells in all stages of growth. If the body's demand for white cells is increased because of an infection, the marrow responds immediately by stepping up production. The same is true if more red cells are needed, as in haemorrhage or with anaemia.

There are two types of marrow, red and yellow. The former produces the blood cells, the latter, which is mainly formed of fatty tissues, normally has no blood-producing function.

During infancy and early childhood all bone marrow is red. But gradually, as we get older and less blood cell production is needed, the fat content of the marrow increases to turn some of the marrow from red to yellow. Red marrow continues to be present in adults only in the flat bones of the skull, the sternum (chest bone), rib, vertebral column, clavicle (collar bone) humerus and part of the femur (thigh bone). However, under certain conditions, as after haemorrhage, nature takes over and yellow marrow in other bones may again be converted to red and resume its cell-producing functions. Marrow is occasionally subject to disease – for instance, leukemia or pernicious anaemia.

Periosteum

Although this is a specialised connective tissue it is so closely linked with bones it is better dealt with here. This is vascular fibrous membrane which forms an outer protective covering and gives attachment to tendons or muscles. In its deeper layers there are bone-forming cells, **osteoblasts**, which are responsible in forming new bone tissue. Periosteum covers most bones of the body, except those parts of bones which participate with freely movable joints, where it is replaced by articular or hyaline cartilage.

Type of bones

There are a variety of shapes of bones but mainly these are classified as follows.

Long bones

A long bone is one whose length far exceeds its breadth and thickness. It has a shaft (diaphysis) and two extremities (epiphyses). The diaphysis is mainly composed of compact bone with a central canal, the medullary canal. The epiphyses are composed of a thin layer of compact bone covered by hyaline cartilage within which there is a cancellous bone tissue containing the red marrow. An example would be the humerus (see Fig. 5.2).

Irregular, short, flat and sesamoid bones

These are composed of a thin layer of compact bone enclosing an inner mass of cancellous bone (with red marrow) and like the long bones they are encased in periosteum (except on their articulating surfaces). Examples of these bones would be:

- irregular bones found in the face and vertebrae;
- short bones found in the wrist and ankle;
- flat bones found in the skull;

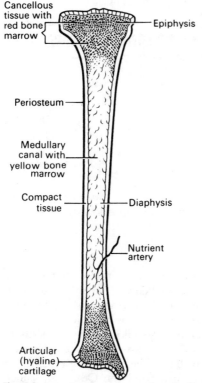

Cancellous tissue with red bone marrow

Epiphysis

Periosteum

Medullary canal with yellow bone marrow

Compact tissue

Diaphysis

Nutrient artery

Articular (hyaline) cartilage

Fig. 5.2 A mature long bone, longitudinal section

- sesamoid bones, being developed in the tendons of muscles, and found in the vicinity of a joint, the patella (triangular bone at the knee cap) being the largest example (see Fig. 5.3).

Bone Surfaces

The surfaces of bone may show projections (or eminences) and depressions. Articular projections are usually smooth and enter into a formation of a joint. They may be called a 'head' if spherical as in the 'ball' of a ball-and-socket joint; or a condyle if oval in shape as in the knuckles; or an epicondyle, which is an eminence above the condyle of the bone.

Non-articular projections are usually rough and form a place of attachment for muscles or ligaments. They have several names, e.g. processes, spines (if pointed), tuberosities (if broad and rough), or tubercles (if small and rough). Depressions or hollows in bones may be called sockets or fossae if rounded and notches or grooves if long and narrow. A crest is usually a projecting structure or ridge on the border of a bone.

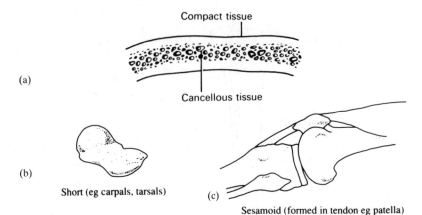

Fig. 5.3 (a) Flat bone (b) Short (e.g. carpals, tarsals) (c) Sesamoid (formed in tendon, e.g. patella)

Development of bones

In very young people, bone develops from cartilage and this accounts for the great flexibility and resilience of the infant skeleton. Gradually, calcium phosphate collects in the cartilage and it becomes harder and more brittle. Some of the cartilage cells break loose, so that channels develop in the bone shaft. Blood vessels enter the channels, bringing with them small cells of connective tissue, some of which become osteoblasts, cells that form true bone. The osteoblasts enter the hardened cartilage, forming layers of hard, firm bone. Other cells called **osteoclasts** work to tear down old or excess bone structure, allowing the osteoblasts to rebuild with new bone. This renewal continues throughout life, although it does slow down with age. Cartilage formation and the subsequent replacement of cartilage by hard material is the mechanism by which bones grow in size. During the period of bone growth, cartilage grows over the hardened portion of bone. In time, this layer of cartilage hardens as calcium phosphate is added, a fresh layer grows over it and it too hardens. The process continues until the body reaches full growth and development is not usually complete until we are about twenty-five years old (see Fig. 5.4).

Function of bones

To sum up the function of bones:

they form a framework for the body;
they give support to the weight of the body;
they form the boundaries for many of the body cavities;
they form a protection for the more delicate organs;
they act as levers, for the movement of the body;
they provide attachment for the voluntary muscles through periosteum, and perform blood-forming functions (due to the red marrow in the cancellous bone).

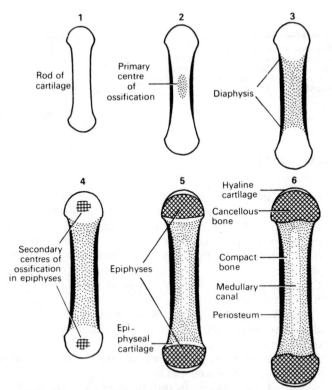

Fig. 5.4 Diagram of the stages of development of long bones

Articulations

Joint (or articulation) is the term used to describe the junction of two or more bones. The main purpose of a joint is to provide flexibility and motion to the skeletal system. However, joints vary substantially from immovable to limited motion to considerable motion. There are three main types.

Fibrous

These are immovable or fixed joints whereby the bones are connected by fibrous connective tissue; for example, the sutures between the flat skull bones (see Fig. 6.1(b)).

Cartilaginous

These joints allow limited movement and, as the name would imply, the bones are united by cartilage, for example, the intervertebral joints of the spine (see Fig. 5.5).

Synovial

These specialised joints permit more or less free movement as they are surrounded by an articular capsule, and these are:

Cartilaginous joints

The bone surfaces are covered by a layer of
cartilage and joined by tough fibrous tissue
embedded into the cartilage, e.g. between
the bodies of the **vertebrae**, and the **pubic
symphysis.**

These joints usually allow a small
degree of movement

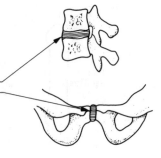

Fig. 5.5 Cartilaginous joint

1. *Gliding* Bones whose surfaces are flat or slightly curved glide over each other in a limited way, for example, at the ankle or wrist.
2. *Ball and socket* Where one rounded extremity fits into a cavity or cup-shaped depression of another bone, allowing much greater freedom of movement than any other type of joint; for example, the shoulder.
3. *Condyloid* This is a reduced ball-and-socket movement which is found at the wrist.
4. *Hinge* Where two or more bones are connected like a hinge of a door but movement is limited to flexion/extension; for example, elbow or knee.
5. *Pivot* Where rotary movement only is possible, for example, in the neck area, between axis and atlas.
6. *Saddle* A joint which can shift in several directions, like a rider on horseback, e.g. at the base of the thumb.

Muscular

The form that the human body takes is largely due to bone and the skeletal muscles and the latter can be divided into groups according to the functions they perform.

1. Flexor muscles bend the parts to which they are joined, or flex a limb.
2. Extensor muscles act to straighten, or extend a limb.
3. Abductor (*ab* = away from) muscles take limbs away from the middle line of the body.
4. Adductor (*ad* = towards) muscles bend limbs towards the middle line of the body.
5. Circumduction combines abduction, adduction, flexion and extension.
6. Rotator muscles enable a rolling movement to take place.
7. Supinator muscles will turn a limb upwards.
8. Pronator muscles will turn a limb downwards.
9. Sphincter muscles are ring-shaped and they close a natural orifice.

Every muscle has an antagonist to reverse its action, e.g. after a flexor muscle has bent a limb an extensor will straighten it (see Fig. 5.6).

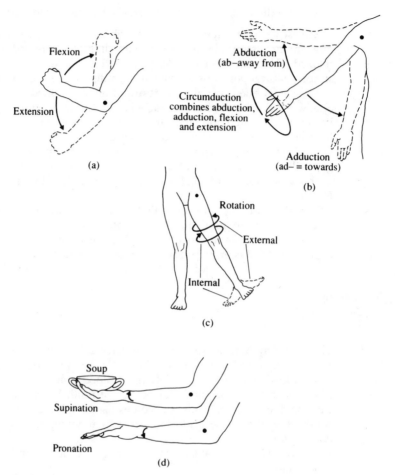

Flexion

Extension

(a)

Abduction
(ab–away from)

Circumduction
combines abduction,
adduction, flexion
and extension

Adduction
(ad– = towards)

(b)

Rotation

External

Internal

(c)

Soup

Supination

Pronation

(d)

Fig. 5.6 Movements

As we already know, muscles are attached to bones by tendons and by connective tissue to other muscles or to skin. When a muscle contracts, and therefore shortens, one of the attachments usually remains fixed and the other moves. We then apply the words:

Origin, which is the term applied to the more fixed attachment; and the *Insertion*, which is the term applied to the more movable attachment.

Muscle fibres vary considerably in length and each has its own supply of glycogen which it uses as fuel for energy. When a muscle contracts several changes occur.

1. It becomes wider and harder as it shortens.
2. The venous blood and lymph flow are accelerated and the arterial blood supply increased.
3. There is a rise in local temperature.
4. Lactic acid, a waste product, is produced from the locally stored glycogen.

5. Carbon dioxide, another waste product, is also produced.

Muscle tone is the term used to describe the normal degree of tension of a muscle, as muscles always remain slightly contracted even when relaxed. The contraction enables posture to be maintained and also the simple, natural positions we take for granted like sitting or kneeling.

Muscle fatigue is usually the result of unaccustomed or excess exercise, when the muscle has contracted so often that its store of glycogen has been exhausted and lactic acid accumulates in the muscle, causing it to ache or become stiff. Sometimes it will cause painful muscular cramp. However, the lactic acid will disperse and the supply of glycogen will be restored. Fat in the muscle can also be used for energy and in this way exercise or electrical therapy can be used to make muscles leaner.

Voluntary muscles are controlled by the conscious part of the brain, so their actions are motivated by the motor and sensory nerves. When a nerve impulse stimulates a muscle fibre its chemical energy changes into mechanical energy, producing muscle contraction.

Circulatory

Blood

This major system carries oxygen, nutrients, hormones and chemicals to the tissues and organs of the body. There are three main types of fluid: blood, tissue fluid and lymph. Blood consists of blood cells, platelets and plasma, the latter being the fluid. When plasma drains through the capillary walls it becomes tissue fluid. In turn, when this fluid leaves the tissues and is collected by the lymphatic system it becomes lymph.

Blood is composed of two parts, 55 per cent plasma and 45 per cent blood cells.

Plasma

This is a straw-coloured liquid and the fluid portion of the blood contains 91 per cent water, 7 per cent protein and less than 2 per cent inorganic and organic substances other than proteins.

Blood cells (also known as corpuscles, Latin for 'little bodies')

1. *Erythrocytes* These are the red blood cells which originate in the bone marrow of the ribs, sternum, skull, pelvic bone (hip bone), vertebrae (spine) and the ends of the long bones of the limbs. The erythrocytes owe their oxygen-carrying ability to haem, which contains iron and also gives blood its red colour. When haem combines with the protein globin and becomes haemoglobin it attracts oxygen in the bloodstream to form oxy-haemoglobin.

2. *Leucocytes* These are the white blood cells, colourless, larger in size than erythrocytes and are developed in lymph glands, lymph tissue, spleen, liver and bone marrow. There are several types of leucocytes,

White cells (*leucocytes*) (defence)
Total count: 4,000 to 11,000 per cubic mm.

Neutrophil ⎤
Eosinophil │ *Granulocytes* (Polymorphs)
Basophil ⎦

Monocyte

Lymphocytes
small   large

Red cells (*erythrocytes*) (O_2 and CO_2 transport)

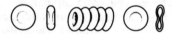

Fig. 5.7 Blood cells

namely lymphocytes, monocytes and granulocytes. The last include neutrophils which are the most numerous, forming up to 70 per cent of the total number and lymphocytes make up approximately 20 per cent of the total. Granulocytes are phagocytic, which means they have the ability to engulf and destroy bacteria. The lymphocytes develop mainly from lymph tissue (i.e. nodes, spleen, liver) and they secrete antibodies which assist in the body's defence mechanism. Monocytes are larger and they can enter and leave the circulatory system at will. They all work together to protect the body against infection and disease (see Fig. 5.7).

3. *Thrombocytes or platelets*   These are small disc-shaped cells, colourless and about one-third size of erythrocytes. They are formed in the red bone marrow and play an important part in the control of bleeding after injury and in the clotting of the blood.

There are approximately 6–9 pints of blood circulating in an average adult and this quantity makes a complete circuit through the body

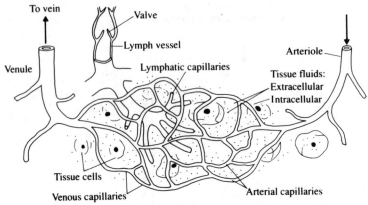

Fig. 5.8 Capillary lake

every minute. In fact, every 24 hours approximately 7,200 quarts of blood flows through the heart.

Therefore, to summarise, blood carries water, oxygen, food and secretions to all cells of the body; it carries away impurities; assists in regularising body temperatures, protecting the body from extreme heat and cold.

The circulatory system consists of the heart, blood vessels and lymph vessels. The heart is a hollow muscular organ which serves as a pump controlling the blood flow. It lies in the chest, slightly left of centre. Division of the heart and its two circuits, pulmonary and systemic and the complete circulatory system are detailed in Volume 2.

The blood vessels are arteries, veins and capillaries. Arteries are the vessels which carry blood from the heart through the main conducting arteries, branching out to distributing arteries. These then diffuse into arterioles (or little arteries) which lead directly to the capillaries, a complex network of simple endothelial tubes, very small, only the diameter of a blood cell. The climax of the circulatory system is sometimes called a capillary 'lake', a mass of tissue fluid, for it is here that the vital work of interchange takes place. Nutrients leaving the blood capillaries permeate the walls of the cells. Waste products of cell metabolism all enter the 'lake' before passing through the capillary walls to minute venules (small veins) then into larger veins, increasing in size. The blood vessels finally divide into two main groups, deep and superficial, carrying the blood back to the heart (see Fig. 5.8).

Lymphatic

Lymph

The lymphatic system is detailed in Volume 2. As mentioned before, nutrients reaching the cells are carried there by tissue fluid which also carries waste products from the cells to the capillaries. The basis of lymph is the extracellular fluid which lies around and between all the cells of the body. Lying in the cellular spaces is the network of lymph vessels which begin as colourless blind-ended lymphatic capillaries. These drain off excess tissue fluid and carry away waste products. From the capillaries the lymph is carried into larger lymphatic vessels which have valves in their walls to keep the lymph moving in the right direction. The lymph nodes are masses of lymphatic tissue set at certain points along the lymph vessels which remove foreign particles and bacteria and also produce lymphocytes and monocytes (white blood cells). Eventually large lymphatic ducts empty into the right and left subclavian veins (situated in the lower neck area) and so return to the circulatory system.

Nervous

The entire nervous system will be dealt with in Volume 2 and the foregoing is a brief description of the main systems.

The nervous system is largely responsible for communication and has two main divisions: the central nervous system and the peripheral nervous system which is subdivided into voluntary (or somatic) and autonomic systems.

Central nervous system

Information or messages are received by the brain and spinal cord via the sensory (or afferent) fibres from the body's sense organs and receptors. Once it has been analysed or filtered, signals are sent out along the motor (or efferent) fibres, producing a response in the muscles or glands. Therefore this system controls the five senses – seeing, smelling, tasting, feeling and hearing. It also controls our muscle actions, i.e. walking, talking and facial expressions.

Peripheral nervous system

From the central nervous system 43 pairs of nerves emerge – 12 pairs of cranial nerves from the brain and 31 pairs of nerves from the spinal cord. These radiate all over the body and form the peripheral system.

This system has two main divisions called the somatic (or voluntary) nervous system and the autonomic nervous system.

The somatic nervous system

This includes both motor and sensory nerves and controls the muscles carrying information to the brain.

The autonomic nervous system

This is involuntary and is concerned with the regulation of the internal organs and glands. This system is further subdivided into two subsidiary systems, the sympathetic and parasympathetic. Briefly, the sympathetic nervous system produces a stimulating effect and the parasympathetic nervous system generally acts as a dampener, so regulating the body's processes.

Nervous fatigue or exhaustion is caused by worry, excessive mental or manual work. There is usually a visual sign that can be gleaned: for example, weariness, irritability, poor complexion of even dull lifeless eyes. Nervous energy in a healthy person is entirely dependent upon a sensible diet, exercise and oxygen.

Self assessment

- how many bones form the skeletal system and what is the composition of bone tissue?
- describe the Haversian system
- describe bone marrow and its chief function
- what is periosteum?
- give an example of:

    a long bone
    an irregular bone
    a flat bone

- name three non-articular projections on the surfaces of bones
- how do bones develop?
- describe the functions of bones
- articulation is the term used to describe the junction of two or more bones, describe the three main types
- what is the difference between a ball-and-socket joint and a hinge joint?
- every muscle has an antagonist, give the antagonists to the following:

    flexor
    adductor
    supinator

- what is meant by origin and insertion of muscles?
- what changes occur when a muscle contracts?
- what happens to a muscle when its store of glycogen is depleted?
- muscles are motivated by which nerves?
- what is plasma?
- explain the difference between erythrocytes, leucocytes and thrombocytes
- explain briefly the circulatory system
- what is lymph?
- which nervous system controls the five senses?
- explain briefly the central and peripheral nervous systems.

6 Anatomy of the head, neck and shoulders (omitting the lymphatic system)

There are terms used in anatomy and physiology which assist in the identification of constituent areas of the body's structure and enable the determination of relative positions and aspects of various body parts.

It is important that these descriptive terms are clearly understood as they indicate the part of the body being treated. The term 'anatomical position' refers to the human body in an upright position (i.e. standing) with arms by the sides and the palms of the hands facing forward. From this position the following descriptive terms apply.

Superior   That which is situated above – i.e. towards the head end of the body or upper surface of an organ or other structure.

Inferior   Situated below or directed downward – i.e. the lower surface of an organ or other structure.

Anterior (or ventral)   Situated at or directed towards the front – i.e. the front of the body when standing upright.

Posterior   Directed towards or situated at the back – i.e. the back of the body when standing upright.

Median line   An imaginary line which runs from the centre of the crown of the head, right through the centre of the body, finishing between the two feet. Therefore medial simply means the mid-line or centre.

Lateral   Describes a part away from the centre or median line, or situated at the side – i.e. the outside of the arm is on the lateral surface of the arm – or it can refer to the point of attachment or origin.

Proximal   The nearest to a point of reference – i.e. to the centre or median line – or it can refer to the point of attachment or origin.

Distal   The furthest from a point of reference – i.e. from the centre or median line – or it can refer to the point of attachment or origin.

Symmetrical   Applies to parts of the body corresponding in size, form and arrangement – i.e. the right and left eyes and ears or right and left limbs.

Bones of the skull

The skull is the bony framework of the head and contains and protects the brain, eyes and organs of hearing, balance and smell. It gives shape to the head and face, contains the teeth and gives attachment to muscles. It consists of two parts, the cranium and the face.

Bones of the cranium

There are eight bones, namely: occipital, frontal, parietal (two), temporal (two), sphenoid and ethmoid.

The **occipital** is situated at the back and lower part of the cranium. It has a large opening called the foramen magnum and on either side are masses of bone which form the condyle of the skull and present articulating surfaces for the atlas (this is the uppermost segment of the spine).

The **frontal bone** forms the forehead and upper parts of the eye sockets.

There are two **parietal bones** – one each side of the head – by which the sides and top of the cranium are formed.

The two **temporal bones** are irregularly shaped, one on either side, forming part of the side and base of the skull and containing the middle and inner ear.

The **sphenoid bone** lies at the base of the skull. It is similar in shape to a bat with wings outstretched, consisting of a body with two greater and two lesser wings. The great wings form part of the sides of the skull anchoring the frontal, parietal, occipital and ethmoid bones. This bone contains the air sinuses which communicate with the nasal cavities and also contains the pituitary gland.

The **ethmoid bone** lies in front of the sphenoid bone and below the frontal bone. It is cubical in shape, light and spongy and is situated at the roof of the nose wedged in between the orbits (eye sockets) so forming nasal cavities and parts of the orbits (see Fig. 6.1(a)).

Between the various bones of the skull there are lines of union and these are called sutures. The parietal bones lie between the sagittal suture and dividing the frontal and parietal bones is the coronal suture. The lambdoidal suture lies between the parietal and occipital bones. Below the parietal bones, either side of the skull over the ear region, are the temporal bones joined to the parietal bones by the squamous sutures (see Fig. 6.1(b)).

Bones of the face

There are fourteen facial bones and these are mainly in pairs, one on either side of the face.

The two **maxillae** meeting in the midline of the face and form the upper jaw. They form the floor of the orbit for each eye, the sides and lower walls of the nasal cavities and support the upper teeth.

The two **palatine** bones join midline (like two Ls facing each other) in the roof of the mouth forming the back of the hard palate and floor of orbits.

The two **lacrimal** bones are located at the front part of the inner wall of the orbits. They contain part of the canals through which tear ducts run.

The two **nasal** bones form the bridge of the nose.

The two small quadrangular bones forming the hard part of the

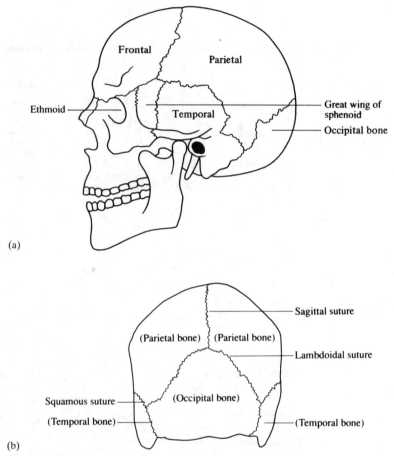

Fig. 6.1 (a) Bones of the cranium (b) Sutures of the cranium

cheeks are called the **zygomatics** (or malar). The zygomatic arches are formed by the zygomatics and temporal bones.

The two **turbinates** (inferior nasal conchae) are thin layers of spongy bone, curled like a scroll, located either side of the outer walls of the nasal cavities. Air inhaled through these is spun around and warmed before being taken into the lungs.

The **vomer** is just a single bone at the back of the nasal septum.

Lastly, the lower jaw bone, the **mandible**, is the only movable bone in the skull. Shaped like a horseshoe it articulates with the temporal bones and has a central portion (or body) which forms the chin and supports the lower teeth. The two portions either side, called rami, point upward from the angle of the jaw. Each **ramus** terminates in two processes, the **coronoid** process in front and the **condyle** of the jaw (or the head of the mandible) which lies behind. This condyle (or mandibular head) articulates with the temporal bone to form the temporo-mandibular joint (see Fig. 6.2).

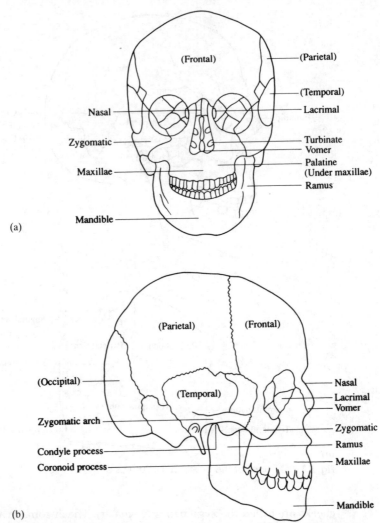

(a)

(b)

Fig. 6.2 (a) Bones of the face viewed from the front (b) Bones of the face viewed from the right side

Bones of the neck and shoulder girdle

The neck

The skeleton of the neck comprises seven vertebrae (i.e. a segment of the spine) known as the cervical vertebrae; the first and second of these are the atlas and axis respectively.

The **atlas** is so named as it supports the 'globe' of the head as Atlas was thought to have supported the world. Although it lacks body or spinous processes it has articulating processes, concave ovals, that act like rocking cradles for the condyles of the occipital bone. This allows nodding movements of the head (see Fig. 6.3).

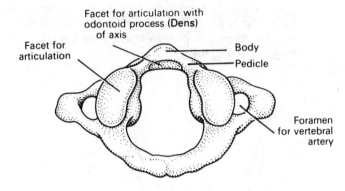

(a)

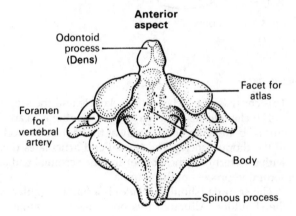

(b)

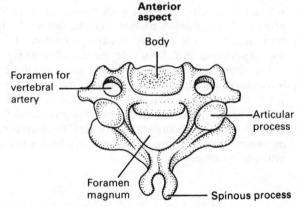

(c)

Fig. 6.3 (a) The atlas viewed from above (b) The axis viewed from above (c) A cervical vertebrae

The **axis** has a toothlike structure, called the dens, which projects upwards to form a pivot upon which the atlas, carrying the head, rotates.

Moving to the front of the neck there is a single U-shaped bone called the **hyoid**. It lies in front of the throat between the root of the tongue and the laryngeal prominence (Adam's apple) and it supports the tongue (see Fig. 6.4).

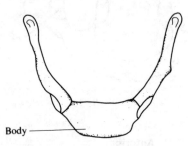

Body

Fig. 6.4 Hyoid bone

The shoulder girdle

This consists of two bones, the clavicle and the scapula.

The **clavicle**, also known as the collar bone, is an elongated, slender, curved bone lying horizontally at the root of the neck in the upper part of the thorax (chest). The sternal end articulates (i.e. united by joints) with the sternum (chest bone) and the acromial end articulates with the acromion process of the scapula.

The **scapula** (shoulder blade) is a flat, triangular bone in the back of the shoulder. Although this bone has three angles, the anterior part is pertinent here as it is the thickest part and forms the 'head' of the scapula. The head presents a shallow articular surface known as the glenoid cavity. The neck of the scapula surrounds the head of the scapula from which arises a thick prominence known as the coracoid process. The acromion process may be felt as the tip or edge of the shoulder. It is the slightly flaring projection at the lateral end of the scapula and articulates with the clavicle (see Fig. 6.5).

The shoulder is a ball-and-socket joint formed by the head of the humerus (the long uppermost bone of the arm) fitting into the glenoid cavity of the scapula. The joint is protected by an arch formed under the surface of the coracoid and acromion process, and synovial membrane and synovial fluid lubricate the socket. The shoulder joint is capable of movement in every direction – forward, backward, abduction, adduction and rotation.

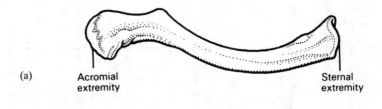

(a)   Acromial   Sternal
        extremity   extremity

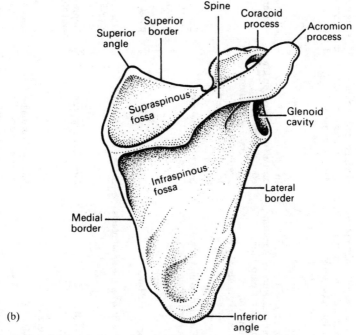

Fig. 6.5 (a) The right clavicle (b) The right scapula: Posterior view

Muscles of the face

These are generally described as muscles of facial expression with the exception of four, which are used for mastication. They can be attached to bones, other muscles or to the skin itself and they vary enormously in shape and strength and also differ in size from one person to another. Muscle contraction is usually the result of external stimuli received by one or more of the five senses and the contraction itself has an effect on the skin. When a contraction – such as frowning – is often repeated, furrows appear very gradually and can become permanent.

For simplicity, the location, origin, insertion and action are detailed in Table 6.1 for easy reference and it is important that these be remembered especially for electrical treatment and massage (see Fig. 6.6).

Table 6.1 The muscles of the face

Name	Location	Origin	Insertion	Action
Occipitofrontalis	Posterior part is occipitalis and anterior part is frontalis connected by an aponeurosis (tendon); forehead, over scalp and down to the nape of the neck	Occipital belly high in the occipital bone – frontal belly, in the aponeurosis	Occipital belly, in the aponeurosis – frontal belly, in the skin of the eyebrows and root of nose	The occipital belly draws the scalp backward. The frontal belly draws the scalp forward; raises the eyebrows and wrinkles the forehead
Orbicularis oculi	Sphincter muscle surrounding the cavity of the orbits	In 3 parts: orbital, centre of the orbit; palpebral, palpebral ligament; lacrimal, lacrimal crest	In 3 parts: orbital, near the origin after encircling the orbit; palpebral – attachment to the zygomatic bone; lacrimal – ligament of the lacrimal crest	Closes the eyelids and wrinkles the skin around the eye
Corrugator supercilli	Small triangular muscle beneath the inner part of the orbicularis oculi, between the two frontalis	The median end of the superciliary arch	Skin of the eyebrow	Draws the eyebrows downward and wrinkles the skin vertically as in frowning
Levator palpebrae superioris	Eyelid	Sphenoid bone	Skin of the eyelid	Raises upper eyelid
Procerus	High in the middle of the nose	Fascia over the nasal bones	Skin of the forehead	Draws eyebrows down, giving an expression of dissatisfaction or annoyance
Nasalis	Nose	Maxillae	Nostril and septum	Depresses the cartilage of the nose and also aids in widening the nostril
Posterior and anterior dilator naris	Very small muscles around the nostrils			Expand and contract nostrils when a person is angry
Quadratus labii superioris	Two levator muscles of the mouth	Maxillae	Skin and cartilage of the nose and upper lip	Raises upper lip and dilates nostril as in an expression of distaste
Levator anguli oris	Lies under quadratus labii superioris	Maxillae	Orbicularis oris and skin at the angle of the mouth	Raises the angle of the mouth
Orbicularis oris	A sphincter muscle of the mouth with no bony attachments, around upper and lower lips	2 parts: labial, whose fibres are restricted to the lips; marginal whose fibres mix with adjacent muscle fibres		Compresses, closes, contracts, puckers or purses lips, e.g. kissing or whistling

Muscle	Position/shape	Origin	Insertion	Action
Buccinator	Principal muscle of the cheek between the upper and lower jaws	From the cavities of the teeth in the maxillae and mandible	Orbicularis oris and lips	Compresses the cheek, also accessory muscle of mastication. Blowing up a paper bag is an exaggerated use of this muscle
Risorius	Triangular muscle in cheek	Fascia over masseter muscle	Skin at the angle of the mouth	Draws the angle of the mouth laterally and gives an expression of grinning
Mentalis	Small thick muscle between lower lip and chin	Incissive fossa of the mandible	Skin of the chin	Wrinkles the skin of the chin or pushes up lower lip. Gives expression of doubt or displeasure
Zygomaticus – major	Extends obliquely from the zygomatic bone to the angle of the mouth	Zygomatic bone	To the angle of the mouth	Draws the angle of the mouth upward and laterally
minor	Extends obliquely from the zygomatic bone to the angle of the mouth	Zygomatic bone	Orbicularis oris and levator labii superioris	Draws the upper lip upward and laterally giving expression of laughing or smiling
Depressor labii inferioris	Lower lip to mandible	External surface of the mandible	Orbicularis oris and skin of the lower lip	Depresses the lower lip, giving an expression of distaste or sarcasm
Depressor anguli oris	Triangular muscle from angle of the mouth to below the chin	Lower border of mandible continuous with the platysma	Orbicularis oris and risorius	Pulls the angle of the mouth downwards and laterally in expression of sadness
Temporalis	Fan-shaped muscle over the side of the head in front of the ear	Fascia of the temporal bone	Coronoid process of the mandible	Closes jaws and draws back lower jaw as it helps with mastication
Masseter – superficial and deep	In the cheeks	Both muscles originate at the zygomatic arch	Ramus of mandible	It raises the mandible and closes the jaws – aids mastication
Pterygoideus medialis (internal)	Runs down from the angle of the mouth towards the chin	Medial surface of the lateral pterygoid place	Medial surface of ramus and angle of mandible	Closes jaw
Pterygoideus lateralis has two heads	To the side of the angle of the mouth	Upper head greater wing of the spenoid; lower head lateral surface of the lateral pterygoid plate	Both enter the neck of the mandible and the capsule of the temporomandibular joint	Moves the mandible from side to side, opens the jaws and also protrudes the mandible

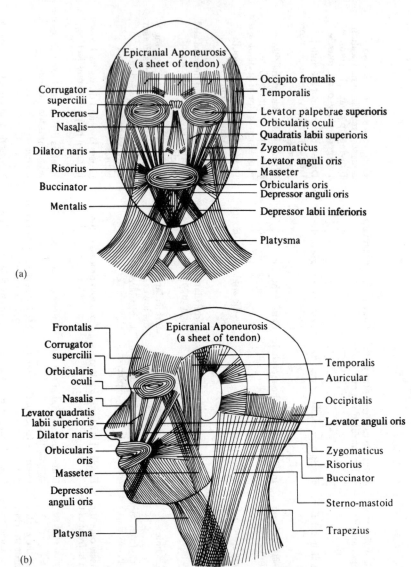

Fig. 6.6 (a) Muscles of the head and neck (front view) (b) muscles of the head and neck (side view)

Muscles of the neck and shoulder girdle

These are detailed in Table 6.2 and Fig. 6.7.

Arteries of the head, face and neck

The aorta, the great artery arising from the heart, branches at the aortic arch into three large arteries: the brachiocephalic trunk, which divides into the right common carotid and right subclavian arteries; the left

Table 6.2 The muscles of the neck and shoulder girdle

Name	Location	Origin	Insertion	Action
Deltoid	Shoulder	Clavicle and acromion process of the scapula	Lateral side of the humerus	Lifts, extends and rotates the arm
Pectoralis	Covers the chest	Clavicle and sternum	Lateral lip of bicipital groove of humerus	Draws arm across the chest and rotates it inwardly and supports mammary glands
Trapezius	Trianguar muscle covering back of neck and upper part of back	Occipital spinous of the last cervical and upper 6 thoracic vertebrae	Clavicle and spine of scapula	Level and poise of the shoulders Draws head backward or to one side. Rotates shoulder blades
Splenius capitus	Deep muscle, side of neck, under trapezius	Upper thoracic and lower cervical vertebrae	Occipital and mastoid process	By contraction head pulled backward in extension
Splenius longissimus	Deep muscle, side of neck, under trapezius	Upper thoracic and lower cervical vertebrae	Occipital and mastoid process	Flexes head, by contraction head is bent, blends with splenius capitus
Sternocleidomastoid	Lies obliquely across side of neck	2 heads, from upper part of sternum and clavicle	Mastoid process of the temporal bone	Draws head forward to shoulder and used in nodding
Platysma	Broad muscle extending from chest to chin	Pectoralis major and deltoid	Mandible and masseter	Depresses lower jaw and lip
Levator scapulae	Side of neck under trapezius	Transverse processes of upper 4 cervical vertebrae	Medial border of scapula	Used in hunching shoulders or extension of neck

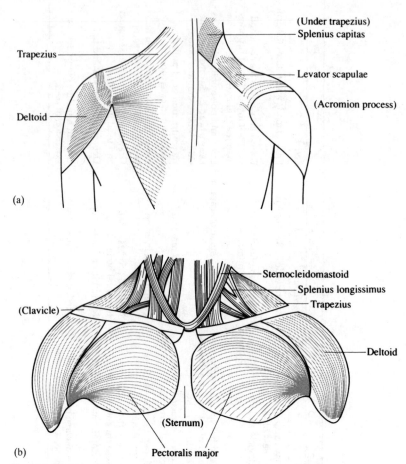

Trapezius

(Under trapezius)
Splenius capitas

Levator scapulae

(Acromion process)

Deltoid

(a)

Sternocleidomastoid
Splenius longissimus
Trapezius

(Clavicle)

Deltoid

(Sternum)

(b)

Pectoralis major

Fig. 6.7 Muscles of the neck and shoulder girdle (a) Posterior (b) Anterior

common carotid artery; and the left subclavian artery. The subclavian arteries then become the axillary and brachial arteries of the arms. The common carotid arteries each divide into an internal and an external branch to supply the head and neck. Table 6.3 and Fig. 6.8 show the principal vessels supplying the general area.

Veins of the head, face and neck

The most important veins lie almost parallel with the arteries and have the same name. The blood from the brain drains in the interior of the skull, into channels formed by the dura mater (a tough covering of the brain) called venous sinuses. From these sinuses the blood returns to the heart by two principal veins either side of the neck. Table 6.4 and Fig. 6.9 show the veins which drain eventually into the external and internal jugular veins. In the neck area these empty into the subclavian or brachiocephalic veins.

Table 6.3 The arteries of the head and neck

Name	Branches	Divides into	Supplies
Internal carotid	Ophthalmic	Supra-orbital	Forehead, superior muscles of the orbit, upper eyelid
		Supra-trochlear	Anterior part of the scalp
		Lacrimal	Lacrimal gland and eyelids
	Anterior and middle cerebral		Brain, forehead and middle ear
External carotid	Superior thyroid		Muscles of the hyoid bone, larynx, thyroid gland and pharynx
	Lingual		Tongue, tonsils and epiglottis
	Facial		Face, tonsils, palate
	Maxillary		Both jaws, teeth, muscles of mastication, ear, nose, palate and paranasal sinuses
	Superficial temporal	Parotid	Parotid gland
		Posterior auricular	Middle ear, auricle and skin of the ear
		Frontal	Forehead
		Parietal	Crown and sides of head
		Transverse facial	Masseter
		Middle temporal	Temples and eyelids
	Occipital	Occipital and sternocleidomastoid	Muscles of the neck and scalp

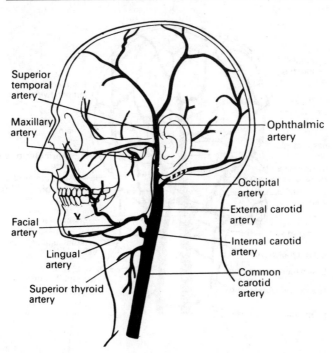

Fig. 6.8 Main arteries of the left side of the head and neck

Table 6.4 The veins of the head and neck

Name	Branches	Position
External jugular	Superficial temporal	Drains lateral part of scalp in frontal and parietal regions and joins maxillary branch to form the retromandibular
	Auricular posterior	Passes down behind the auricle and joins the retromandibular
	Auricular anterior	Passes in front of the auricle to join the superficial temporal branch
	Retromandibular	Passes behind the neck of the mandible and runs directly into the external jugular
	Maxillary	Drains areas of jaws, ears and nose before joining the superficial temporal to form the retromandibular
	Anterior jugular	Arises under the chin and passes down the neck to join the external jugular
Internal jugular	Facial and deep facial	Drains areas of face, tonsils and palate joining the internal jugular
	Transverse facial	Passes just below the zygomatic arch and drains into the retromandibular
	Angular	Passes between the eye and root of the nose to join the facial branch
	Lingual	Follows the lingual artery and joins directly into the internal jugular
	Thyroid middle and superior	Drains the area of the thyroid gland and joins directly into the internal jugular

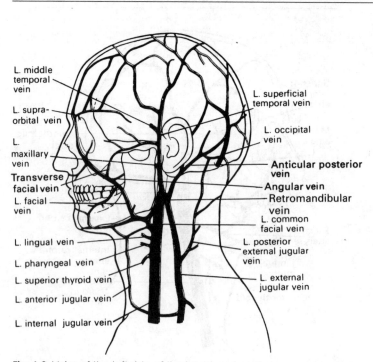

Fig. 6.9 Veins of the left side of the head and neck

Nerves of the head, face and neck

There are twelve pairs of cranial nerves and these are detailed in Tables 6.5–6.7 and Figs 6.10 and 6.11. Although all of them should be remembered, the fifth, seventh and eleventh cranial nerves and the cervical nerves originating from the spine are the most important when giving facial treatments.

Table 6.5 The twelve pairs of cranial nerves

Name	No.	Type of nerve	Function
Olfactory	1st	Sensory	Nerve of smell
Optic	2nd	Sensory	Nerve for the sense of sight
Oculomotor	3rd	Motor	Controls the muscle of the eye
Trochlear	4th	Motor	Nerve to the corrugator muscle
Trigeminal	5th	Sensory	Nerve to the scalp and face
		Motor	Nerve to muscles of mastication
Abducent	6th	Motor	Nerve to one of the muscles moving the eyeball
Facial	7th	Motor	Nerve to muscles of facial expression and part of the scalp
		Sensory	Nerve to the tongue
Auditory	8th	Sensory	For the sense of hearing and it also maintains body balance
Glossopharyngeal	9th	Sensory	Nerve of taste
		Motor	Nerve to the muscles of the tongue
Vagus	10th	Sensory	Nerve to respiratory and digestive organs
		Motor	Nerve to the above and to the heart
Accessory	11th	Motor	Nerve to sternocleidomastoid and the trapezius muscles
Hypoglossal	12th	Motor	Nerve to the muscles of the tongue

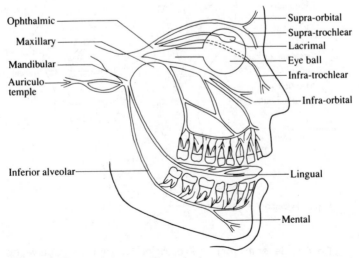

Fig. 6.10 Fifth cranial nerve, Trigeminal

Table 6.6 The fifth cranial nerve – trigeminal

This is the largest cranial nerve, the chief sensory nerve of the face and supplying most of the skin. There is a small motor nerve supplying the muscles of mastication. It arises from the brain and in front of the ear it divides into 3 parts.

Name	Branches	Function
Opthalmic	Supra-orbital	Affects the skin on the forehead, scalp, eyebrows and upper eyelids
	Supra-trochlear	Affects the skin between the eyes and the upper side of the nose
	Infra-trochlear	Affects the membrane and side of the nose
	Nasal	Affects the tip and lower sides of the nose
	Lacrimal	Affects the upper eyelids and tear ducts
Maxillary	Zygomatic	Affects the temple, side of the forehead and skin of the upper part of the cheek
	Infra-Orbital	Affects skin of lower eyelid, skin of the nose, upper lip and mouth
Mandibular	Anterior	Affects muscles of mastication, buccinator and the skin of the cheeks
	Posterior in 3 parts	
	Auriculotemple	Affects the ear and skin above the temple to the top of the skull
	Inferior alveolar	Affects all the teeth along the lower jaw
	Mental	A branch of the inferior alveolar affecting the skin of the lower lip and chin

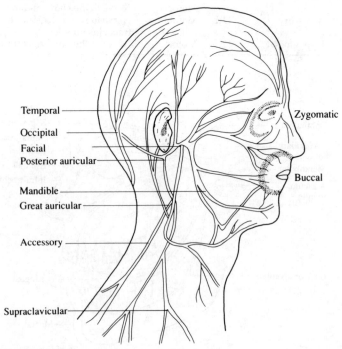

Fig. 6.11 Seventh cranial nerve, facial. Eleventh cranial nerve, accesory, cervical nerves

Table 6.7 The seventh cranial nerve – facial; eleventh cranial nerve – accessory; and cervical nerves

Seventh cranial nerve – facial

This is the chief motor nerve of the face. It emerges near the lower part of the ear and its branches supply and control the muscles of facial expression and extend to the muscles of the neck area.

Branches	Function
Posterior auricular	Affects the sternocleidomastoid, auricularis posterior and occipitalis
Temporal	Affects the temporalis, auricularis anterior, zygomaticus, orbicularis oris and corrugator
Zygomatic	Affects the zygomaticus
Buccal	Affects the buccinator quadratus labii superioris, obicularis oris
Mandibular	Affects the quadratus labii inferiors, triangularis, mentalis, orbicularis oris and platysma

Eleventh cranial nerve – accessory

This nerve extends over the neck and upper part of the back. It has two branches, one internal and one external. The external branch affects the sternocleidomastoid and trapezius.

Cervical nerves

These nerves originate from the spinal cord and supply the muscles of the back of the head and neck

Branches	Function
Greater and lesser occipital	Both affect the occipitalis
Greater auricular	Affects the sternocleidomastoid, auricularis posterior and anterior
Supraclavicular	Affects sternocleidomastoid and platysma

Self assessment

- an anatomical position refers to the body in an upright position, explain the following terms:

    superior
    anterior
    median line
    symmetrical

- name, or give a diagram of, the 8 bones of the cranium and the 14 bones of the face
- explain the movements of the atlas and axis
- how does the clavicle articulate with the scapula?
- the scapula is the shoulder blade, explain its three angles and say which type of joint is formed with the humerus
- give the location, origin, insertion and action of the following muscles of the face, neck and shoulder girdle:

    orbicularis oculi
    masseter
    orbicularis oris

corrugator supercilli
zygomaticus major
temporalis
pterygoideus lateralis
trapezius
levator scapulae
platysma
sternocleidomastoid
pectoralis
deltoid

- which branches of the external carotid artery supply:

    (a) the ears, nose and teeth, and
    (b) the temples and eyelids?

- name the corresponding veins which drain the blood into the external and internal jugular veins
- the trigeminal nerve is the largest cranial nerve, name the branches which supply the forehead, scalp, eyebrows and upper eyelids, the skin of the lower lip and chin
- which is the chief motor nerve of the face, name the 5 branches and describe their function
- which nerve affects the sternocleidomastoid and trapezius muscles.

7 Structure and functions of the skin

The skin, like other organs, is made up of muscle, connective tissue, blood capillaries, lymphatics and epithelial cells. As it is the external covering of the body it is liable to more forms of irritation than other organs.

The skin is constantly being worn away and replenished by new cells from below. It varies in thickness on different parts of the body; for instance, it is thinnest on the eyelids and lips and thickest on the soles of the feet, palms of the hands and buttocks.

The attachment of the skin to the structure underneath varies with the density of areolar and adipose tissue present; on the buttocks, for example, where areolar tissue is compact or where fat is plentiful, the connection is firm. On the eyelids and joints where greater mobility is required the aerolar tissue is loose, so the connection is slight.

The skin is divided into two layers, epidermis and dermis.

Epidermis

This is a laminated, slightly elastic membrane composed of stratified epithelium and consists of five layers. It contains no blood vessels and has very few nerves. It is pierced by hair follicles and the ducts of the sweat and sebaceous glands. It is marked by minute furrows which represent the depressions caused by the papillae in the dermis (see Fig. 7.1). Outward from within these five layers are:

Stratum germinativum (or basal layer)

In this layer there are cells from which new epidermal cells are constantly being produced. The cells are packed closely together and form the first layer or two of cells which rest on the papillae of the dermis. The cells of the deepest layer are conical in shape and as they multiply, the cells previously formed are pushed towards the surface (being in turn components of the different layers). This cellular multiplication is known as 'cellular regeneration' and it may be increased or decreased by a number of factors, such as age or state of health. This layer contains pigment-bearing cells known as melanocytes which produces melanin. This in turn determines the colour of the skin.

Stratum Malpighii

This layer can be referred to as stratum aculeatum or stratum spinosum. It is composed of several layers of nucleated cells which vary in

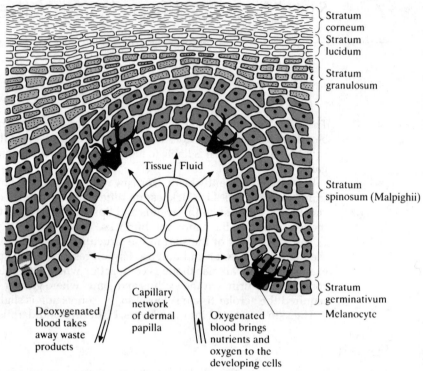

Fig. 7.1 The layers of the epidermis

size and shape. It is the upper portion of this layer which is known as the stratum spinosum or the prickle-cell layer. This is because the cells are linked by fine threads and their projections give a prickly or spiky appearance.

Stratum granulosum (granular layer)

This has between one and four layers of flattened cells well defined and containing nuclei. As the cells from the layer beneath ascend to the surface they become progressively larger and accumulate granules containing a substance called keratohyalin, which plays an important role in the production of epidermal keratin, the latter being a scleroprotein, a strong fibrous protein in the epidermis. Soft keratin is a component of the epidermis and hair follicles, whereas hard keratin is found in nails, the cortex and cuticle of the hair and the organic matrix of the enamel of the teeth.

Stratum lucidum

A narrow transparent layer with an indistinct outline and no nuclei lying immediately beneath the stratum corneum. It is sometimes regarded as a 'junction area' between this and the stratum granulosum. In this layer the cells are almost at the end of their life-span. They are becoming dehydrated and the keratohyalin granules present in the stratum granulosum are gradually formed into keratin.

Stratum corneum (horny layer)

This is the external layer composed of several strata (15–20) of flattened irregular-shaped cells. They assume this flattened form from the evaporation of their fluid contents, and the horny epithelial scales consist almost entirely of keratin. This layer is the protector of the skin, preventing excessive dehydration of the skin tissues. As the cells near the surface they desquamate (shed) or are rubbed off during normal wear and tear of the skin. The outer layer is sometimes called the squamous layer or stratum disjunction.

It takes about three weeks to a month for cells to activate from the stratum germinativum to the stratum corneum and shed.

Dermis

This is the true skin situated immediately below the epidermis, sometimes called corium or cutis vera. It is a highly sensitive and vascular layer of connective tissue and contains blood vessels, lymph vessels, nerves, sweat and sebaceous glands, hair follicles, arrector pili muscles and papillae. It has two layers and contains 60 per cent of the water circulating in the skin.

Papillary

This lies directly under the epidermis containing small cone-shaped projections of connective tissue which protrude into the epidermis. These projections are called papillae. Some of these papillae contain looped capillaries, others contain nerve endings called tactile corpuscles. This layer, together with the stratum germinativum, represents the most active area of the skin. It consists of stationary cells called fibroblasts forming a network of fibrils (minute filaments) and migrating cells called phagocytes which resemble leukocytes of the blood.

Reticular (deep layer or corium)

This layer is continuous with the papillary and consists of a highly sensitive and vascular layer of connective tissue. The elements forming the bundles of the connective tissue are:

1. *collagenous fibres* composed of an albumnoid protein called collagen;
2. *elastic fibres* which are composed of a protein, elastin.

These fibres maintain the skin's tone and elasticity (see Fig. 7.2).

The principal functions of the dermis are to provide nourishment to the epidermis and to be a supporting framework in the cutaneous tissues. Therefore you will appreciate that all beauty treatments involving

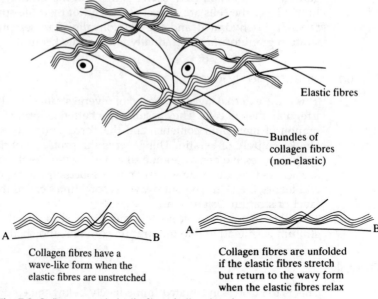

Fig. 7.2 Collagen and elastic fibres in the dermis

stimulation and nourishment of the skin should affect the dermis as well as the epidermis.

Hypodermis (or subcutaneous)

This is a thick layer consisting of fatty connective tissue found below the dermis. Adipose and aerolar tissue are present in this layer and the latter act as 'shock absorbers', supporting delicate structures, such as blood vessels and nerve endings. The fatty tissue varies in thickness according to the age and general health of the individual.

Vascular system of the skin

Blood

The arteries supplying the skin form a plexus (network) in the subcutaneous tissue from which ascending arterial branches supply blood to the hair follicles, sweat glands and sebaceous glands. These arterioles also branch horizontally to form the sub-papillary plexus just beneath the papillary layer of the dermis. Ascending vessels from this plexus supply the capillary networks in the dermal papillae.

Venules form descending branches to the sub-papillary plexus and then to the subcutaneous plexus taking waste products away from the skin. Venules also collect blood from the capillaries around follicles and glands and return it to the subcutaneous plexus.

Lymph

The lymphatics are numerous in the dermis and generally accompany the veins. Lymph vessels are found around the dermal papillae, glands and hair follicles.

Nervous system of the skin

The skin has two different types of nerve fibres, sensory and motor (see Fig. 7.3).

Sensory

The sensation of touch resulting from the stimulation of the nerve endings in the skin varies with the type of nerve ending stimulated. Certain spots exist in the skin called sensory spots and some of these are sensitive to cold, some to heat and some to pain. Therefore sensory nerves do not end in the same way. They are located in the papillary (by the papillae) and reticular of the dermis. Sensory nerves terminate into:

1. free endings, which supply the various strata of the epidermis but always beneath the stratum granulosum;
2. tactile corpuscles, which are specialised in as much as they can be divided in corpuscles sensitive to heat, cold, pressure, etc. Complex sensations, such as vibration, seem to depend on a combination of both these nerve endings.

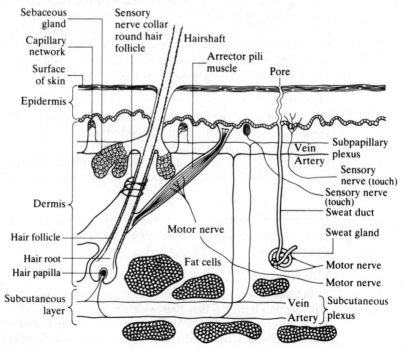

Fig. 7.3 Section of skin

Motor

These are distributed to the blood vessels and to the arrector pili muscles of the hair follicles. Stimulation of these nerves to the blood vessels results in an increase or decrease of the blood flow in the capillaries. Stimulation of the arrector pili muscles results in the erection of the hair and formation of a 'goose pimple' at the mouth of the follicle.

Appendages of the skin

These are the hair, nails (a separate chapter is devoted to these), sebaceous glands and sweat glands (see Fig. 7.3).

Hair

Hairs are a peculiar modification of the epidermis, varying in length, thickness and colour. They are found in every region of the body except the palms of the hands, soles of the feet, mucous membrane of the genitals and the lips (see Figs 7.4 and 7.5).

Hair follicle

This is a pore-like indentation in the skin in which a hair develops from the matrix at the base. A hair follicle is formed as a downgrowth of the epidermis into the dermis, the follicle wall or outer sheath being continuous with the Malpighian layer of the epidermis. While in the follicle the hair itself is enclosed and protected by an inner root sheath which grows along with the hair but degenerates at about the level of the opening of the sebaceous gland. When a hair is plucked the inner root sheath is removed along with the hair. The whole follicle is enclosed in a connective tissue sheath which is continuous with the corium and is highly vascular and well supplied with nerve fibres.

Hair root

This part of the structure of the hair which lies in the follicle and the enlarged base of the root (a club-shaped formation) is known as the hair bulb. The latter surrounds loose connective tissue called the dermal papilla which is rich with blood and nerve supply, thereby contributing to the growth and regeneration of the hair, but is not part of the follicle.

Hair shaft or scapus

This extends above the surface of the skin and is composed of keratinised cells.

Hair structure

In the main there are two main classifications of hair, vellus and terminal. Lanugo hair is foetal hair which is replaced by vellus hair in the same follicles before birth. Vellus hairs are usually found on the cheeks and elsewhere where hairs are downy and soft. Terminal hairs are much coarser and grow on the underarms, pubic region and of course

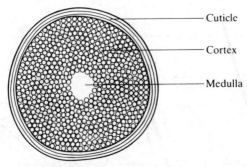

Fig. 7.4 Section of hair shaft

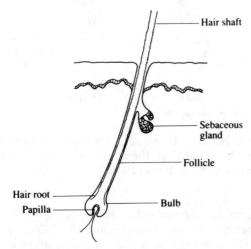

Fig. 7.5 Hair follicle, root and shaft

the scalp. Vellus hair lacks pigmentation and although it may share the same opening as a sebaceous gland it always has its own follicle. It is unusual for a vellus hair to become a terminal hair but it may occur if it is stimulated by an increase in glandular activity; for instance, terminal hair may replace vellus hair in the same follicles in the beard area of males at puberty. It may also occur by what is known as 'topical' irritation, plucking or depilatory waxing. Sometimes then a vellus hair will turn downwards and over a period of time become a follicle of a terminal hair. Terminal hairs have a well-developed root and bulb and are composed of cells in three layers (see Fig. 7.4).

1. **Cuticle** is the outside layer, composed of transparent, overlapping protective scale-like cells pointing towards the shaft end.
2. **Cortex** is the inner layer which gives strength and elasticity to the hair. It is composed of elongated cells and contains the pigment giving hair its colour.
3. **Medulla** is the marrow of the hair shaft which is composed of round cells. It may not be present in very fine hair.

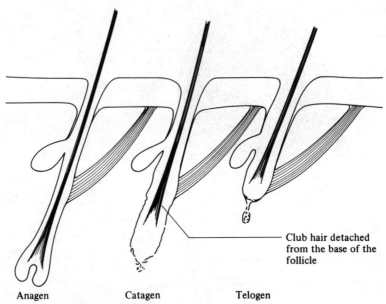

Club hair detached
from the base of the
follicle

Anagen   Catagen   Telogen

Fig. 7.6 Growth cycle of the hair follicle

The shape of the hair usually assumes the shape and size of the follicle, for instance, for straight hair the follicle is round; for wavy hair it is oval and for curly hair it is almost flat.

Hair growth

The lifetime of terminal hairs varies but the average growth rate of hair is about a half-inch per month and approximately 25–50 scalp hairs are shed each day. The growth cycle of hair is divided into three stages – anagen, catagen and telogen (see Fig. 7.6).

1. **Anagen** is the period of active growth which only ends when the hair becomes loose from the papilla and not able to receive nourishment from the dermal papilla.
2. **Catagen** is the transitional stage and very short-lived where the follicle begins to shrink or a new hair begins at the base of the follicle as the old hair moves up the follicle to rest or shed.
3. **Telogen** is the final part of the resting period; how long the follicle rests is dependent on the individual or the type of hair.

Arrector pili

This is a minute involuntary muscle, controlled by the sympathetic nervous system, attached at an angle to the base of the follicle. Eyelashes and eyebrows do not have these muscles (see Fig. 7.3).

Sebaceous glands

These are small saccular glands found in the dermis. Their ducts are usually connected to hair follicles. These glands are oval in shape and are most numerous in the scalp and face (around the nose, mouth and ear) but they do not occur in the skin on the palms of the hands or soles of the feet. Both gland and duct are lined with epithelial cells. Changes in these cells result in a fatty secretion called sebum which is composed of fat and epithelial cells of the Malpighian layer. Adequate sebum is important, it gives lustre to the hair and keeps the skin soft and supple. Secretion varies with age and state of health and it is also subject to the activities of certain endocrine glands. Secretion is slight in the young until puberty, increases in the adult and decreases with age. Inadequate secretion of sebum causes the hair to become dull and brittle and the skin to become dry. If dry patches on the skin irritate, they can become infected through rubbing or scratching.

Excess secretion of sebum (seborrhea) causes an oily skin and hair. Although not a direct cause of blackheads, if left on the skin, the excess sebum will attract dust and trap dirt and block the pores of the sweat glands. The amount of sebum present on the face is one factor which will decide the choice of treatment or cosmetic preparation and advice to the client.

Sweat glands (or sudoriferous glands)

There are approximately two million of these glands in the body. The active secretion, sweat, from these glands is under the control of the sympathetic nervous system. It is essentially a salt solution containing water, sodium chloride, small amounts of urea and lactic acid. It also has anti-bacterial substances which help the body's defence against infection. If the liquid evaporates without the skin becoming visibly wet, insensible perspiration is taking place. If the skin becomes wet, sensible perspiration is taking place. There are two types of sweat gland:

1. **Eccrine gland**: most of the glands are of this type and open on the surface of the skin. Their function is to regulate body temperature

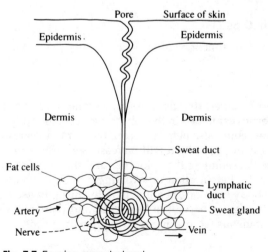

Fig. 7.7 Eccrine sweat gland

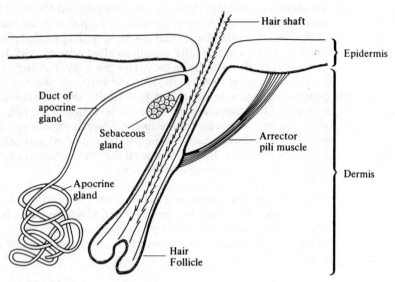

Fig. 7.8 Hair follicle with apocrine gland

and help eliminate waste products. Normally one or two pints of liquid are eliminated daily through the sweat pores. Practically all parts of the body are supplied with sweat glands but they are more numerous on the palms of the hands, soles of the feet, forehead (see Fig. 7.7).

2. **Apocrine glands** are connected with hair follicles but are only found in the genital and underarm regions. They produce a more fatty type of secretion than the eccrine glands. Breakdown of the secretion by bacteria leads to body odour under the armpits and in the groin. Their activity is increased by heat, exercise, emotions and drugs of a certain type (see Fig. 7.8).

The functions of the skin

To summarise the functions of the skin:

Protection

The dead horny layer, *stratum corneum*, together with the slightly anti-septic properties contained in the sebum, protects the body against bac-teria. Natural sebum also helps to screen the ultra-violet rays of the sun. Melanin pigment production will increase with exposure to the sun's rays and the darkening of the epidermis and this provides a protection to the true skin. Perspiration or sweating, which has a cooling effect, protects the body from overheating. Finally, the body itself is protected by the skin's sensory nerves, to heat, cold and pain, and by its horny layer and cutaneous fat, making it virtually waterproof.

Absorption

Having said that one of the skin's most important roles is to provide a protective waterproof covering, how then can we expect cosmetics to penetrate the epidermis? The medical profession has proved that certain drugs, such as iodine, antibiotics or copper sulphate and oil can be introduced into the skin, minimal amounts of water will also penetrate the epidermis. Therefore it must be assumed that there is a degree of absorption by the skin, albeit small, by the sebaceous glands, the hair follicles and vellus hairs.

Regulation of body temperature

The circulatory system regulates the body's temperature. For instance, if the outside temperature drops, the body is able to respond because the nerve endings near the skin sense the change and communicate it to the hypothalamus (portion of the brain). Certain cells of the hypothalamus then signal to increase the body's heat production. On the other hand the body will conserve its heat by constricting the arterioles so that less blood will flow near the surface of the skin. On a hot day, sweat is released and evaporates and the skin cools. Body temperature varies at the time of day, being slightly higher in the evening, immediately after eating, excitement or exercise. The temperature of a healthy adult is normally 98.6 °F (37 °C).

Excretion and secretion

Excretion is minimal and concerns the removal of waste products by the sweat glands. Secretion concerns the production of sebum through the sebaceous glands to keep the skin supple and add lustre to the hair.

Sensation

The nerve endings in the skin are responsible for this and enable us to be aware of pain, pressure, pleasure, heat or cold. Many books have been written on 'touch' therapy, but for the therapist it is the hands which are the most important communicating role. The ability to feel the texture of the skin, the structures of the body and the type of tissue present all indicate the correct treatment and advice. It is worth mentioning here that the therapist's hands should not be sticky or hot or be like 'blocks of ice'. They should be cool, flexible and light, transmitting comfort and reassurance.

Note: One square centimetre of skin contain 1 yd (0.9 m) of blood vessels, 4 yds (3.6 m) of nerves, 200 nerve endings, 100 suderiferous glands, 15 sebaceous glands and 10 hairs.

Self assessment

The epidermis has 5 layers, explain these from the basal layer to the horny layer and say how long it takes for a new cell to be shed

- explain the principal functions of the cutis vera and name the two layers
- where would you find collagenous and elastin fibres?
- in which layer would you expect to find adipose and areolar tissue?
- describe how blood is circulated in the skin
- where would you find the lymphatics in the skin?
- where are sensory nerves located and how do they terminate?
- how are motor nerves distributed to the skin and what is their action?
- hair is an appendage of the skin, explain the structure of the hair and its growth cycle
- where would you find sebaceous glands and where are they most numerous in the scalp and face?
- sebum, the secretion from sebaceous glands, is important as it keeps the skin soft and supple, but explain what happens when the glands become either under-active or over-active
- which nervous system controls the sudoriferous glands?
- what is the difference between

  (a) eccrine glands, and
  (b) apocrine glands

- summarise the functions of the skin by explaining how:

  it is protected
  cosmetics can penetrate the epidermis
  the skin can help to regulate the body temperature
  sensation can be felt?

8 Factors influencing skin condition

There are many factors which have a temporary or more lasting effect on the skin, some beneficial others detrimental. Before dealing with each specific type, consider first what will affect the skin.

A nutritious diet for the reproduction of healthy new skin cells should include certain vitamins, taken in their natural state, such as:

1. *Vitamin A*, found in milk, cheese, eggs, butter, spinach, broccoli, carrots, offal and fish oils. It helps to repair body tissue and prevent skin dryness and ageing. It is a fat-soluble vitamin (which means that it can be stored in the liver and does not need replenishing daily) but if taken in excess can be detrimental.
2. *Vitamin B*, found in yoghurt, wholemeal bread, wheatgerm, yeast, cereal, green leafy vegetables and offal. It improves circulation and therefore skin colour and is essential to cellular oxidation which directly affects the skin.
3. *Vitamin C*, found in citrus fruits, strawberries, blackcurrants, potatoes, cabbage, broccoli, sprouts and watercress. It is essential for healing and its main use is to maintain levels of collagen.

Both vitamins B and C are water soluble and should be taken daily as excess is excreted in the urine.

This is only a partial list of vitamins; most are detailed under 'Nutrition and diet' in Volume 2. The old adage 'You are what you eat' still holds true as the skin is a barometer of general health. Despite all the claims made by cosmetic manufacturers about 'feeding' the skin, there is only one way the skin can be nourished (in the literal sense of the word) and that is from the blood. It takes a healthy body to have a healthy skin.

Water is essential, preferably a pint daily. It aids digestion and helps to flush the kidneys and prevent a build-up of toxicity in the body's system.

Rapid weight loss, either as a result of illness or excessive dieting, will deplete the skin of its water (hydric balance) causing dehydration. Fad or crash diets rarely contain all the nutrients necessary for good health and therefore a healthy skin.

Sleep is the most important beauty treatment. The amount required varies with each individual but sufficient deep sleep is essential to mental and physical health. A good night's sleep will help to make the eyes sparkle and the skin glow.

Stress and tension, the single most destructive factor in our emotional and mental lives today. It causes lines around the eyes, furrows on the forehead and as the skin is a very sensitive indicator it often reacts and produces an abnormal skin condition, e.g. shingles, eczema and even boils. As a beauty therapist you cannot alleviate your client's personal problems but you can help to relax the neck and shoulders, mouth, eyes and forehead with a few basic exercises (see Table 8.1). You can ensure relaxing treatments are given and have a sympathetic attitude towards your client.

Table 8.1 Exercises to relax the neck, shoulders, mouth, eyes and forehead

Neck and shoulder	For tension in the shoulder area, sit the client comfortably and let the head drop on to the chest and rotate very slowly to one side; let the head drop backwards and to the other side and finally on to the chest again. This can be repeated three times to the left and three times to the right.
	Pick up one shoulder to the ear and let it drop. Repeat several times and then rotate the shoulder forward and backward. The other shoulder can then repeat the exercise.
	Finish with both shoulders rotating together forward and backward
Mouth	Pretend to be blowing up a balloon or blowing a trumpet and relax.
	Stretch the mouth sideways as if saying 'eee' and relax.
	Lift the left corner of the mouth to the eye, using the cheek muscles and relax and repeat with the right side
Eyes	Open them very wide and relax.
	Rotate both eyeballs very slowly to the right, look up to the left and then look down.
	This can be repeated the opposite way and finish with closing the eyes for a second or two
Forehead	Lift the forehead up into wrinkles and relax several times.

Fresh air and exercise are vital to overall health. Exercise promotes good circulation, increases oxygen intake and blood flow and is therefore important for the skin as the dermis relies entirely on the blood supply for nutrients.

Hormones play an important part in the condition of the skin. During puberty the hormonal balance is responsible for the coarsening of the pores and the sex hormones stimulate the glands. Deep cleansing must play an important role in maintaining a clear complexion and care should be taken not to over-stimulate the skin.

At the onset of the menstrual cycle various sequences occur which are controlled by two hormones, oestrogen and progesterone. Occasionally the skin will erupt. Advise clients of a suitable healing and drying product and emphasise the importance of cleansing the skin to prevent the possibility of infection. You may also suggest using less make-up for this short time as it tends to accentuate puffiness and lines caused by tension and stress due to discomfort.

During pregnancy pigmentation changes are common but these usually disappear after birth. The pigmentation may worsen if exposed to ultra-violet rays, it is one reason why the sun-bed is a contra-indication during pregnancy.

The menopause has an effect on the skin as the body undergoes a hormonal change. The normal supply of oestrogen is greatly reduced and eventually stops. HRT (hormone replacement therapy) is available which certainly helps to keep tissues healthy and control some of the ageing effects. In the salon you will have clients suffering from emotional changes due to the menopause when they are nervous, apprehensive and often weepy. A sympathetic ear and relaxing treatments are important and at this stage electrical treatments should be avoided. They may suffer 'hot flushes' where the face becomes red and there is excessive sweating. You can only make the client comfortable by using cooling treatments, i.e. cool facial sprays and fresh eye pads. Once the sweating has subsided, a very light facial massage may be given, followed by a cooling mask, spray and moisturiser.

For post-menopause clients advise regular care of the skin to keep the epidermis soft and supple.

The pill has a high oestrogen content and its effect on the skin is individual. Most women say that there is no obvious change; some say their skin improves whereas others say it worsens. Occasionally the pill causes brown pigmentation on the face, but usually the client will seek further medical advice. Dermatologists have prescribed the pill (instead of antibiotics) to acne sufferers with good results.

Skin colour not only varies in different parts of the body but from person to person, mainly depending on hereditary factors, hormones and climactic environment. Melanocytes (melanin-forming cells) are found in the germinative layer of the epidermis. Their function is to produce granules (or grains) containing the pigment melanin and to distribute these via the dendrites of the melanocytes to the prickle-cell layer (stratum spinosum). Melanin itself is the brown pigment and is formed by the oxidation of the amino acid, tyrosine, under the influence of an enzyme called tyrosinase. The function of melanin is to absorb harmful ultra-violet rays from the sun.

Heredity seems to play an important role in determining the colour of the skin. Experts believe that four to six pairs of genes exert the primary control over the amount of melanin formed by melanocytes. Therefore, heredity must determine how light or dark one's basic colour will be. Other factors will modify this effect, i.e. sunlight and hormones. The excess secretion of MSH (melanocyte-stimulating hormone) from the anterior pituitary gland will increase melanin production.

In white-skinned races, through enzyme action, melanin is normally broken down as it reaches the stratum lucidum. However, exposure to ultra-violet rays causes the melanocytes to be stimulated to increase melanin production. In dark-skinned races, the number of melanocytes is not thought to be any greater, but their activity is increased, producing larger quantities of melanin and they are more efficient in providing protection against ultra-violet rays.

Melanin is not the only skin pigment. There is also carotene, the natural yellowish pigment of the epidermal cells themselves.

Basically, there are three colour groups – black, yellow and white – but within each group there are considerable variances of skin shades. Afro-Asian skins will vary from blue-black to pale olive; Chinese skins have a yellow tinge; Japanese skins are creamier.

Skin colour can also change without any change in melanin. It can often alter through a change in the volume of blood flowing through the capillaries. If the blood vessels dilate, as they do in blushing, the skin appears red due to oxyhaemoglobin in the red blood cells. If the vessels are constricted, e.g. by the cold, the blood flow decreases and the presence of de-oxygenated blood makes the skin appear blue. In general, the sparser the pigments in the epidermis the more transparent the skin is and therefore the more vivid the change in the skin colour will be with a change in blood volume. Conversely, the richer the pigmentation, the more opaque the skin, resulting in less colour change with a change in skin blood volume.

The environment

The **environment** in which we live can have an adverse effect on the skin.

Climate

With clients now travelling to and from countries further afield, you need to know how the skin is affected by associated climates.

1. Desert climates are hot and dry during the day and in some areas the temperature drops to nearly freezing at night. The humidity (i.e. the degree of moisture in the air) is low and if the skin is uncared for it will dry and age. The highest protection from the sun is needed and a wide-brimmed hat to protect the delicate facial skin. Advise clients to use moisturisers and night creams to prevent skin water loss.
2. Tropical climates have a very high humidity content as well as being exceedingly hot. This will result in an oily skin where the pores are continually open and the sweat never evaporates. White skins look sallow, greasy and unhealthy. Dark skins are much better adapted as they are rich in pigments, sebaceous glands, sudoriferous glands and venous and arterial capillaries.

   Air-conditioned houses and offices provide respite from the heat but bring their own problems. Air conditioning lacks moisture or humidity and the skin becomes dehydrated. Cleansing is still important to keep the skin clear of bacteria. Showering and moisturising the body and face well before sitting in air-conditioned rooms helps prevent water loss from the skin. A container of fresh water daily with herbs added provides some moisture for the room.
3. Sub-tropical climates are obviously slightly cooler and the humidity less with more variation in temperature. Although the skin looks healthier it remains oily with enlarged pores. Cleansing is again necessary to prevent bacteria spreading. With less humidity care

should be taken to ensure the sun does not dry out the top layers of the skin. Protect with sunscreens and moisturisers.

4. Arctic climates with their sub-zero temperatures cause excessive dryness and the cold can burn more quickly than the sun.

5. Temperate climates have few extremes of temperature and humidity. The four seasons are very distinctive and this makes it easy to plan seasonal skin-care regimes. The British complain about their weather but it is the humidity content in the air that keeps the skin from dying out quickly. In this climate offices and homes are often centrally heated in winter. From an artificially hot atmosphere created by a heating system the air is dehydrated and moisture is lost from the skin at a faster rate than it can be replaced. To humidify the air, place a container of water near a radiator or vent. Humidifiers or vaporisers are of benefit if they are cleaned daily with detergent. Water residue in a humidifier can build up a fungus that is dispersed into the air with the moisture which is eventually inhaled and can produce harmful mycoses (disease). However, research has shown that the new ionisers (now available) producing negative ions do have an advantageous effect on physical and mental capacity.

The weather can have an effect on the skin, a warm humid day will stimulate the sebaceous glands and a hot day will stimulate the sweat glands. Extremes of hot and cold will dry out the skin. When cold winds blow advise the use of a chap stick, barrier creams and under eye cream as added protection.

Pollution

This is one of the most difficult adverse elements to avoid, especially for those who live in or near cities. Waste gases from chimneys, vehicle exhaust fumes, etc. contaminate the skin's natural protective film. In order to avoid skin problems caused by bacteria, advice should be given for extra deep cleansing and for the use of a fine film of moisturiser on its own or under make-up.

The sun or ultra-violet rays

These are definitely factors that can have a temporary or more lasting effect on the skin, being both beneficial and detrimental. Either through sun-beds or the sun, ultra-violet rays (which are explained in Chapter 36) can help decrease excess oil secretion and, in some cases, improve acne. They also act on sterols in the epidermis to produce vitamin D, which is absorbed into the bloodstream ensuring good maintenance of bone tissue and the proper utilisation of calcium and salts.

However, too much exposure to these rays causes dryness, promoting surface facial lines but more importantly it is responsible for the breakdown of elastin and collagen in the skin. Collagen reacts to sunlight by hardening; without its gel-like quality, the skin loses its soft, supple texture. So in addition to dryness, wrinkles and sagging skin are the inevitable results. The effect is irreversible and unfortunately it is not immediately obvious as the damage occurs in the dermis.

There is no doubt that a natural sun-tan makes most people not only look better but feel healthier. Your advice to your client to tan safely is paramount. A large number of tanning lotions or gels incorporate sun-screens, the most commonly known being PABA (or para-aminobenzoic acid), to absorb or block the sun's damaging ultra-violet rays. There will also be an SPF (sun protection factor) on the label/bottle (see Table 8.2). To determine the number to advise, you will not only need to examine the client's skin but find out how long he or she can sit in the sun before the skin begins to redden, i.e. if the redness appears in 15 minutes, suggest the sunscreen No. 4, which will allow the client 4×15 minutes – an hour – before the skin begins to burn.

Fair skins should never be given more than $1-1\frac{1}{2}$ hours direct exposure to the sun each day and you should suggest sun-tan creams rather than gels. Advise application 20 minutes before exposure and re-apply every hour. Medium skins rarely burn but advise clients to re-apply the sun preparation every hour. Dark skins still require the same protection even though they appear to tan easily.

To protect delicate or sensitive facial skin suggest a high sun-protection factor or a complete sun block. One can always apply a tan make-up and blusher to give the illusion of a tan to the face. The use of an after-sun preparation or a moisturiser will counteract the inevitable drying effects of the sun. You could also suggest physical barriers, such as large hats to screen the face, cover ups on the beach and large sun glasses with side panels to protect the delicate eye area.

Skin cancer

One of the most serious forms of skin damage caused by excessive sun exposure is skin cancer. It is developed through repeated UV exposure particularly to UBV rays which damage the DNA in keratinocytes and melanocytes. Although the body has a complex system of DNA repair, with repeated and intense exposure it becomes ineffective and mutations occur leading to such conditions as carcinomas. With the world-wide incidence of melanoma, which is an aggressive and deadly form of cancer that attacks the melanocytes it is important to recognise the warning signs in your client's skin, always check for sudden changes in colour, size and texture in warts, scars, birthmarks and moles, for instance:

- if a mole becomes painful, tender or it itches
- if a mole has a hard lump in it, or if it is scaly, or bleeding and does not heal quickly
- if the skin surrounding the mole has become discoloured or lost its pigmentation.

Early diagnosis of melanoma is easily and readily cured by simple surgical removal, so it is important that you do not alarm your clients but put them at ease and encourage regular self-examination or advise them to see their own doctor.

Skin cancer is preventable by taking sensible precautions by using the correct sun-screening products and avoiding long periods of

Table 8.2 Guide to sun protection factors

Skin type		Initial Exposure SPF	Subsequent Exposure SPF
Very fair			
Always burns easily	face	15	15
Rarely tans	body	15	15
Sun sensitive			
Fair, with freckles			
Burns easily	face	10	10
Tans gradually	body	8	5
Normal			
Tans easily	face	6	6
Sometimes burns	body	5	2
Olive			
Tans easily	face	6	4
Rarely burns	body	4	2

exposure to the sun, especially between the hours of 10.00 am and 3.00 pm. See Table 8.2 which gives a guide to sun protection factors.

Alcohol can have a dehydrating effect on the skin. Excess consumption of alcohol causes blood vessels to dilate, thereby encouraging thread-like veins to appear on the cheeks and nose.

Smoking, apart from being a major cause of emphysema, bronchitis, lung cancer and heart disease, also increases blood pressure, constricts blood vessels and therefore affects the complexion. Nicotine is a poison which affects cells and destroys the vitamins B and C in our bodies which are so important for a healthy skin. The smoke exhaled not only pollutes the pores of the skin and dulls the hair, but the action of smoking will increase lines around the mouth and eyes.

Drugs in the form of marijuana, hashish, cocaine or heroin are the subject of considerable concern today. The massive increase of addiction over the past few years has forced governments to take action and now there is readily available information and advice. The effect on the skin is disastrous, colour recedes leaving a dull muddy complexion and premature wrinkles are evident. The eyes become yellow and blood-shot and the hair loses its shine.

Medicated drugs can also have an effect on the skin but no doubt the client will seek further advice if this happens.

Ageing – the natural process of wear and tear – naturally affects the skin. At puberty, adjustment to increased hormonal activity usually manifests itself on the skin of the adolescent. By the age of twenty (approximately) the systems of the body should be fully grown and developed. If the body is healthy, the skin should be at its best, glowing, firm and without lines or wrinkles.

It is from the mid-thirties that the facial skin starts to lose its firmness and fine lines and wrinkles appear and, if there is any loss of muscle tone, there is sagging of the skin.

In the forties and fifties the lines of expression and furrows in the forehead deepen and loss of muscle tone will cause further sagging of the skin on the cheeks and neck. This is largely due to the subcutaneous fat and connective tissue losing its elasticity and becoming less firm. The papillary part of the dermis flattens out so that the skin is finer and thinner. During menopause the activity of the sebaceous glands is reduced and the skin becomes drier.

As we grow older the cells' capacity to reproduce, grow and renew themselves decreases; therefore, in the older person cell regeneration slows down due to the lack of nourishment as the arterioles thicken and venous circulation is impaired. Over the years sebaceous glands and hair follicles atrophy and there is a general loss of colour and thinning of the hair. More keratin is produced and the skin becomes dry and looks dull. Skin tags may appear and age spots can occur, especially on the backs of hands.

No one can put back the clock, but as a beauty therapist you can give advice and help at all ages and possibly delay the ageing process of the skin.

Self assessment

- a nutritious diet should include vitamins A, B, C. Under each vitamin make a list of the foods (in which the vitamin can be found) and give the main benefits for healthy cell renewal – explain why –

    drinking water is essential
    crash diets are unhealthy
    sleep is important
    stress and tension should be avoided
    fresh air and exercise are vital

- hormones influence skin conditions, explain what happens

    at the onset of the menstrual cycle
    during and after the menopause

- what factors determine the colour of the skin?
- climate will affect skin condition, what advice would you give your client going on holiday during the summer months to the Mediterranean?
- how can you humidify the air in centrally heated rooms?
- what causes pollution? and what advice can be given to the client to protect the skin?
- explain what happens to the skin when it is over-exposed to ultraviolet rays?
- how would you determine which SDF to give to your client?
- what happens to the skin when alcohol is taken in excess?
- we know that smoking is dangerous to health but how does it affect the skin?
- what visible signs would alert you to the fact that your client may be taking drugs?
- how does cell renewal slow down as we get older?

9 Skin lesions, diseases and tumours

There are some skin disorders or diseases that you will encounter in your work and it is important that you are able to recognise them. In some cases, treatments in the salon may not be performed and should be referred to a specialist.

Basic understanding of skin lesions

A lesion is damage to a tissue whether caused by injury or infection and these are listed as follows.

1. A **macule** is a stain or a spot, especially a discoloured spot on the skin which is level with the skin surface, e.g. a freckle.
2. A **papule** is a solid elevated lesion of the skin where the skin is not broken but which often develops into a pustule.
3. A **pustule** is a pus-containing lesion of the skin which is visible. Inflammation of the surrounding tissue is usually evident.
4. A **cyst** is a sac containing a liquid or semi-solid substance. Most cysts are harmless, but where possible they should be removed as they may occasionally change into malignant growths or become infected or obstruct a gland.
5. A **scar** is a mark left after a wound has healed.
6. **Erythema** is redness of the skin due to dilation of blood capillaries just below the epidermis.
7. A **wheal** is a localised area of oedema on the surface of the skin.
8. A **vesicle** is a small sac-like blister above the skin although situated in or just below the epidermis. It contains a clear liquid called serum.
9. A **comedo** or blackhead is an abnormal mass of keratin and sebum within the dilated orifice of a hair follicle.
10. **Milia** or whitehead is the result of sebum being blocked in a duct, the top of which is closed. It lies under the skin as a small, hard, pearly white spot.
11. **Skin tags** are small growths of fibrous tissue which stand up from the skin. They are sometimes pigmented black or brown.

Skin diseases caused by micro-organisms

The micro-organisms causing skin diseases include bacteria, viruses and fungi.

Skin diseases caused by bacteria

Bacteria are one-cell organisms only visible through a microscope. There are many varieties, many are useful, most are non-pathogenic (harmless) and only some cause disease. Bacteria are classified in three basic groups according to their shape (see Table 9.1), e.g.

1. bacilli – rod shaped
2. spirilla – spiral shaped
3. cocci – dot shaped; cocci may appear in pairs – diplococci; or like strings of beads – streptococci; or in clusters (like bunches of grapes) – staphylococci.

Table 9.1 Classification of bacteria

Type of bacteria	Forming		Diseases
Bacilli (rod shaped)			Diphtheria, typhoid
Spirilla (spiral shaped)			Venereal diseases
Cocci (spherical) 1. streptococci	Chains		Impetigo, sore throats
2. staphylococci	Bunches		Boils
3. diplococci	Pairs		Pneumonia

Most bacteria co-exist quite happily with mankind and can even be helpful. Some obviously exist in the intestines and they feed on other organisms that could be harmful to us. They also produce some vitamins including vitamin B complex and vitamins C and K.

However, the harmful organisms produce toxins. The body's defences fight back by rushing leucocytes and anti-toxins to the area of infection. The extra blood supply contributes to the inflammatory process.

Staphylococci are generally found on the surface of the skin and they can invade the body tissue through a cut or wound.

Streptococci may spread through the bloodstream and disease is more serious.

Bacilli may have fine hair projecting from their surfaces, with which they can propel themselves through liquids, or they may have spores which can survive high temperatures.

So for growth, bacteria needs moisture, the right temperatures, food and usually oxygen. Therefore in the salon to combat bacteria you must disinfect your implements with either chemical disinfectants, e.g. hypochlorites, or the use of an autoclave. On the surface of the skin they may be controlled by antiseptics or antibiotic ointments.

Boils

When bacteria, staphylococci, enter the skin, the infection usually settles in the hair follicles or sebaceous glands. Despite all the body's defences a local infection may occur, showing on the surface of the skin as a red tender swelling containing pus, a boil. Treatment is given by the client's doctor.

Impetigo

This infectious disease, caused by streptococci entering breaks in the skin, can be seen as small blisters filled with clear liquid, which later becomes thick and forms a yellow crust. The disease occurs most frequently in children, especially in the mouth area. It is spread by direct contact with the moist discharges of the lesions and is readily passed from person to person either by touching the infected area or using infected towels.

Seborrhoea

This is formed by an excessive discharge from the sebaceous glands. The skin appears greasy and the over-abundance of sebum becomes blocked in the sebaceous glands and follicles. This can cause black-heads and can also be the forerunner to acne vulgaris. Staphylococci, which are always present in hair follicles, may well multiply in the sebum plug and, as with acne vulgaris, a pustule will form and if pus develops, the condition must be treated as infectious.

Seborrhoeic dermatitis is an inflammatory condition of the skin of the scalp, commonly known as dandruff. It may spread to other areas of the face, neck, central part of the trunk and the axillae (armpit). There are both greasy and dry conditions. The greasy condition is recognised by the excessive oiliness of the scalp and hair and there may be redness of the scalp and itching. In the dry form of the condition, patches of small dry scales are evident on the scalp and the hair is dry and brittle. Often the dry scales are seen falling from the scalp on to the clothing around the neck and any accumulation of these scales on the skin of the scalp provides breeding areas for bacteria. It is accompanied by itching and, if the skin is broken, bacteria will enter and cause infection.

Acne

This is the most common form of dermatosis and is recognised by spots or eruptions of varying kinds. Generally, the type affecting young people from their teens to early twenties is called *acne vulgaris*. Statistics show that 60 per cent of all girls and 80 per cent of all boys are affected, therefore, you may know of its misery.

First of all, how does it start? The sebaceous glands, as you already know secrete through the pilo-follicle measured amounts of sebum about every three hours which lubricates and softens the skin. With the hormonal disturbance at the onset of puberty, the glands enlarge and produce an excess of sebum. It should also be remembered that the pilo-follicle has a minute orifice capable of receiving bacteria, which in turn produces certain enzymes which can act on the sebum and result in irritating acids causing the walls of the follicle to thicken. The continual excess flow of sebum, if not kept scrupulously clean begins to form a waxy plug (comedo) in the orifice. If it is open at the top of the epidermis, and therefore exposed to the air, the contents become oxidised and turn black and you have a blackhead. However, if the top of the orifice is closed over and oxidisation cannot take place, it becomes a whitehead. To go one step further, the sebum is still pumping into the follicle and because it cannot escape, the walls of the duct break down and the sebum and some of the fatty acids leak into the surrounding tissue. Here then is the beginning of a pimple with the surrounding tissue becoming irritated and inflamed.

Pustula acne occurs when the body's defence mechanisms – leucocytes – rush to the area and invariably cannot cope, the result is a pustule, or, where more than one follicle breaks down, a cyst is formed. Although the plug causing the acne is not infectious, if pus is evident, this condition must be treated as an infection.

Dirt is not the determining factor. The reason for cleansing well and often is to rid the skin of the excess sebum and film of oil and keep the follicles clear. Poor hygiene can often lead to secondary infections. Any attempt to pick or squeeze an unsightly blemish may spread infection to the surrounding tissue and the end result will be more pimples and possible scarring. Often hereditary factors will play a part in acne vulgaris. Severe cases of acne require more intensive and complicated treatment which only a doctor may prescribe. Tetracyclin still seems to be the most popular oral antibiotic and some of the topical agents used are benzol peroxide which has bacterial effects and vitamin A jelly which is an acid and an irritant producing an increase in lesions initially. This in turn causes peeling and thinning of the stratum corneum and therefore assists in the removal of blackheads.

Your liaison with the doctor or dermatologist is very important as you will need to know if any drugs have been prescribed and if the doctor concurs with the treatment you propose to give. Acne, fortunately, is not contagious as such, but advice as to the use of a fresh towel daily should be given and a towel should not be shared with other members of the family. A soft tissue to pat the skin dry is preferable as this can be thrown away. Hair which is oily and falls across the face will aggravate an acne condition. You should suggest professional advice from a hairdresser to improve the condition of the hair and a style to prevent contact with the face. Diet is a debatable point, and the avoidance of all fatty foods , sweets and nuts etc. used to be advised. Acne is an individual problem and rarely are two cases alike. It is a question of trial and error, but obviously fresh fruit and vegetables and a well-balanced diet effects the blood which in turn affects the skin, but it cannot alter a glandular disturbance. Acne does not confine itself to the adolescent. Nervous tension and emotional factors or a change of climate can cause a flare-up of this complaint in an adult. Women who take the contraceptive pill may find their acne condition improve or worsen.

This is a very brief outline of a disturbing dermatosis and you should read the many articles already written in depth on the subject. As acne-related research continues and further clinical tests are made, advanced data will be available to help in this field.

Acne rosacea

This is recognised by its 'butterfly' pattern affecting the centre of the forehead, nose and cheeks. The red and crusted papules usually result from hormonal or vasomotor disorders. Clients are usually fair-skinned and middle-aged, as it is rare for this type of acne to appear before the age of thirty. It usually affects the above areas and sometimes the chin. Clients will consult their doctor and they will probably be given antibiotics or hormone therapy. Often this distressing acne is caused by stress, and tranquillisers may be prescribed,

Skin diseases caused by viruses

A virus is a minute infectious agent, smaller than bacteria, which multiplies inside a living cell. Viruses are so elusive they can only be observed by the electron microscope. Viruses not only destroy the cells in which they live, they are parasitic. When they invade a living cell, the cell proceeds to make changes and assembles a unit into complete viruses, so that when the cell dies it releases countless viruses that can invade other cells. They are the cause of a variety of infectious diseases, including the common cold, influenza, chicken-pox, measles, mumps, herpes simplex and warts.

Herpes simplex

This is an acute infectious virus disease with groups of watery blisters on the skin and mucous membranes most commonly around the lips or nose, i.e. cold sores. These later form crusts oozing moisture. Although they can disappear in a few days they tend to recur, especially in times of stress, as the virus remains in the skin.

Herpes zoster (shingles)

This is an acute virus disease which attacks the sensory nerve endings. Small yellow blisters usually appear on one side of the midline and eventually dry into a thick crust. This normally starts on the body but does reach the neck and facial area. The disease can be caused by the virus of chicken-pox or triggered by trauma or injection of certain drugs. There is a possibility of scarring, so early medical advice should be sought and analgesics will be given to relieve pain and lotions prescribed to dry the blisters.

Warts

A wart is a small hard abnormal growth on the skin and, apart from being unsightly, is also contagious. In more than half the cases, warts disappear without treatments; others remain for years. Clients may object to them on the hands of the therapists, so it is advisable to have them removed by a doctor. A wart develops between one and eight months after the virus becomes lodged in the skin. There are several types of wart:

1. **Plain or juvenile warts** are usually seen on the hands, face, knees

and legs of children. They take the form of small papules of normal skin colour, irregular in outline, with a flat smooth surface.

2. **Common warts** are seen mostly on the fingers, hands and knees and are slightly rougher and larger than plain warts. A common location is near and beneath the nails.
3. **Plantar warts** occur on the soles of the feet. The main body of the wart is beneath the skin surface and the condition becomes sensitive, even painful, due to pressure. Clients should seek the advice of a chiropodist.

Skin diseases caused by fungi

Fungi are a group of plants, to which mushrooms and moulds belong and they contain no chlorophyll (green colouring matter). Those living on the skin are parasitic. As fungi are unable to obtain food from the carbon-dioxide of the air or water, they take nourishment from the body's waste products of dead skin and perspiration. The fungus consists of a mass of long, threadlike cells called a mycelium. The threads penetrate the epidermis and attack the skin, nails and hair with a digestive enzyme.

Ringworm (tinea)

Some forms of ringworm, usually found in children, are often traced to infected domestic pets. Ringworm attacks the scalp and exposed parts of the body, particularly the arms and legs.

Ringworm of the scalp (tinea capitis) is seen as round, scaly patches with hairs broken off. This is caused by fungus digesting the hair keratin; as a result the hair shaft weakens and breaks. Infection of the bearded parts of the face and neck is called tinea barbae.

Ringworm on the body (tinea corporis) appears as reddish patches, often scaly or blistered. They often become ring-shaped as the infection spreads and there is always itching and soreness.

Ringworm of the hands causes them to become red and infected, resembling patches of rings and often very irritating. This is usually due to exterior damage coming into contact with infections through animals, gardening and even nursing. It is a persistent and virulent type of fungus which can attack the nail plate (tinea unguium), matrix (end of the nail bed) and eventually destroys the nails.

Athlete's foot (tinea pedis) is another type of ringworm associated with the feet. It can be seen between the toes as thick white skin or watery blisters. It can appear on the soles of the feet and spread to the nail walls and infect the nail bed. It is usually spread from person to person, for example while walking barefooted at swimming pools and in changing rooms.

The fungi are highly contagious and are spread by humans and animals and even objects, such as combs, brushes and towels. No salon treatment may be given to anyone suffering from ringworm. If you have touched hands or feet with this disease, wash your hands well in an antiseptic solution, dry them on a paper towel and wipe the hands with surgical spirit.

Infestations caused by animal parasites

A parasite in this case is an animal which lives in or on another organism from which it gains its nourishment. **Endoparasites**, which include various worms, live inside the body and may inhabit the digestive tract. **Ectoparasites** live outside the body, usually on the outer surface or just beneath the skin and the presence of a number of these parasites is known as an **infestation**. Although this is not an infection in itself, if the skin is broken by a bite of the parasite, or scratching, bacteria can enter the skin and cause a secondary infection, such as boils or impetigo.

Pediculosis

This is an infestation by lice that live on human blood that is obtained from biting the skin. The area bitten itches and may become sore and infected from scratching. Head lice lay eggs in silvery oval-shaped envelopes that attach themselves to the shafts of hairs, and a female can lay about 300 eggs, which are called **nits**, in a life of 4–5 weeks. Treatment is simple but should be referred to a doctor as lice are easily passed from person to person by direct contact or from infected brushes or towels.

Scabies

This is a contagious skin disease caused by the **itch mite** which burrows into the epidermis. The female digs a short tunnel parallel to the surface and lays its eggs. These hatch after a few days and the baby mites find their way to the surface of the skin. There is considerable itching and a slight skin discoloration where the burrows can be seen as dark lines. Blisters or pustules may occur as a secondary infection and cause boils and impetigo. As the infection is easily passed from person to person medical advice is required.

Tumours

Tumours, although classified in different ways, are either benign or malignant. Benign tumours rarely endanger life and benign tumours of the skin are frequently encountered. Generally these can be classified under three headings:

viral tumours	e.g. verruca or wart
chemical tumours	e.g. skin tags
naevi	e.g. epidermal and or dermal, including seborrhoeic warts and cellular naevus (see Chapter 10)

Malignant tumours are composed of poorly differentiated cells that grow so quickly, and in such a very disorganised manner, that the nutrition of the cells becomes a problem and so they invade surrounding tissue and spread.

Squamous cell carcinoma

Originating in the epidermis, particularly the prickle layer, it is also known as skin cancer and the causes are attributed to certain by-products of petroleum: chemicals, i.e. asbestos, arsenic, nickel, coal tar: some substances found in insecticides; some synthetic dyes and especially prolonged exposure to sunlight. It can be seen as a lesion with a crust-covered crater as in sores or ulcers that do not heal. Sudden changes in colour, size and texture in moles, warts, scars and birthmarks should be referred immediately to the medical profession.

Basal cell epithelioma (rodent ulcer)

This malignant tumour consists of dark staining epithelial cells which can invade the dermis and begins as a small pearly white lesion, but when it enlarges the centre becomes depressed and ulcerates.

Malignant melanoma

This is encountered more frequently in women than in men, and usually manifests itself between 40 and 50 years of age. Rarely is there a pre-existing lesion so it is believed that it develops from cell 'nests'. It is an invasion of a mass of new, abnormal tissue of the cells of the epidermis producing melanin (i.e. germinative layer). The malignant cells break through the basement membrane and go down through the connective tissues into the lymphatics. The tumour cells contain melanin granules and can evoke a marked inflammatory reaction. However, a tumour can appear as a painless lump, i.e. breast cancer or a nodule with ulceration or crusting.

Self assessment

- you know that a lesion is damage to a tissue, itemise those which would be contra-indicated for facial massage.
- it is important to know the classification of bacteria but what name is given to the bacteria, usually found on the surface of the skin, which can penetrate through a break in the skin, hair follicles or sebaceous glands?
- what do bacteria need for growth? how would you control bacteria in the salon and on the skin?
- how would you recognise seborrhoeic dermatitis?
- what is acne, how does it start and what happens to cause this condition to become infectious?
- what advice would you give to a young person suffering from acne vulgaris?
- how would you recognise acne rosacea?
- what happens when a virus invades a living cell?
- explain the difference between herpes simplex and herpes zoster
- where would you find common warts and plantar warts and what advice would you give to the client?

- describe a mycelium and explain how a fungus is spread
- what are tinea capitis, tinea unguium and tinea pedis?
- explain the difference between endoparasites and ectoparasites
- how would you recognise

  (a) pediculosis, and
  (b) scabies. How would you deal with a client with either of these infestations?

- give examples of a benign viral tumour and a chemical tumour
- malignant tumours are rarely seen in the salon, but if you noticed a mole or scar change colour, size or texture, how would you advise the client?

10 Non-infectious diseases and pigmentary disorders

Non-infectious diseases

Psoriasis

This is a chronic, recurrent skin disease, the cause of which is not known and unfortunately at present there is no known cure. The fact that it seems to occur in families with a previous history of this disease does seem to suggest a hereditary factor. It is recognised by bright red patches covered with silvery scales. Again this is a medical condition affecting many parts of the body, i.e. scalp, knees, elbows, palms of the hands and soles of the feet.

It may respond to salt baths or ultra-violet rays. If there are cracks and the area – i.e. the hands or feet – is sore, a light massage with wheatgerm and two drops of pure lavender oil, followed by covering the area with paraffin-wax, may help.

Alopecia

Alopecia is a general term meaning total or partial loss of hair. It applies to both men and women and is often hereditary. It can also be caused by illness, scalp infections, or nervous tension or stress.

- **Alopecia capitis totalis** is the loss of all hair from the scalp.
- **Alopecia areata** is hair loss in defined areas, usually the scalp.
- **Alopecia universalis** is the loss of hair from the entire body.

You should be sympathetic and understanding when giving treatments if wigs or toupees are worn.

Dermatitis

Dermatitis is inflammation of the skin which can result from various irritants, i.e. animal, vegetable and chemical substances, or from heat or cold, certain forms of malnutrition or from an infectious disease. There may be redness, itching, blisters or crustiness evident. One of the most common forms of this disorder is **contact dermatitis** which results from contact of the skin with various irritants. There are two types:

Primary irritant dermatitis

This is due to a direct irritating effect on the skin resulting in inflammation. It is often caused by chemical, physical or mechanical agents.

Chemical agents include acids, alkalis, petroleum products and mineral dusts. Physical agents are excessive cold or heat, which can either result in chilblains or sunburn. Mechanical agents, such as pressure, chafing or scratching, are other common causes of dermatitis. A primary irritant causes inflammation on its first contact with the skin and usually manifests itself within 48 hours.

There may be an occasion when the client is introduced to a new skin product containing a chemical agent, and it could cause an almost immediate reaction resulting in redness. Remove the product immediately and use plenty of water to remove the irritant.

Allergic contact dermatitis

This is produced by an external agent which is a sensitiser or allergen. Many substances may be the cause of an allergenic reaction and these include paint, rubber, plastics, industrial chemicals, poisonous plants, insect bites and stings, costume jewellery and cosmetics. A person may be exposed to any of these substances and no visible cutaneous change will occur initially but will induce certain changes in the skin, so that after a period of days, weeks or months, further contact will result in dermatitis. Therefore, that person is said to be allergic to the substance and should avoid it where possible. The symptoms of dermatitis may be a mild, slight reddening of the skin or result in serious swelling of the tissues, or even blistering and cracking of the skin.

It is important to find out from the client if she has any allergies, especially to cosmetics. Often a client will refer to products from well-known cosmetic manufacturers. This allergy is probably due to some of the products having a highly perfumed content or having an alcohol-based content to which the client is allergic. It may only be the lipstick due to the eosin (the red colouring matter) or the nail enamel due to the plastic resin present. Cosmetic formulations are becoming more and more complex and before purchasing cosmetics you should find out from your supplier the content of their formulations. Should a client disclose any allergy, knowing the content of your own products, you will be able to advise if they are not suitable. The hypo-allergenic cosmetics on the market today screen out some of the sensitising elements that cause irritation.

Eczema (atopic)

This is frequently caused by an allergenic sensitivity to food and substances which are inhaled, i.e. eggs, milk, fish or to dusts and pollens. Eczema will often disappear if the root cause in the diet is found and eliminated. It usually appears on the face and neck and in the folds of the skin at the elbows and knees. Occasionally it can become severe when it is complicated by skin infections. Someone who suffers from eczema as a child is often prone to hay fever or asthma as an adult.

The symptoms are a skin rash characterised by a scaling of the skin, itching, swelling and blistering.

Urticaria (also known as hives)

This is caused by a temporary exudation (escape) of fluid into the dermis, causing a vascular reaction of the skin. Raised patches or wheals can be seen and these are redder or paler than the surrounding skin. It is often caused by:

1. drugs, i.e. aspirin, codeine;
2. foods, i.e. eggs, milk, nuts, fish, tomatoes;
3. heat, cold, exertion or emotion;
4. certain plants and more usually biting and stinging insects (i.e. bees, wasps). It is useful to have an antihistamine cream or tablets in the salon, especially during the spring and summer.

Its onset is quite sudden and any swelling or lesions may only last a few hours.

Pigmentary disorders

Ephelis or freckle

This is a very small pigmented area usually found in abundance on the face, arms and legs in fair-skinned or red-haired people. When exposed to the sun the pigmented areas join together making larger patches. Occasionally clients may feel that freckles are cosmetically unattractive and you can advise the use of bleaching creams to lessen the intensity of colour and suggest that they do not expose themselves to ultra-violet rays.

Lentigo

This again is a pigment spot on the skin due to increased deposition of melanin and an increased number of melanocytes with a lightly raised appearance, smooth, flat and dark brown. They vary from 0.04–0.2 in (1–5 mm) in diameter and, unlike freckles, they are unaffected by sunlight.

Chloasma

This is the hyperpigmentation of the skin where discoloration is found on the cheeks and nose mainly during pregnancy. This will probably disappear quite quickly after the baby is born. If it still persists, biological skin peeling will help.

Vitiligo

A condition due to the failure of melanin formation in the skin which produces loss of colour in the hair and skin. On the skin it looks like milky-white patches with hyperpigmented borders, and as the cells no longer produce melanin, the areas should be protected from the sun or ultra-violet rays. Cosmetic camouflage can conceal these areas on the face, neck and hands so alleviating embarrassment.

Naevi

In the range of skin blemishes you will find two types of naevi. One is cellular, as in a mole or wart, and the other is vascular as in a port-wine stain.

Cellular naevus

This is a common form of mole, a small, flat, elevated lesion of the skin, pigmented or non-pigmented, with or without hair growth. Naevi vary in colour, either black, brown or flesh-coloured, and can appear anywhere on the face or body. Usually they are not disfiguring – in fact some women will colour a mole on the face and highlight it as a beauty spot! However, it must be emphasised that if there is any change in size, colour or texture of a mole, or any itching or excessive bleeding, the client must seek medical advice. Naevi seldom become cancerous, but if they do it is usually caused by irritation.

Seborrheic warts

These are very common especially over the age of 40, but mainly appear on the body rather than the face. They project above the skin normally brown or dark grey in colour and their size varies from a few millimetres to 0.78 in (2 cm). They can be treated medically.

Dermal naevi

These include skin tags which are made up of loose fibrous tissue and which look very much like small warts. They are quite common and are usually found on the neck, chest and axillae area. Middle-aged and elderly clients are more prone to this skin condition. They are a nuisance as they can catch in clothing, causing soreness. They can be removed by diathermy coagulation by a skilled electrologist but medical agreement should be obtained first.

Hairy naevus

This is a pigmented naevus with hairs growing from the surface. Generally speaking the hairs should always be cut with sterilised scissors and never plucked. They can be removed by diathermy under medical supervision.

Hemangioma

This is the name given to benign tumours made up of newly formed blood vessels grouped together and these include the following:

Naevus flammeus

A port-wine stain, this is a large, poorly defined area of dilated capillaries varying in colour from pink to a dark bluish red and is normally present from birth. The stain is normally found on one side of the face and as the skin texture is quite normal, cosmetic camouflage is the best way to conceal this very embarrassing blemish

Naevus strawberry

As the name would imply, it is strawberry in colour and can be seen at birth or very soon afterwards. This stain is usually superficial and can often disappear of its own accord as a person grows older.

Naevus arachnoideus (spider naevus)

It is composed of dilated blood vessels radiating from a point in branches resembling the legs of a spider. It is often called 'broken veins' and these are usually found on the upper cheek and eye area. A skilled electrologist will be able to perform diathermy coagulation treatment. Otherwise a green concealment under the make-up can be used to hide the red area.

Self assessment

- what is

    (a) psoriasis and
    (b) alopecia?

- explain the difference between primary irritant dermatitis and allergic contact dermatitis
- what would your initial advice be to a client with atopic eczema?
- give a brief description of:

    ephelis,
    lentigo,
    chloasma,
    vitiligo,

- explain the difference between cellular and vascular naevi and give examples of each.

11 Skin analysis and skin types

Skin analysis

This is an in-depth evaluation of the skin and the success of any treatment is largely dependent on the therapist's ability to recognise the skin's condition, taking into account some of the factors outlined in previous chapters. A true analysis can only be assessed after the skin has been well cleansed and gently blotted with a toner.

Invaluable aids are either a magnifying glass, which obviously magnifies the skin or a Wood's light. The latter is an ultra-violet lamp with a nickle-cobalt filter which allows only certain wavelengths of ultra-violet rays to pass through and it has the peculiar quality of inducing fluorescence. Table 11.1 shows how the fluorescences appear when the epidermis is exposed to this light.

Table 11.1 Wood's light

Skin type	Colour of fluorescence
Normal skin	Blue-violet
Dry skin	Pale violet
Moisturised skin	Deep violet
Thick, keratinised skin	Whitish
Slightly keratinised skin	Dark
Small boils and acne	Greenish white
Psoriatic desquamation	Chalky white
Thickening of the stratum corneum	Bright silver white
Normal scalp	Violet-grey
Dandruff	Quite white
Bleached hair	White

If you are using any of these aids, remember to cover the client's eyes with cotton wool *before* switching on the light to examine the skin. It is also beneficial to darken a room when using Wood's light.

Apart from taking age into account, the most important factors to look for are the temperature, moisture and texture of the skin, the acid or alkali balance (pH) and any imperfections or pigmentation.

Temperature

The temperature of the skin can be seen as well as felt. If the epidermis is fine and the dilation of the surface capillaries can be seen, the skin will have a pink appearance (indicating a higher temperature) and it can be easily stimulated. On the other hand, if the epidermis is compact and surface capillaries well covered, the skin will have a creamy appearance (indicating a lower temperature). The temperature of the skin may change temporarily, perhaps due to nervousness or even embarrassment. It is, therefore, important to reassure and calm the client before making an assessment.

Moisture

Generally, the moisture in the skin (or its hydric balance) is maintained by the amount of water in the body. We know that some moisture is lost from the stratum corneum as well as sweat from the pores of the skin and that it should be replaced naturally from the dermis. However, as age advances there is a much lower retention of moisture in the dermis to replace any epidermal loss. The hydric balance can also be altered by excessive dieting and over exposure to the sun and the effect of cold winds leading to loss of moisture.

Texture

The texture of the skin is mainly dependent on the rate of secretions from sebaceous glands and the moisture level in the skin. Correcting the balance of these two elements must be your aim when giving treatments.

The acid or alkaline balance

The pH value of the skin (pH is merely a symbol for the hydrogen ion concentration) expresses the degree of acidity or alkalinity. The pH range extends from 1–14. Acid pH values are those below 7 whereas alkaline pH values are those above 7. The combined activities of the keratinisation of the epidermis, the secretions from the sebaceous glands and the sweat glands form an *acid mantle* over the entire skin surface. This mantle is important as it protects the skin from bacteria. A healthy stratum corneum has a pH value between 5 and 5.6, thereby showing a slightly acidic reaction and any decrease in acidity often results in an uneven texture skin. The male skin does have a more acidic skin surface and this should be taken into consideration when giving grooming treatments to men.

Imperfections or pigmentation

These have been covered in previous chapters but they should be noted on the skin-analysis card. If there is a contra-indication always give an explanation to the client, as to why the treatment may not be given, e.g. any infectious skin condition.

```
West End Beauty Clinic

Mr/Mrs/Ms  Surname ................................................. Forenames ................................

Address .........................................................................................................................

Skin temperature ........................................................................................................

    moisture ................................................................................................................

    texture .................................................................................................................

    imperfections or pigmentation ...........................................................................

    ......................................................................................................................

Skin type      Normal      ☐    Dry      ☐    Greasy        ☐    Combination ☐
(tick box)
               Sensitive    ☐    Mature   ☐    Dehydrated    ☐    Dark         ☐

               Temporary imbalance ...........................................................................
```

Reverse side of card

```
Recommendations to improve:

Skin tone .................................................    Moisture ...........................................

Texture ...................................................    Sensitivity .........................................

Ageing tendencies ................................    Dehydration .....................................

Muscle tone ...........................................    Seborrhoeic condition ...................

Recommended salon treatments:                                                 Date:

...................................................................................................    ..............

...................................................................................................    ..............

Recommended retail products:

Cleanser............................. Toner ................................ Moisturiser ...................

Specialised products:      Day .................... Night .......................................

Advised by: (name of beauty therapist) ....................................................................
```

Fig. 11.1 Suggested skin analysis card (attach to client's record card)

Skin types

Normal or balanced skin

This type is becoming rare, mainly due to pollution and congested living in industrial areas. The skin is evenly supplied with oil and moisture, it has a slightly acid reaction and the epidermis is fairly thick. It is flexible, soft, almost velvety to touch and should leave a very faint trace of moisture on the tissue when blotting the skin. The colour of the skin would be creamy rather than pink.

Under a magnifying glass this skin would appear fine-grained, containing very slight irregularities and under a Wood's light it would present a blue-violet fluorescence.

Salon treatments are few. Choose your products carefully, cleanse the skin well, tone, follow with a facial massage and a suitable mask. After you have studied aromatherapy, essential oils, e.g. lavender, camomile, geranium in a carrier oil, e.g. wheatgerm or avocado oil, may be used for the massage and similar oils can be used in the mask to maintain this ideal skin type.

Ampoules are available which contain biological ingredients, e.g. cactus flower or orange etc., and if chosen with care these can be used for this skin type. Always check with your skin-care house for the appropriate ampoules for any skin type. They can be used over the face and neck either manually or with a galvanic current. Occasionally, a treatment with the faradic current (see Chapter 22) could be used to maintain muscle tone.

Home care advice to the client, as with all skin types, is important. Recommend cleansing with a milk or cream, night and morning, a suitable toner, e.g. rose water to close the pores and a moisturiser to be worn under make-up during the day. If the client does not wear make-up stress the importance of the moisturiser. There are tinted moisturisers available which may be used instead of foundation and others which include a protection against UV-A and UV-B light giving a supple film to the skin. Explain that the main function is to prevent loss of moisture already present in the epidermis and dermis. Advise the use of light cream at night and explain some of the facial exercises that can be performed (see Table 8.1).

Even with this ideal skin, skin care for the eyes and neck, should be emphasised. The delicate skin around the eyes is very fine and can become dry easily. An eye gel or eye cream is beneficial, using it around the eye, i.e. above and below the eye, but avoiding cream on the eyelid. With movement of the lids, there will be sufficient cream above to maintain moisture on the eyelid itself. Necks also need attention as so often they are neglected and become dehydrated and wrinkled. The dermis and epidermis are quite thin and there is a lack of melanocytes, therefore little protection from the UV-A and UV-B rays is afforded. There are specific neck creams available to help firm the tissues and combat wrinkles and sagging.

Unfortunately, as we get older, skin tends to dry out and this skin type does not last many years.

Dry skin

Eighty per cent of women have this skin type. The epidermis is thinner and therefore the skin appears fine and transparent. There are often creases and fine lines around the eyes, mouth and neck. It wrinkles easily and often prematurely. There will be evidence of open pores, the surface is frequently powdery or scaly and can also have a tendency to sensitivity and couperose (capillary damage). It will leave no trace of moisture on the tissue when blotted and the colour of the skin is normally pink.

Under a magnifying glass a dry skin will appear as a coarse squamous formation and under a Wood's light it will appear pale violet.

The drying out of the skin is caused by many factors and there are varying degrees of dryness, you will even find dry patches on the zygomatics of teenagers. It can be caused by an external or internal disorder, over exposure to the sun's rays, a glandular disturbance or the insufficient activity of the sweat and sebaceous glands. Dryness, is of course, inherent with ageing simply because of the slowing down process already explained in Chapter 8. Milia (whiteheads) are usually associated with fine textured and dry skin.

Salon treatments are varied but the objective must be to stimulate blood circulation, lymph action and glandular activity in the dermis. Dry skins require cleansing with an oily or cream-based cleanser, toned with rose water followed by a cream-based moisturiser. A steamer may be used to increase circulation but any dilated arterioles must be covered with dry cotton wool. Heat therapy (infra-red explained in Chapter 36) oil masks and paraffin-wax treatments will soften the texture of the skin. Vacuum massage and hand massage will assist the lymph flow and glandular activity. The use of galvanic and/or high-frequency currents (see Chapter 22) will increase blood circulation and soothe nerve endings.

The use of essential oils, e.g. patchouli, camomile, rose, sweet basil or lavender in a carrier oil, e.g. sweet almond oil for massage and in the mask, will encourage the growth of new cells. Ampoules containing collagen or elastin are helpful to prevent premature ageing. There is considerable controversy as to whether collagen or elastin present in ampoules or creams are beneficial other than to superficially soften the surface tissues. Manufacturers recognise that collagen and elastin molecules are too large to penetrate the skin so the molecules are hydrolysed. This is a process whereby the molecules are broken down into their original amino acid form so that they can easily be absorbed by the skin. Other ampoules used may contain royal jelly or some vitamins, all are claimed by the skin-care houses to combat the loss of skin elasticity and avoid the appearance of wrinkles. These can also be used over the face and neck either in manual massage or with a galvanic current.

Home care advice to clients with dry skins should include oil/cream-based products for more penetrating abilities. In the morning, cleanse the skin, use a gentle toner (again rose water is ideal), a moisturiser and a creamy type foundation. At night, recommend cleansing with an appropriate cleanser for dry skin, eye make-up remover, toner, the use of a rich night cream, eye cream and a nourishing neck cream. Advise against products containing alcohol as these can be drying and also that extremes in temperature should be avoided.

Greasy skin

This type of skin is normally thick, with a coarse uneven texture due to enlarged pores. Fatty secretions from the sebaceous glands are normally abundant at the corners of the nose, chin or forehead and are subject to comedones (blackheads), papules and pustules. This skin is sallow in colour and it feels moist to the touch. Grease marks will be left on the tissue when the skin is blotted.

Under a magnifying glass the skin will appear thick grained and under Wood's light it presents a whitish fluorescence.

Many women will say that their make-up 'slides off' and this actually happens! However, a greasy skin, with good skin-care routines, will stay younger-looking longer because of its lubrication. In Chapter 7 sebaceous glands were explained, in that they secrete sebum which lubricates the skin and it is the over-activity of these glands which cause a greasy skin.

This type of skin is often the result of internal changes as the sebaceous glands are regulated by the action of certain sex hormones. This is why it is often found at the onset of puberty. Emphasis must be placed on the gentle cleansing of the skin, keeping the enlarged pores clean and removing the excess film of oil on the face. Dirt or grime in itself is not the important factor, if it were we would have toddlers in the salon! Diet is quite important, recommend green vegetables, fruit, salads, some dairy products, lean meat, fish and drinking plenty of water. An oily skin will often go hand-in-hand with greasy hair, so advise that this is kept away from the face.

Salon treatments should include steaming, deep cleansing and comedone extraction, i.e. using a comedo extractor gently, never squeeze with a tissue. Exfoliators, face washes and brush cleansing are useful. A low alcohol content toner with an approximate pH factor of 5.3 should be applied with cotton wool. Vacuum suction and facial massage are good for loosening the blocked sebum in the ducts. Galvanic desincrustation will stimulate the sluggish or congested skin. The direct method of high frequency and the use of the ultra-violet lamp have a germicidal effect (see Chapter 22).

Certain essential oils, e.g. camomile, camphor, cypress, or lemon in a carrier oil, e.g. grapeseed oil, may be used in the massage, followed by a deep cleansing non-oily mask. Again selective biological ampoules are beneficial, containing for example, extracts of grapefruit, lemon, seaweed, bio-sulphur or vitamin B complex. These are usually applied to the face only, either manually or by using a galvanic current. An alternative essential oil (e.g. geranium) or extract (e.g. collagen) is used for the neck area where the epidermis requires nourishing. However, it must be mentioned here that repeated cleansing, whatever the method, will excite the sebaceous glands. Restrict salon treatments to once every 10–14 days.

Home care advice to the client should include the dietary factor. Recommend cleansing with a mildly medicated soap, cleansing bars or face wash and rinsing well with water, paying particular attention to the corners of the nose, chin and forehead. Suggest a cleanser that does not contain fat, preferably a lotion with a mild antiseptic agent. If the client lives in a hard-water area, toilet soap, which is usually alkaline, may not lather and a film of impure matter will lay on the skin and pores will obviously be blocked. This is where your advice is important.

Advise against the use of a flannel or towel, suggest patting the face dry with a tissue. A suitable tonic or witch-hazel is effective to close the pores. Emphasise that spots or blackheads should not be squeezed as the surrounding tissue will be damaged and may cause permanent scarring or spreading of infection. With squeezing, a little of the surface blackhead may come out, but it is more likely that the rest will be pushed down. Before make-up suggest a medicated lotion and a suitable moisturiser all over the face and neck area. For make-up, advise a liquid foundation, to be applied with a damp sponge, this will last longer than a cream foundation. There are several cosmetic houses that can supply medicated cover sticks for blemishes on the skin. Well applied lipstick and eyeshadow will draw attention away from blemished skin. At night use the cleanser and toner for a greasy skin, eye make-up remover, eye gel and a suitable night cream. Gentle exfoliators, i.e. facial scrubs can be used but these should be limited to twice a week. The neck rarely becomes greasy and a nourishing cream should be applied.

Combination skin

As the name would imply, a mixture of dry and greasy skin. It is usually recognised by a greasy triangle, stretching from the forehead to the chin, yet the cheeks and sides of the face are dry. It is a fairly common skin type and requires patience and time. Ideally two types of products are needed for both dry and greasy areas. Although this can be carried out in the salon and the client advised on the use of them at home, it is unlikely that the advice will be heeded, mainly due to lack of time! There are some skin-care houses that recognise this problem and have products which apparently help the greasy panel without drying out the rest of the face and neck.

Salon treatments for a combination skin include steaming, face masks, high frequency, vacuum suction and massage. Again, the use of essential oils (e.g. thyme, rosemary, lavender or camomile) and a suitable mask. When giving specialised treatments for the greasy area protect the dry areas with cotton wool. Galvanic iontophoresis will help to correct the pH balance and rehydrate the skin.

Home care advice would be the use of a cleanser which is non-irritant to the dry areas and yet can deal with the greasy panel. If this is not adequate, two cleansers should be used (i.e. cream based for the cheeks, sides of the face, eyes and neck area and a medicated cleanser for the centre panel) and then use a toner/tonic and a light moisturiser all over the face and neck. For make-up suggest a water-based foundation. At night, the same cleanser and toner may be used, eye make-up remover, eye gel or cream, corrective night cream for the centre panel and a light nourishing cream for the dry areas and neck.

Sensitive or delicate skin

This is a type of skin which is normally hypersensitive and can be easily recognised. Although the skin can be pale and delicate to the touch, it reddens very easily with stimulation, has many dilated capillaries and has dry and flaky patches. Sometimes there are small acid spots around the mouth and this type of skin can also be prone to allergies. Many allergic reactions are caused by anxiety and stress and this should be taken into account when performing treatments.

Sensitive skins should be treated with great care, the epidermis is very thin and any treatment should be light.

Salon treatments should not include any heat therapy or vacuum suction. Massage by hand would preclude tapotements, petrissage, friction or pinching movements (described in Chapter 19), using only light effleurage and vibrations on the face. Use products that are suitable, i.e. cleanser, toner and moisturiser for a sensitive skin. The facial massage and mask should contain ingredients to calm the skin. Essential oils, e.g. lavender, rose or sandalwood in a wheatgerm or avocado oil for massage and a mask containing camomile, are very useful. Ampoules containing collagen or elastin can be manually applied to good effect. Masks are also available for the eye, neck or face containing 100 per cent insoluble collagen impregnated with a high percentage of soluble collagen which are apparently absorbed via osmosis into the skin to help plump out fine lines and maintain water balance of the skin.

Usually it is the dry skin types which are prone to becoming sensitive, therefore the advice given for this category should apply. Emphasise the importance of a moisturiser for protection under make-up and if no make-up is worn it should be applied twice a day.

Home care advice should include a cleanser, toner and moisturiser for a sensitive skin during the day. For make-up suggest a creamy foundation. At night, the same cleanser and toner can be used, eye make-up remover, eye cream and a light night nourishing cream for the face and neck.

Dehydrated skin

This skin is lacking in moisture and appears dull and may have a crêpey texture. By talking to the client the cause may be diagnosed as excessive dieting, a recent illness or certain drugs which all deplete the body fluid and therefore reduce the water in the tissues. Over exposure to ultra-violet rays will also dehydrate the skin. It may be a temporary condition and you can help and advise methods to effect a skin recovery. However, if it is ascribed to ageing, help should be given to hydrate the skin to improve the texture and suppleness.

Salon treatments can be given to improve the hydric balance of the skin, increase sebaceous secretion and cellular function. These include the use of a steamer (cover any dilated capillaries with dry cotton wool), massage, warm oil masks, collagen and ginseng masks, indirect high frequency and galvanic iontophoreses. Essential oils, e.g. camomile, geranium or lavender in a carrier oil, e.g. avocado oil or jojoba oil will improve dehydration. Ampoules and products containing ginseng, collagen or elastin will help to improve the skin's elasticity and firmness.

Home care advice should include a cleanser, toner and moisturiser for this skin type, and for make-up suggest a creamy foundation. There are many products on the market today which include collagen or elastin and these can be used during the day and at night. Prescribed essential oils, i.e. a pure oil in a base oil, can be given to the client for use at night. If your knowledge of essential oils is limited choose a suitable blended oil which is available from either the skin-care house or manufacturer. Emphasise the use of an eye gel or cream and a nourishing neck cream.

Mature skins

These are normally associated with ageing. However, it is a gradual process which can be slowed down and in some cases reversed. This applies mainly to premature ageing where usually there is a fundamental cause, i.e. illness or poor health; general neglect; stress and over exposure to the sun. Although the age of the client should be taken into consideration, premature ageing can begin as early as 30 years of age. In young skin the collagen fibres are well hydrated and flexible but with advancing years hydration and elasticity diminishes and the skin loses its firmness. Lines and wrinkles become obvious, the contours around the jaw line sag and there is loose skin on the neck. Dilated capillaries may be present on the cheeks and nose and often super-fluous hair appears above the lip and on the chin.

Salon treatments can be given to improve the skin's condition. The use of a steamer, massage, stimulating or warm oil masks, vacuum suction, faradic and galvanic treatments should be considered. It is important to clear the surface of dead cells and encourage new cell growth. Exfoliators, in the form of 'scrubs', are creams containing abrasives obtained from either natural or synthetic sources, e.g. crushed walnut stones or a derivation of styrene (i.e. an oily liquid which is hardened to form granules). These are recommended for non-sensitive skins to give a brighter, clearer look. Essential oils, e.g. clary sage, cypress, lavender or myrrh in a carrier oil, e.g. jojoba oil will undoubtedly improve the texture of the skin. Again products or ampoules containing collagen, elastin, vitamins A and E will help to revitalise and firm the tissues.

For an older client, when the skin has atrophied, a warm oil mask or paraffin-wax mask (with the protection of dilated capillaries) followed by lymphatic massage to avoid stretching the skin further will be of benefit. Also use the products mentioned above which will help to retard further ageing.

In general (due to the age group range) treatments will vary considerably and your expertise will decide the treatment to be given and the products to be used.

Home care advice to the client should include the night and morning cleanse routine with a non-alkaline cleansing lotion or emulsion. Exfoliators can be used (again it depends on the age of the client and the skin condition). The skin should be refreshed, possibly with witch-hazel in the toner/tonic. Moisturisers are important to prevent any further loss of moisture. For make-up suggest a creamy or semi-fluid foundation with good covering properties. At night, as with dehydrated skins, the use of products containing active ingredients should be used, eye make-up remover, eye cream, a firming cream for the face and a nourishing cream with vitamin E for the neck.

Dark skin

As you know, the colour of the skin varies enormously and, although mainly hereditary, light plays an important role. The darker the surface of the skin the more absorption of light, whereas a white surface will reflect practically all the light.

A dark skin is shiny and velvety to touch and generally thicker and tougher. This is mainly due to three factors:

1. The sudoriferous glands are larger and more numerous. The excretory duct opens at the skin surface into a longer and more obvious 'pore'.
2. The sebaceous glands are also larger and more numerous and a large number of them (one-tenth) open directly on to the epidermis.
3. The horny layer of the epidermis is much thicker and the dark skin desquamates easily.

Pigmentation plays an important role. *All* skins appear to have the same number of melanocytes which produce melanosomes (granules containing melanin as described in Chapter 8). The melanosomes pass into the cells of the prickle-cell layer via the dendrites of the melanocytes. The keratinocytes then containing melanosomes move upwards towards the surface of the skin.

In white skins the melanosomes are small and are destroyed by enzymes by the time they reach the stratum lucidum; whereas in dark skins the melanosomes are larger and more widely dispersed and remain in the keratinocytes until they are shed from the stratum corneum. By absorbing visible light these melanosomes give the skin its brown colour. There are colour differences from one ethnic group to another and they are only due to the variations in the degradation of the grains.

As pigmentation in a coloured skin may be intense it can hide flaws or alter the colour of lesions, i.e. erythma is red on a white skin but can be purple on a dark skin.

Vitiligo (explained in Chapter 10) is characterised by a total disappearance of the melanocytes in patches on the skin. On a white skin this disorder is very easy to camouflage but on a dark skin, although not a major problem, it is psychologically disturbing. Doctors try to stimulate melanin production by using ultra-violet rays.

Other disorders affecting white skins, i.e. cellular or dermal naevi or hemangioma (see Chapter 10) rarely affect a healthy dark skin. It is also unusual to see adolescents with acne vulgaris even though the coloured skin contains more sebaceous glands. The sebum does not form comedones (as in a white skin) but small cysts can be felt under the skin.

Unfortunately, dark skins do have a tendency to develop keloids. These are scar-like growths that rise above the epidermis as a benign tumour, usually resulting from a scar after injury or surgery. The surrounding fibrous tissue regenerates very quickly and forms keloidal tissue which continues to grow and harden.

Under a magnifying light, erythema, not easily seen on a dark skin, will appear as dark purple areas (i.e. darker than the skin itself) and will alert you to the fact that these areas are very sensitive.

Dark skins maintain a youthful appearance and rarely age before 60 years and then quite suddenly.

Salon treatments will include a thorough cleansing of the skin and the use of electrical brush applicators and exfoliators give good results on firm skins with a thick horny layer. Cleansers, toners and moisturisers from plant extracts should be used unless you are able to find a skin-care house that specialises in products for the darker skin. The use of a steamer, iontophoreses and bio-peeling will help to clear away excess dead cells and brighten the colour of the skin.

Small vacuum suction ventouses can be used to help clear any small cysts felt under the skin. It is very important that you do not break the skin in an attempt to remove these, as any small injury may develop into a keloid.

Massage is very beneficial using natural products, e.g. essential oils, geranium, lavender or sandalwood in a carrier of sweet almond oil. The massage could include small pincement and friction movements.

Masks may be used to brighten the complexion but be careful not to use those which can leave a whitish residue on the skin. Again these can be made from natural ingredients, e.g. avocado or papaya.

Home care advice to the client is to cleanse, tone and moisturise the skin every morning. Gentle exfoliators can be used fairly regularly. At night, after the cleanse/tone routine, use an eye gel or eye cream and a night cream containing plant extracts or enzymes for the face and neck.

The colour and type of skin varies from the Mediterranean, Latin, Asian, Oriental through to the Afro-Caribbean. As the world seems to be shrinking and ethnic groups moving from one country to another it is important to know how to recognise and give treatments to all types of skin.

Summary

Make-up can hide a multitude of flaws and it may be necessary to cleanse twice before making an assessment. After examination of the skin, note the type on the skin-analysis chart. Talk to the client, propose the type and number of treatment sessions required and the skin-care products you suggest for home use. Discuss the cost and dovetail your suggestions to be well within a price range the client can afford.

Self assessment

- what are the most important factors to look for when examining the skin?
- what is the purpose of an acid mantle?
- what home care advice would you give to a client with a well-balanced skin?

- how does the skin dry out?
- what salon treatments would you consider beneficial for a greasy skin?
- explain how you would recognise a combination skin
- explain the difference between a sensitive skin and a dehydrated skin
- a mature skin is associated with ageing, what salon treatments would you suggest?
- explain the difference between a fair skin and a dark skin
- what is a keloid?
- what home care advice would you give to a client with a coloured skin?

12 Product knowledge, manual cleanse, tone and moisturise

Product knowledge

Some product knowledge is essential and the following gives brief descriptions of the various components used in creating lotions or creams. All creams in their various forms, thick or thin, can be described as emulsions.

Emulsions

An emulsion is the fine dispersal of one liquid in another. In cosmetics the basis of emulsions are mixtures of various oils and water with numerous additives, which are also either oil and water soluble. The type of emulsion will be dependent upon the proportion of water and oil, the emulsifier and sometimes the method of manufacture. If the oil is dispersed in water it is known as an oil-in-water (O/W) emulsion, the oil being the *dispersed phase* and the water being the *continuous phase*. However, if water is dispersed in the oil phase it is a water-in-oil (W/O) emulsion. This is quite important as it is the continuous phase which makes contact with the epidermis more easily than the dispersed phase. However, if water is the external phase it will rapidly evaporate leaving the oil phase in contact with the skin. Each has its own function:

water – dissolves and removes water soluble dirt
 – supplies moisture to the skin
 – by evaporation, it produces a cooling effect, and
oil – dissolves and removes oil soluble dirt
 – has a lubricant effect and acts as an emollient
 – delays water loss from the skin

Therefore, an emulsion is a mixture of two immiscible phases stabilised by an emulsifier system.

The components of an emulsion are:

1. *Emollients* The primary function of a skin-care emulsion is the delivery of its emollients. These are moisture barriers, lubricants, feel, modifiers, conditioning agents etc. Oils – both vegetable and mineral, esters and lanolin derivatives are examples of these, i.e.

   Vegetable oils which are derived from plants, e.g. almond oil, jojoba oil, avocado pear oil, grapeseed oil, wheatgerm oil, etc.

   Mineral based oils, in their various forms are obtained from petroleum products, e.g. petrolatum (petroleum jelly), liquid paraffin and paraffin wax and are used in cosmetics as they are good grease solvents and good barrier products. However, in skin-care products there is renewed interest in natural oils and greater expectation from a product's efficacy, mineral oil has been replaced in many products by natural oils and esters.

Esters are the result of reacting a fatty acid with an alcohol and are used in skin-care products for their spreading properties and 'dry' oiliness. They reduce the greasy feel of mineral and vegetable oils, giving a lighter, more pleasant skin feel and they often improve skin-penetrating properties because of their solvent powers allowing them access through the epidermis by intercellular absorption.

The words 'lanolin derivatives' have been mentioned and this may cause a few eyebrows to be raised! As you probably know lanolin is the equivalent of human sebum and acts as the waterproof material on the wool of sheep, usually known as wool wax. Unfortunately, a decade or so ago, some people developed an allergic reaction to the use of lanolin. It was unlikely to have been from the sebum itself but more from the insecticide residues from sheep dipping or the strong surfactant residues used in the cleaning process. It became a known sensitiser, which meant that any product containing lanolin had to be clearly stated so on the label. This is not the case now, many lanolin derivatives are used in cosmetic products and specific labelling is not necessary.

2. *Humectants* Humectants attract the moisture that the emollients help to retain and retard evaporation, glycerine (glycerol), propylene glycol, sorbitol are examples.

    The water content in the cream will evaporate as it is spread on the skin or if the jar/container is left open. Loss of water from a product can also result in its deterioration, so you will appreciate the importance of closing containers immediately after use.

3. *Emulsifiers* Emulsifiers ensure that the incompatible components of an emulsion can be blended together to produce a stable and consistent product. Triethanolamine soaps and beeswax-borax soaps are mainly used in cleansers and lotions. Most emulsifiers are non-ionic, such as ceteareth-20, polysorbate-20, sorbitan esters and many others. Glucose chemistry is a current favourite as it uses natural renewable resources and the results are nice as well. Examples would be methyl gluceth-20 disterate which is an O/W emulsifier and methyl glucose sesquistearate which is a W/O emulsifier. Silicone emulsifiers are also popular although some manufacturers find the results a little disappointing.

    Stabilisers or secondary emulsifiers, such as fatty alcohols balance and support the emulsifying system and sometimes give added cosmetic properties to maximise the benefits of the formulation.

4. *Thickeners* Thickeners are used primarily to build viscosity and improve stability. They include:

    - natural gums, i.e. acacia, guar, karaya and tragacanth

- mineral thickeners, i.e. refined naturally occurring silicate clays such as bentonite, magnesium aluminium silicate
- modified celluloses, e.g. methyl cellulose
- synthetic polymers, e.g. polyvinylprrolidone
- waxes, i.e. paraffin wax, beeswax, ozokerite and derivatives of lanolin.

5. *Active ingredients*   There are a multitude of active products added to a formulation and these are dependent upon the purpose for which they are intended, such as for antiperspirants, antiseptics, sunscreens and tints. One such active ingredient could be alcohol (ethanol) which is in itself an antiseptic. When it evaporates off the skin superficial blood vessels contract and this makes the skin feel fresh and cool. It is used in some toners and in the compounding of fragrances.

   Many other 'active' ingredients will be recognised from the claims attributed to a specific product, e.g. anti-wrinkle, anti-inflammatory, anti-ageing, anti-cellulite, rejuvenating, tanning accelerators, skin lighteners etc. or from the mention of specific ingredients, e.g. proteins, vitamins, herbs, liposomes or AHA.

   The cosmetic industry generally avoids the use of active ingredients that can fall into the category of 'drugs' in order to comply with the controls enforced by countries throughout the world.

6. *Vehicles*
   Water   Although the principle function of an emollient lotion is to promote water retention, water in such formulae serves mainly as a vehicle. It delivers water-soluble functional ingredients (e.g. humectants, preservatives, cleansers) and the emulsified oils, but is quickly lost after application.

   Oil   The oil phase of a lotion is rich in emollient or moisture barrier materials and also serves to deliver other oil-soluble functional materials, parts of the emulsifier system and fragrance, etc.

7. *Fragrances*   A mixture of natural oils and aromatic chemicals make up this category to create the right odour. For instance essential oils can be used. These are obtained from flowers, fruits and leaves etc., of different types of plants cultivated in many countries. Although the chemistry of the oils is complex, they usually contain alcohols, esters, ketones, aldehydes and terpenes (see Chapter 15, Volume 2 on Aromatherapy). Many essential oils are said to have antiseptic and healing properties and are very useful in cosmetic creams.

   Compound fragrances have been developed to such an extent that it is now possible to recreate any odour or scent required.

8. *Preservatives*   All emulsions require preservatives to control bacterial growth and mould originating in raw materials, manufacturing process, containers and user handling. However, these are kept to a minimum and are strictly controlled by legislation.

9. *Colours*   Colours are used extensively in cosmetics. Any colouring matter must be non-irritant and non-toxic with special emphasis on

eye make-up and lipstick. This is because these areas are very sensitive and can be easily inflamed and with lipstick there is the additional hazard of colour being digested and entering the blood stream.

All colours are covered by legislation, in America, in the EEC and also in other countries. Although not all legislation agrees, there are very strict controls on what colours may be used and where they may be used:

- *dyes*, are coloured compounds soluble in water, alcohol or oil and are said to be soluble colours. They rarely occur naturally and most are synthetic dyes.
- *true pigments*, which are also coloured compounds, are not soluble in any of the above solvents and are therefore termed insoluble colours. The range of true pigment colours is limited whereas the range of dye colours is vast and so to take advantage of the dye colour range, they have to be made insoluble. This is done by treating soluble dyes with metal oxide or hydroxide and the result is known as a *lake*.
- *inorganic pigments* are used extensively in eye make-up, nail enamel and as the non-staining colour in lipsticks. They are obtained from metallic oxides, e.g. iron, for black, brown, yellow and red; chromium for green etc. White titanium dioxide is added to the pigments to produce lighter pastel shades.

Cleansers

Cleansing preparations must be able to remove:

- all make-up effectively
- surface dirt and grime
- skin debris, i.e. cleansing the horny layer and removing dead cells (thereby aiding desquamation)
- excess sebum and help to unblock congested enlarged pores.

Apart from being able to do all this, the product must be suitable for the client's skin, i.e. without causing sensitivity or removing the skin's natural protective layer. The skin-care house will advise which products to use for certain skin types.

There are numerous cleansing products available, e.g.

Soap acts as an emulsifying agent dissolving grease and dirt and water will dissolve any water-soluble substances on the skin and finally you have a fresh clean skin. However, it can be drying, especially if the sebaceous glands take time to produce the sebum required to restore the acid mantle. Vegetable oils or glycerine may be added to soaps to help combat dryness. In the main it is the client with an oily skin who is able to use soap without irritation.

Cleansing bars are blocks of cleansing cream with the addition of a soapless surfactant (triethanolamine lauryl sulphate). Cleansing bars are also known as 'syndet' bars – synthetic detergent – and properly formulated they can match the pH of the skin and be very mild.

Although they lather up well with water they are not so good at removing make-up.

Cleansing milks or lotions are very similar. Their descriptions are determined by the terminology used by either the skin-care house or cosmetic manufacturer. They are either O/W or W/O emulsions and, dependent upon the type of emulsion, they can be formulated to suit most skin types. Some will contain a surfactant to facilitate the removal of oil and dirt.

Medicated lotions or gels are generally non-greasy water-based preparations. Sometimes they are structured into a gel with an astringent together with other active ingredients, e.g. triclosan, to act as an anti-bacterial agent.

Facial scrubs (or exfoliators) resemble creams with very fine exfoliating particles, i.e. granules obtained from either natural or synthetic sources, e.g. ground walnut stones or a derivation of styrene. They cleanse the skin gently, removing dead cells and impurities leaving the skin soft and smooth. As these scrubs usually contain a surfactant, they can be used at least twice a week for a greasy skin but less often for a normal to dry skin.

Cleansing creams, although formulated as either O/W or W/O, they are usually W/O emulsions. This means that the water content is reduced and evaporates and cools the skin; the oil content is increased dissolving sebum and make-up and it also helps the cream to spread evenly over the skin. These creams are ideal for dry, dehydrated and mature skins.

Liquefying creams contain mineral oils and waxes but no water. As they only remove greasy products they are very useful after make-up competitions, fashion shows, photographic sessions and theatrical make-up.

Eye make-up removers are usually very light, non-oily products containing cocoamphocarboxyglycinate (a very mild surfactant) which also has a conditioning effect. The skin around the eye is thin and delicate and should not be stretched in any way. An oil-based product which acts as the solvent may contain a mineral oil and will remove waterproof mascara.

Toners

Skin-care houses use different names for different purposes, i.e. toners, tonics, astringents, freshener or bracers and to make life more complicated they do not always agree with each other, e.g. one is labelled 'a mild tonic' another 'a gentle toner' both having the same ingredients! However, the purpose of using any of these is to:

- ensure a complete removal of all cleansing products
- remove any traces of a face mask left on the skin
- restore the acid balance of the skin after cleansing
- close the pores
- freshen the skin

Most contain alcohol (ethanol). Their strengths vary according to the alcohol content which can range from 2 per cent to 10 per cent.

Greasy skins which have no apparent signs of sensitivity can accept a product with a higher alcohol content, e.g. 10 per cent with a 5 per cent astringent, e.g. witch-hazel which can also cause contraction and help to close the pores. This is also known as hamamelis water as it is extracted from the leaves and bark of the bush of the same name. It is a mild astringent with soothing and healing properties. For this skin type other ingredients may be added, e.g. active sulphur and propylene glycol.

Normal skins will accept a product with a reduced alcohol content, e.g. between 8 per cent to 10 per cent, together with a mild astringent. Other ingredients are added, e.g. glycerine, sodium lactate to adjust the pH factor and essential oils.

Dry skins will tolerate a product with up to 8 per cent alcohol without any drying effects, but sensitive skins will need a much lower alcohol content, i.e. from 2 per cent to 5 per cent. Some products for this skin type do not contain any alcohol. Other ingredients would also include glycerine, sodium lactate and essential oils.

Dehydrated or mature skins should have a product which consists mainly of purified water, e.g. rose- or orange-flower water with a few active ingredients, e.g. allantoin. A few ingredients may also be added as for dry skins.

It should be possible to find out from your skin-care manufacturer the alcohol content and other ingredients suitable for specific skin types.

Moisturisers

The main functions of moisturisers are to:

- slow down the rate of evaporation of moisture in the skin
- act as a 'barrier cream' to prevent dehydration, often caused by central heating, sun exposure, extremes in temperature, e.g. cold winds and hot weather
- soften and lubricate the skin
- facilitate the cleansing of the skin
- act as a balancer, so that make-up does not change colour through oil or perspiration
- provide a smooth base for make-up
- prevent the pigments in cosmetics permeating the pores.

The preparations come in various forms from creams to lotions.

The oil or wax contained in the emulsion remains on the skin after the evaporation of the aqueous phase and this helps to preserve the moisture level in the skin. As explained before, this part of the emulsion is called the emollient and is essential for the texture and softness of the skin. For greasy skins the moisturiser should contain about 15 per cent emollient content but for drier skins it should be increased to as least 25 per cent. The ingredients in the moisturiser would include emulsifiers, waxes, emollients, humectants, oils and possibly essential oils.

Cream moisturisers should be worn by clients with dry, dehydrated or mature skins, under make-up or by itself. There are tinted moisturisers which can be worn as an alternative to a foundation.

Moisturising lotions (or milks) have a higher content of water and are lighter in texture. The ingredients would be similar to those in creams and are often preferred by younger clientele.

Other types of moisturising products.

These include eye creams and gels, neck creams, night creams which are mainly retail items, i.e. for the client to purchase for a home care routine.

Eye creams for use during the day are usually O/W emulsions which are easily absorbed by the skin. At night a richer W/O emulsion is used to hydrate and soothe the area. These normally contain active ingredients, e.g. vitamin E, and regular use helps to prevent lines and wrinkles. Again any excess must be blotted with a tissue.

Eye gels cool, soothe, firm and tighten the skin around the eyes, which means that they are useful for puffy eyes or loose skin. They contain a mild astringent, e.g. witch-hazel together with plant or herbal extracts and they are non-greasy.

Eye lotions are useful for compresses, i.e. when applied to cotton-wool pads and placed on the eyes. They usually contain a very mild astringent and plant extracts. As an alternative, slices of cucumber will refresh tired eyes and thin slices of raw potato will help to reduce puffy eyes.

Neck creams are essential especially after the mid-twenties. The epidermis and dermis of the neck is thin; its hydrolipidic film is inadequate and cannot ensure hydration; it lacks melanocytes, so has virtually no protection from UVA/UVB rays. The neck is very sensitive to external aggressions and ages early when neglected. Neck creams are W/O emulsions and should be massaged gently into the area to increase cellular activity and the humectant properties will help to retain moisture in the skin.

Night creams also known as nourishing creams or skin foods are also essential from that mid-twenty age group. They are W/O emulsions using different oils/waxes and other ingredients to formulate different textures, i.e. a soft solid cream or a thick liquid cream. They usually contain a fairly high oil content, as much as 75 per cent for a dry skin but only 40 per cent for a greasy skin, which enables the cream to be gently massaged on to the face.

Their purpose is to balance and refine skin texture and delay moisture loss from the surface of the epidermis. Some creams are easily absorbed by the skin and others are adsorbed (i.e. leaving a thin protective film on the skin) enabling the emollient properties to preserve the moisture level.

Technological advances in skin-care products increase every year and are tested for performance and safety. Collagen has become an increasingly popular ingredient in skin care as it is said that it can firm and smooth the texture of the skin. When used in cosmetic products, it is either obtained from animals (i.e. a by-product from skins, bones and other meat-processing sources) or derived from wheat protein.

Collagen implanting has now become accepted as the collagen used is not a foreign substance but a natural protein and, when injected by a surgeon, it is accepted by the collagen fibres of the skin. It plumps out depressions and is mainly used for naso-labial lines (nose to mouth) and glabella (forehead) furrows and small vertical lines above and below the lips. The effect is temporary, lasting approximately one year but that is rather dependent on the age of the client.

Ampoules containing 'active' biological ingredients are supplied by some skin-care houses and they include collagen, elastin or various extracts from herbs, plants and fruits. These are usually applied to the skin during salon treatments.

Also available are tissue extracts and these are obtained from either the skin, ovaries or placenta of young animals. No one seems to know exactly how the tissue extracts work, but their actions appear to have a temporary rejuvenation of the skin. There is still suspicion that clients have been influenced by hope and expectancy!

Hygiene factors

Your working surfaces must be kept clean, using a disinfectant (e.g. chloroxylenol (Dettol) or surgical spirit), to wipe them down after each client.

Cotton wool, not in use, should be kept in a closed container or jar. It must be thrown away immediately after use.

Spatulas must be used to remove any product from a jar/container. These can then be sterilised or thrown away after use. If you drop anything on the floor, do not use it again until it has been properly cleaned.

Always use clean towels, couch papers and headbands/caps for each client.

Preparation

This section deals with the general preparation of the client and should not be confused with preparation for more concentrated treatments.

You should have ready, prior to arrival of your client:

- a bowl containing clean water (if you do not have a washbasin near by)
- sterilising solution (e.g. for spatulas)
- clean towels
- tissues
- cotton wool in a container, with some pieces cut into 4 ins (10 cm) squares. Some of the squares should be put into water, surplus squeezed out between the palms of your hands and divided into thin squares and placed in a clean bowl. Circular cotton-wool 'wipes' may also be used in the same way.

- cotton buds
- spatulas
- crêpe bandage as a headband or disposable head cap
- skin-care products
- a waste bin at the side of the chair/couch.

Ideally it would be better if the client could remove her clothes to the shoulder area to enable you to cleanse the entire neck area. This is not always possible, especially if the beauty section is within the hairdressing salon and cannot be screened off. However, it is pointless to give this treatment if the client is wearing a polo-neck sweater!

Put on a disposable cap and tuck all the hair inside and/or wind a crêpe headband around the head at the hairline and secure it within itself or use a safety-pin. Relax the client, either in a chair at a semi-reclining position with the feet on a footstool or lying on a couch with the back raised. Protect her clothing with a towel/paper tucked in the clothes in the lower neck region. Remove all jewellery, i.e. ear-rings, necklaces and put these away safely within view of the client. If contact lenses are worn, the client may wish to remove these before you commence the cleanse.

Your client will probably arrive wearing make-up and if she is a new client you will have to make sure that you use a cleanser which would visibly suit her skin. Consider the following factors:

- take into account her approximate age
- does she have a flawless complexion?
- does she looked flushed or have a blotchy skin?
- does she have a shiny nose, blackheads or pimples?
- has she obviously been in the sun?
- are there any cuts or abrasions on the face?

Only with experience will you know immediately the cleanser to use, but surprises and mistakes can always be corrected with a second cleanse.

Wash your hands thoroughly and dry them with tissues or paper towels.

Manual method of cleansing the skin

Most clients will prefer manual cleansing – perhaps it is the computer –machine age which is affecting the preference where the personal approach is concerned or it may be that clients are wary and afraid that the skin's natural protective barrier may be stripped or over stimulated. Therefore, use electrical rotary brushes for your younger clientele but take into account their temperament. Highly strung or nervous clients will find brush cleansing irritating. Sensitive or delicate skins will become aggravated (see Chapter 23).

Commence your cleanse with the eyes and then the lips as the make-up for these features is usually more dense in colour than for the remainder of the face.

1. Put a little of the eye make-up remover on the back of your left hand

and place the left third (ring) finger at the outer corner of the left eye to steady the tissues there while you work. With the ring finger of the right hand take a small amount of the remover and start at the upper inner corner of the eye. Sweep across the lid, around and under the eye towards the nose to complete a circular movement (see Fig. 12.1). This movement should be widened to follow the corrugator and orbicularis oculi muscles. The touch should be light to avoid dragging the delicate eye tissue.

Take damp cotton-wool pads – you will find it easier to clean the inner corner of the eye if a pad is folded into a triangular shape. Wipe gently so that there is no pressure on the eyeball itself. The pad is then turned and the area under the eye is wiped clean towards the nose. Remember to support the skin at the outer corner of the eye. Movements are the same as those used with the cleanser (see Fig. 12.2).

Heavy mascara is better removed with its own cleanser, i.e. an oil or cream which is commercially available, on a cotton-wool bud or a small piece of cotton wool. Place a damp cotton-wool pad under the bottom lashes and stroke both upper and lower lashes down on to the pad (see Fig. 12.3). This will avoid irritation to the eye itself and also ensure that the area under the eye (which has been cleansed) is not smeared with mascara. To clean the lashes, a clean area of the bud or pad is used for each movement. When finished, request the client to open the eye to ensure the lashes and corners are completely clear of the cleanser. Reverse hands and repeat for the other eye.

If the eyes show any discomfort you can take about a third of the thickness of dry cotton wool and divide this into two – it should be sufficient to cover both eyes – dampen these with an eye lotion and place them on the eyes for a cool, refreshing effect.

2. To clean the lips, place the left ring finger at the side of the mouth and take a little cleanser from the back of the hand, making sweeping movements across the lips, from left to right two or three times. Take two squares of the dampened cotton wool; fold in two (one in each hand); hold one side of the mouth so that the lips are not distorted and wipe across the lips (see Fig. 12.4). Reverse the hands and repeat ensuring that both corners of the mouth are clean. Try to ensure that the client is relaxed, if not lips may be pursed or held tightly together making it difficult to cleanse, especially the corners of the mouth.

3. For the neck and remainder of the face, where possible, the palmar surface of the hands (as well as the fingers) should be in contact with the skin, so that your hands are 'moulded' as it were, to the client's features. Take sufficient cleanser and spread evenly over the palms of your hands and fingers.

(a) Starting with the left hand at the sternal end of the clavicle, stroke up the platysma to the mandible, followed immediately with the right hand (see Fig. 12.5(a)). The left hand starts again a little to the right of the beginning of the previous stroke, sweeping up to the mandible and again the right hand follows simul-

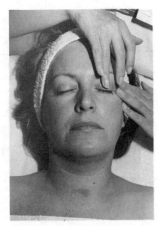

Fig 12.1 Cleansing of the eye with cream

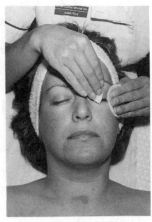

Fig 12.2 Removing cleanser with damp cotton wool

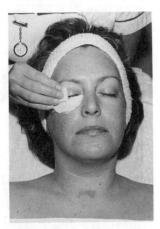

Fig. 12.3 Removing mascara

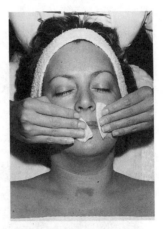

Fig. 12.4 Removing lipstick with damp cotton wool

taneously. Each hand should follow the other with light strokes. Anatomically you are cleansing the skin covering the platysma and part of the sternocleidomastoid muscles. Follow the contours of the neck avoiding any pressure on the trachea. This movement is repeated until your hands have reached the right ear. Continue across the neck to the left ear and back to the centre of the neck, finishing just below the mandible.

(b) Divide the hands and make a stroking movement along the mandible towards the ears and slide the hands lightly back to the chin (see Fig 12.5(b)). Repeat, but this time separate the index finger and place this above the mouth before stroking towards the ears. Slide the hands back to the chin. These two movements can be repeated two or three times.

(c) Divide the hands again and stroke up to the zygomatic arch and slide them lightly down the cheeks (see Fig 12.5(c)). Repeat two

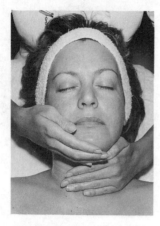

Fig 12.5(a) Cleansing the neck

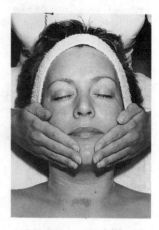

Fig 12.5(b) Cleansing the mentalis, buccinator and orbicularis oris

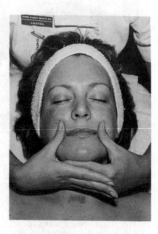

Fig. 12.5(c) Cleansing the masseter and zygomaticus

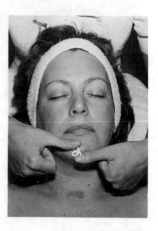

Fig. 12.5(d) Thumb frictions around the chin

or three times ensuring that the entire cheek and sides of the face are covered.

(d) Keep your fingers under the chin and give light thumb frictions around the chin area (see Fig 12.5(d)), finishing with the thumbs stroking up the naso-labial lines (see Fig. 12.5(e)).

Note: Check the eye pads if these have been used, as they may have dried out and are likely to fall off. In which case remove them.

(e) Make light finger frictions at the sides of the nose, working alternately, otherwise the client will have both nostrils closed at the same time, then stroke over the bridge of the nose to the forehead.

(f) The entire forehead is then cleansed with circular finger movements transversely across the frontalis to the temporalis. Also

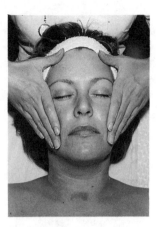

Fig. 12.5(e) Thumbs stroking naso-labial lines

cover the upper border of the orbicularis oculi, procerus and corrugator and with a sweeping movement to the temple, finish with very light pressure.

During part of the facial cleanse the client's eyes may have been covered, therefore it is important that your hands remain in contact with the skin at all times. Relaxation for the client is lost if hands suddenly touch the face without warning or if movements are performed in a jerky manner. Knowledge of the product will ensure that the amount of cleanser on your hands at the beginning is sufficient for the whole face and neck. Removing the cleanser with damp cotton wool is more gentle that with paper tissues. The latter are made from wood fibres and although minuscule they do subtle damage to the skin. Sponge pads are very convenient but, to avoid the risk of cross-infection, they must be washed thoroughly and sterilised before being used again.

(g) With a square of damp cotton-wool pad in each hand, use the same basic movements for the neck and wipe the area clean, turning the pads or using fresh ones as necessary. Progress to the mandible and chin areas. Move on to the cheeks working upwards, so lifting and not dragging the tissues. Clean the sides and bridge of the nose thoroughly. Finally the forehead, with sweeping movements from the centre to the sides, finishing with that very light stroke around the orbicularis oculi, procerus, corrugator and pressure at the temples.

There are other schools of thought as to the method of cleansing the skin, this is just one example of covering the entire neck and face.

It is quite possible that you will have to repeat part or whole of the cleanse again as it is important that the skin be clean so that an accurate analysis can be given. If you have made a mistake in your choice of product now is the time to make a correction.

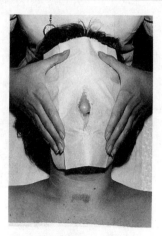

Fig. 12.6 Blotting the toner
with a tissue

Method of toning the skin

1. Choose the toner to suit the skin type
2. For a manual tone, pour a little of the liquid on to two pads of damp cotton wool. With one pad in each hand, gently wipe the face and neck area (using similar movements to the cleansing routine) removing all traces of the cleanser.
3. There are aerosol and electrical sprays available for toning the skin. Explain to the client that a fine mist will be directed on to the face and neck. Ensure that the eyes are closed and spray from about one foot (30 cm) away. Whichever method you use, blot lightly with a tissue (see Fig. 12.6).

Method of moisturising the skin

Moisturisers are better applied when the skin is slightly damp. To apply cream moisturisers, place small 'dabs' on the neck, chin, cheeks and forehead and a little on your fingers. Using upward and outward movements (similar to those used when cleansing) and circular movements around the eyes, using only the third (ring) finger, always towards the nose under the eyes. Lightly blot any excess with a tissue, as excess moisturiser will only evaporate on the skin and make it drier.

Self assessment

- what is the difference between an oil in water and a water in oil emulsion?
- what is the purpose of an emulsifier and a stabiliser?
- give an example of a humectant
- emollients are skin softeners, explain their purpose and give examples
- why are thickeners used in products? and again give examples

- why are preservatives used in products?
- how would you prepare your client for a cleanse, tone and moisturise treatment?
- what should a cleansing preparation be able to achieve?
- describe the difference between soap and facial scrubs
- what cleansers would you use for greasy, normal or dehydrated skins?
- how would you clean heavy mascara?
- what is the purpose of using a toner?
- give the percentages of alcohol content in a toner for greasy and dry skins
- what are the main functions of a moisturiser?
- what is the difference between an eye gel and eye cream?
- why are neck and night creams so important after the mid-twenty age group?

13 Cosmetic products and simple make-up sequence

Cosmetics

Concealer creams and sticks

Creams are coloured foundations containing waxes, such as carnauba wax, mineral waxes (e.g. ozokerite), powders, i.e. talc (magnesium silicate) and kaolin (known as china clay or alumino-silicate or diatomaceous earth) and pigments. These creams are used to conceal blemishes, e.g. a cream with a green pigment can be applied to the nose or cheeks to disguise a high colour, or a cream with a hint of pink/lilac will help to brighten a sallow skin. They should be used after the moisturiser but care must be taken not to 'move' the concealer cream when applying the foundation.

Sticks are solid creams. These contain a higher proportion of waxes, mineral oils, powder and pigments than concealer creams. They come in various skin-tone shades to suit most clients and can be used on isolated blemishes, e.g. simple moles or freckles and small scars or to smooth out the colour on dark skins.

Foundations

The main purpose of foundations is to even out, possibly hide minor imperfections and improve the appearance of the skin. All foundations are in the main O/W emulsions containing mineral oil and wax. The range of colours is extensive to suit all skin types, e.g. from white (to suit Chinese complexions) through to dark tones (to suit Afro-Asian skin types). This is dependent upon the type of inorganic pigment used. They are also produced in varying consistencies.

Cream foundations contain mineral oil, wax, humectant and powder and are thick and creamy which makes them slide easily over the face. They do need blotting very lightly with a tissue and usually need a covering of loose powder. This type of foundation is well suited for the drier skin type.

All-in-one foundations are very popular and consist of a cream foundation with powder, e.g. talc and kaolin to give a matt finish.

Liquid foundations have a lighter texture and this is because, although they may have similar ingredients to cream foundations, they contain a higher percentage of water and a lower content of oil. Some manufacturers include gamma-orizanol (from rice husk extract to act as a UVB filter), chitin (a marine product) and tocopherol acetate (vitamin E). They provide a light protective film and are suitable for all skin types. There are liquid foundations which are oil free and these are generally used for oily/combination skins. However, these rarely contain sufficient density to cover blemishes.

Medicated liquid foundations contain antiseptic agents, e.g. triclosan, and these can be applied over acnegenic skins.

Gel foundations are simply liquid foundations containing gelling agents. Most gels are based on carbomers, which are synthetic thickening agents. These foundations give a natural glossy look to the skin with a translucent film of colour and are suitable for all well-balanced skin types.

Cake foundations are usually compressed creams with the addition of mineral oil, carnauba wax, pigments and powder. They do have high covering power and are useful for greasy skins and for concealing minor imperfections.

Cream rouge/blushers, highlighters and shaders

These follow the foundation and are produced as creams, liquids or gels. They are usually formed from mixtures of mineral oils, petroleum jelly and waxes (e.g. beeswax, carnauba or candelilla wax). Inorganic pigments, which are dissolved in water together with thickening and wetting agents are added for colour.

Rouge/blushers come in various shades of red, pink or peach and give colour and glow to the cheeks. They should blend in and be lighter than the lipstick and look very natural but can be slightly more dense in colour under artificial light.

Highlighters are light colours, e.g. cream or beige and are used to emphasise good features, whereas shaders are darker colours, e.g. dark beige to light brown and are used to reduce facial defects.

Powders

Loose powders are used to 'set' the make-up. The ingredients are talc, kaolin for covering power, magnesium stearate or zinc stearate for adhesion purposes and precipitated chalk which provides bloom. Derivatives from natural amino and fatty acids are often used to give softness, tolerance to pigment, smoothness and to prevent irritation.

Face powder can be translucent, natural or lightly pigmented and at different weights. Generally, light weights are used for dry to normal skins and medium weights for greasy skins. If you use a powder with a colour, it should be the same colour as the foundation or a shade lighter but never darker.

Pressed powders have similar ingredients to loose powders with an increase in magnesium stearate. Titanium dioxide or zinc oxide can be added to increase covering power. These are usually retail items and are mainly used by clients to re-touch their make-up during the day.

Powder rouge/blushers, highlighters and shaders

These have the same ingredients as powders and are coloured by inorganic pigments or lakes to give a specific colour. They are usually manufactured in cake form and this is made possible by adding an increased amount of magnesium stearate.

Eye-shadows

Cream eye-shadows usually contain selected pigments in an emulsion or a mixture of oils and waxes (e.g. isopropyl mysristate, ozokerite and ceresin). Polyamide powder is used to facilitate easy application. Some cosmetic companies use 'Mother of Pearl' to give sheen and to reflect colour.

Powder eye-shadows contain talc, mineral oil (and/or isopropyl mysristate), magnesium stearate and inorganic pigments for colour.

Gel eye-shadows are generally suspensions of pigments in water and thickened to gel-like consistency by adding methyl cellulose or a carbomer. These are mainly used for the younger eyelid.

Water paints are in cake powder form and come and go as fashion changes. They are good for staying power but like powders they can be drying.

Eye-liners

Liquid eye-liners contain beeswax and inorganic pigments suspended in water together with a gum solution, e.g. methyl cellulose.

Pencil eye-liners consist of oils and waxes with organic pigments added.

Kohl pencils consist of a black antimony sulphide which is made into a black waxy pencil by the addition of various waxes.

Cake eye-liners have a similar formulation to powder eye-shadows containing mixtures of talc, mineral oils (and/or isopropyl mysristate) inorganic pigments and magnesium stearate.

Mascaras

Liquid mascaras, rather like eye-liners, contain beeswax, carnauba wax and inorganic pigments suspended in water (or water and alcohol) together with a thickener, e.g. methyl cellulose. Today's market includes many mascaras having certain merits, i.e. waterproof, smudge proof, extra thickening and protein enriched properties which are obtained by the addition of synthetic resins, e.g. polyvinyl acetate, with castor oil added to prevent the film of mascara left on the lashes becoming brittle. Lash-building ingredients include microcrystalin wax (a natural wax) and short filaments of rayon or nylon.

Cake mascaras are gaining popularity again, especially in the salon as they can be applied with a brush which is easy to clean and sterilise. They consist of a mixture of waxes (beeswax or carnauba wax) and pigments in a soap base, e.g. triethanolamine stearate.

Eyebrow pencils

These help to define and strengthen colour to the eyebrow hairs. The colours are fairly limited to be compatible with the colour of the client's own hair, e.g. black, brown or grey.

Lipsticks

Stick lipsticks which are the most popular contain waxes, e.g. carnauba wax, to give hardness, lanolin for emollience, petroleum jelly to enable the lipstick to spread and castor oil which acts as a solvent for the dyes. Colours which vary from the palest pink through to chocolate and the pigments used may be organic or inorganic in origin. All the ingredients must be harmless, non-toxic and non-irritant and should soften on contact with the skin.

Liquid lipsticks are either water based or water/alcohol based with colouring matter. Gums or methyl cellulose are added to thicken the liquid.

Cream lipsticks have more or less the same ingredients as stick lipsticks but the proportion of waxes is lessened and oils are added.

Lip gloss or gels contain mineral oils which are made into a gel by adding bentonite clay. They give a glossy appearance to lips but as they give minimum colour they are usually applied over stick lipstick.

Lip balms are very useful to moisten chapped or dry lips. They are made with hard waxes and oil and some will contain sun-screen agents.

Hypo-allergenic lipsticks avoid known sensitisers, e.g. eosin (a bright red dye) lanolin and perfume.

Lip pencils are used to give a distinct outline to the lips. They have similar ingredients to stick lipsticks but have an increased amount of hard wax to form a crayon.

Simple make-up sequence

The following is a simple make-up excercise but with experience your skills will improve. Remember to take your costings into account including the amount of time it will take you to complete the cleanse, tone and make-up and charge accordingly. Most salons allow half-an-hour, but longer if a make-up lesson is required by the client.

It is assumed that you have cleansed, toned and moisturised the skin and make-up can now be applied. Hygiene factors and preparation are more or less the same as the previous chapter but you should also have ready a make-up tray/stand (see Fig. 13.1) which should include the following:

- concealer creams/sticks
- selection of foundations
- highlighters, shaders rouge/blushers in cream and powder form
- different types of face powder
- eye-shadows, various types
- eye-liners, eye pencils and mascaras
- selection of lipsticks, lip liners, lip gloss and lip pencil

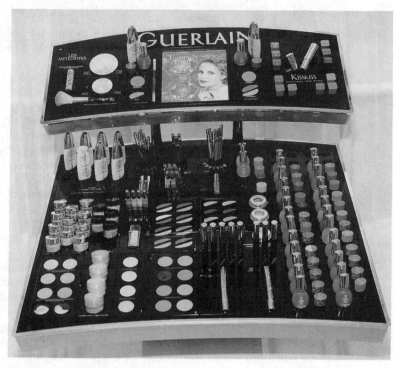

Fig. 13.1 Make-up tray/stand

You should also have sterilised brushes ready for applying make-up, i.e. for concealers, blushers, contours, powders, eye-shadows, eye-liners, eyebrows and lipsticks (see Fig. 13.2). Small dishes or palettes, clean cosmetic sponges, cotton wool, cotton buds and tissues should also be to hand. Ensure good lighting and a large mirror.

Discuss with your client her make-up. First of all decide the shape of the face including bone structure, then take into account the age of the client and the texture and colour of the skin. It is also important to find out the occasion for which the make-up is being worn, be it for the day, to wear with certain colours in her clothes, evening or for a wedding.

Clients rely on your expertise and are interested to watch you apply their make-up. Preferably seat the client to face a mirror. If the make-up is to be worn for the day, natural daylight is best, but if this is not possible, use day-light fluorescent lamps. Evening make-up should be applied in artificial light; a white warm light is sufficient providing it does not cast shadows.

Decide whether the chosen foundation will hide any obvious flaws in the complexion. If the client has small pimples, a redness (probably due to dilated capillaries) or shadows under the eyes, concealing creams should be used at this stage. Before commencing a make-up, wash your hands.

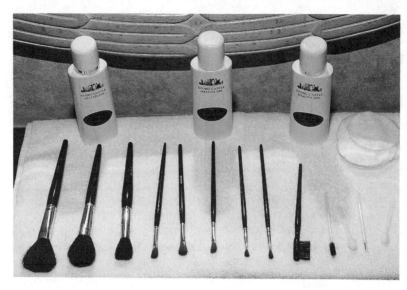

Fig. 13.2 Selection of make-up brushes

To apply concealer creams and sticks

Skin tone concealer creams can be used to lessen the effect of ageing facial lines, e.g. crow's feet or naso-labial lines and to lighten dark circles under the eyes but it is not suitable for dark puffy eyes. Remember to use the concealer under puffy eyes otherwise you will be highlighting rather than hiding the puffiness! Use a corrective cream lighter than the proposed foundation, place a tiny amount on the back of your hand and with a small brush, thin it out, and apply the cream to the lines/furrows or under the eye, again making sure that it is only in the hollow areas (see Fig. 13.3). To use a green corrective cream, again put a little

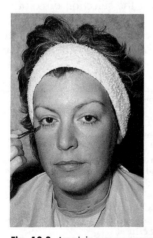

Fig. 13.3 Applying a concealment to the crow's feet area

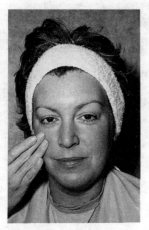

Fig. 13.4 Applying a green concealment to highly coloured areas

on the back of your hand, thin it out and lightly press and roll with your fingertips over the red areas (see Fig. 13.4).

To use a concealer stick, take a small amount on to a spatula and apply thinly to the blemish. Two thin coats are better than a thick one which could show through the foundation.

Medicated sticks can be applied under a medicated foundation on spots or blemishes in the same way as a coloured concealer stick.

To apply foundation

Foundations are the base for all other cosmetics, therefore your choice of texture and colour is important.

The texture will depend on the skin type and Table 13.1 is a rough guide.

Table 13.2 is a general guide for the selection of colour dependent upon the client's own skin tone.

Remember that the pink or peachy shades can hot up and go orange after they have been worn for a while, especially if used on an oily skin,

Table 13.1 Guide for type of foundation

Skin type	Foundation
Normal	Most types
Dry	Cream or oil based
Greasy	Liquid, water based or cake
Combination	Liquid, oil free or all-in-one
Blemished	Medicated liquid or cake
Dehydrated	Cream
Mature	Cream, light aerosol mousses or liquid
Hypersensitive	Hypo-allergenic, i.e. all known irritants screened out, e.g. perfume

Table 13.2 General guide for selection of colour

Skin tone	Foundation colour
Fair	Peach, soft pink/beige or cream
Medium	Peach, beige with pink tint or honey beige
Dark	Dark beige, light olive with a pink tone, or deep peach or golden
Suntanned	Bronze
Olive	Light olive with a pink tone, dark beige or bronze

also the oil on the skin and the air will conspire to darken the shade chosen. Take into account the colour of the hair, eyes and neck. Where the skin is florid use a flat beige foundation as this will soften the reddish tone and it can be applied before the main foundation – this is useful if a concealer cream is not being used. A pale or sallow skin will come alive with a medium pink/beige tone foundation.

If the foundation is in a tube, squeeze sufficient on to the back of your hand; if in a jar, use a spatula; for liquid foundation, pour a little into a small dish or palette.

For a cream foundation, place small dabs on the chin, cheeks and forehead and a little on your fingertips. Liquid foundations can be taken from the palette and, dependent upon the consistency, you can use fingers or a clean sponge. For day wear do not cover the neck as this will rub off on the client's clothing. Use foundations sparingly, blend evenly all over the face, fading it away at the hairline and under the chin. Use upward and outward movements on the face and inward circles around the eyes.

When using a cake foundation, dampen a clean sponge and take sufficient foundation on one side of the sponge to cover the entire face. Use the other side of the sponge to smooth out and make even. Always be careful not to apply too heavily under the eyes, as it can make tiny lines look deeper.

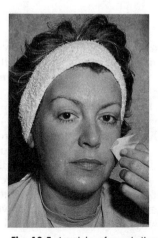

Fig. 13.5 Applying foundation with a sponge

You may find some areas will absorb more foundation than others, possibly the nose or chin and here you can add a little more. Just adding more foundation of the same colour will not alter the colour. The object is to have an even overall appearance and be as natural looking as possible. Foundations can also be used as corrective make-up (see Chapter 14). For evening make-up use two layers, i.e. one very light application and allow it to dry followed by a second application and this will definitely last all evening!

These are very broad guidelines as each cosmetic house has its own range of products, which vary in colour and consistency from one to another. Also the cosmetics themselves are always changing, new discoveries are being made and ingredients are added or taken away. Presently perfumes and chemicals are being discouraged and hypoallergenic ranges have been introduced. Essential oils and herbs are playing a greater role and moisturisers are being added to foundations and powders.

To apply cream rouge/blushers, highlighters and shaders

With clean spatulas or orange-sticks place a little of these on to the back of your hand. Start with the colour for the cheeks and blend in well, but not too far in towards the nose. In some cases it may be difficult to define the cheeks, but if you place your index finger along the upper edge of the zygomatic arch and your thumb underneath, it should resemble an egg. This is the area to place your rouge/blusher fading it away down to the ear lobe. Then add the highlighter or shader to the required areas and ensure that these are faded into the foundation or the colour on the cheeks. It is better to stand in front of the client as you will see more easily that the colours are even and that there are no lines of demarcation.

It will probably be necessary to wash your hands now.

To apply face powders

If the client is wearing contact lenses care should be taken, when using any powder product, to avoid particles of powder entering the eye.

With a clean piece of dry cotton wool take the powder from the container and press firmly, starting upwards from the throat, outwards from the nose and across the forehead. If you need more powder use a fresh piece of cotton wool (see Fig. 13.6).

With a clean powder brush, lightly brush across the forehead, inwards under the eyes, down the nose and the remainder of the face and throat. This is the only time you work down the face, the reason being that there are tiny hairs on the face and if you were to brush upwards, the smallest particle of powder would adhere to the fine hairs and these would be visible. Avoid applying face powder when there is excessive facial hair growth or if the skin is dry and flaky (see Fig. 13.7).

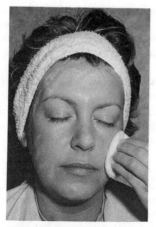

Fig. 13.6 Applying face powder with cotton wool

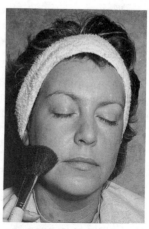

Fig. 13.7 Using a face powder brush

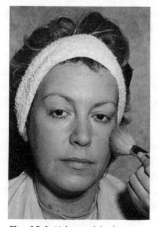

Fig. 13.8 Using a blusher brush

To apply powder rouge/blushers, highlighters and shaders

Charge a clean blusher brush, getting rid of the excess on the back of your other hand and stroke across the cheeks (see Fig. 13.8) making sure the colour is faded away at the edges. Always use the excess from your hand, do not recharge the brush from the cake.

Powder highlighters and/or shaders can be added at this stage if required. Use clean brushes and apply in a similar manner to the blusher.

To apply eye-shadow

Eye-shadow follows, either in powder, cream or gel form and its purpose is to make the eyes more expressive. It should be lightly applied during the day but can be more sophisticated for evening wear.

Women who have dark hair and eyes can use adventurous eye make-up until their late thirties, but blondes with fair skins need a more subtle eye make-up, avoiding the bright blues and greens. You can suggest soft greys, pale turquoise, browns, lemons, apricot and pink shades.

To apply powder, charge a small brush well and get rid of the excess on the back of your other hand. If applying from the front, to steady your hand, the edge of it can rest on the cheek area; if applying from behind the client, the edge of the hand may rest on the forehead. To avoid disturbing the make-up already applied, use a tissue beneath your hand (see Fig. 13.9).

Request the client to close her eyes. Starting from the inner corner of the eye, use a long sweeping stroke along the upper eyelid. This can be repeated with more powder taken from the excess left on your hand. Pay particular attention to the outer corner of the eye – the colour should fade away. If fashion dictates, clients may wish eye shadow beneath the eye. This should be applied from the outer corner to the middle of the eye, sweeping towards the nose. Using clean brushes, complementary deeper or paler shades can be added to the area beneath the eyebrow. It may be necessary to use several brushes especially if there is not enough excess powder left over for the other eye. You should ensure that the brush which has touched the client is not re-charged from the powder in the container. There could be bacteria present and by returning the brush to the container, be it for cream or powder, you could infect the unused make-up and cause a cross-infection.

To apply cream eye-shadow, use an orange-stick to take a tiny amount of the cream on to the back of your hand. With a small brush, soften the cream and apply very light strokes across the eyelid using the same procedure as for the powder. Other colours may also be applied beneath the eyebrow. These are excellent for the young eyelid, but tend to crease in the tiny folds of an older lid. Pressing a natural

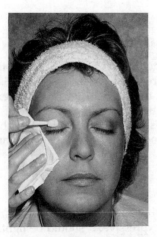

Fig. 13.9 Applying powder eye shadow

face powder on to the cream will help it to stay 'put' for a little longer. If the cream tends to crease or move, a powder shadow should be used.

Applying water paints is rather more time consuming. They are in cake-powder form, so remove a little with a hoof stick into a palette and mix with a drop of water. Apply as for powder or cream. Have another small palette handy with a little clean water. As water paints can leave a harsh line, dip the brush in the clean water, shake away excess, and fade away the edge of the colour. Mix other colours for the area under the eyebrow. Now check the powder rouge/blusher, highlighter or shader applied as the skin has had time to absorb the colour. You can add more or tone it down.

To apply eye-liners

These are in and out of fashion but it is necessary to know how to apply them and you will need a great deal of practice to perfect a very thin line on the edge of the upper and lower lids. Eye-liners come in a few colours and these should complement the eyes, eye-shadow or mascara.

To apply a liquid eye-liner use a very thin sterilised brush. You can rest the edge of your hand over a paper tissue on the cheeks or forehead. Request the client to close her eyes and, starting at the inner corner of the eye, apply a very thin line along the top lashes of both eyes. When this is dry, request the client to open her eyes and apply a very thin line along the edge of the lower lashes. A client, unfamiliar with the use of a lower eye-liner, will be inclined to blink. With a tissue under your finger, gently lift and hold the eyelid until you have completed the line and it is dry.

Coloured pencils and Kohl pencils are the easiest to use, providing the point is kept sharp, wiped with alcohol and placed in a container or kept in an ultra-violet cabinet when not in use. A line can be drawn

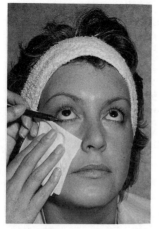

Fig. 13.10 Applying eye-liner with a pencil

with a coloured pencil and these are soft enough to be blended in with the eye-shadow if a distinct line is not required (see Fig. 13.10). They are very useful for the older client. Kohl pencils are used on the inner rim of the lower eye-lid to enhance the white of the eye. If it is used on the rim of the upper eye-lid as well it does tend to make the eye appear rounder and smaller.

Cake eye-liners are applied in a similar way to eye-shadow water paints, i.e. to remove a little into a palette and mix with a wetted brush before application. These can create a harsh effect if the line is too thick and should be avoided for the older client.

To apply mascara

The purpose of mascara is to make the lashes appear longer and thicker. There are a few colours to complement the eyes or eye-shadows. Spiral brushes are available but these should be avoided in a salon *if* they are part of the mascara container. For reasons of hygiene the brush should not be returned to the container to be re-charged. There are disposable spiral brushes available which can be used once in the container, then given to the client or thrown away.

With a clean brush mix a little cake mascara with a drop of water or use a drop of the liquid from the container into a palette. Place a small piece of paper tissue under the lower lashes (see Fig. 13.11), and request the client to close her eyes. Brush down the lashes, open the eyes to brush up the top lashes and brush down the lower lashes. The tissue will prevent any mascara touching the skin under the eye.

Two coats may be applied, allowing time for the mascara to dry between each application. Repeat for the other eye. When the mascara is completely dry, take a small stiff brush and stroke the lashes downwards and upwards to separate the hairs as mascara tends to make them adhere to one another.

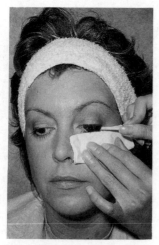

Fig. 13.11 Applying mascara

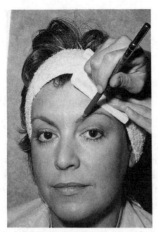

Fig. 13.12 Using an eyebrow pencil

To apply an eyebrow pencil

Before using the pencil, take a small stiff brush and stroke the eyebrow hairs up and down to remove any face or eye shadow powder. The most hygienic way of applying colour is to take a small amount of crayon on to your hand with an orange-stick and use this as a pencil. However, most therapists use a pencil and sterilise it afterwards. If the hairs are strong and the eyebrow has a good line, the hairs may be lifted and stroked up and then down. The pencil can also be used to make a line, to correct the brow or fill in where the hairs are sparse (see Fig. 13.12).

To apply a lip pencil

These come in a few colours and you should use a pencil colour slightly darker but which also complements the lipstick. The pencil must be well sharpened and a fine line should outline the lips. The outline can

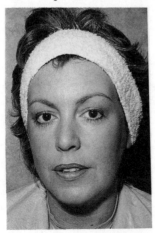

Fig. 13.13 Lip pencil applied

be blotted and repeated if necessary before filling in with the chosen lipstick. Lip pencils are very useful if the lipstick is inclined to 'bleed' (see Fig. 13.13).

To apply lipsticks

As they come in a variety of colours, choose one which will blend in with the rest of the make-up and certainly no lighter than the cream/powder rouge/blusher. Light or pearlised shades add fullness to the lips and dark shades have the contrary effect. If your client has difficulty in maintaining the colour of the lipstick on her lips – and this often happens with the lighter shades – use a white lipstick first, blot well with a tissue and then use the colour of her choice. If the lips are slightly chapped, use a medicated lipstick first and blot well. Do this twice before applying a colour.

Advise clients who have a high colour to avoid using a lipstick with a blue tone as it tends to emphasise the facial colour and, vice-versa, those who have a sallow complexion should avoid a lipstick with an orange tone.

To apply, take a little from the container with an orange-stick and place on the back of your hand. With a small brush outline the lips from the centre to the corner of the mouth. Try to create a balanced look and straighten out crooked lip lines. With a little more on the brush fill in the lips. Blot well with a tissue and repeat (see Fig. 13.14). Blot again if a matt look is preferred. A lip gloss can now be applied if desired.

Evening make-up

Make-up for the evening can be accentuated as colours will be subdued under artificial light. Rouge/blushers, highlighters or shaders can be enhanced but not to the extent that the client feels conspicuous! For the

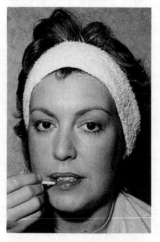

Fig. 13.14 Applying lipstick

younger clientele, glitter can be applied and eye make-up could include gold and silver shades.

Make-up for darker skins

Make-up choice for the darker-skin types is improving, but as the colour of the skin ranges from a pale olive through to a blue-black, there are very few manufacturers able to provide a complete range of colours to satisfy all requirements. Fortunately these skins have a superb natural bloom and quite often do not require a foundation or powder. After toning the skin look for the undertones. These may be yellow, olive, grey or even slightly red.

If a foundation is required, it should not be oily but be resistant to heat and moisture of the skin. Often a colourless base or tinted gel will be sufficient to form an invisible film over the skin. If there are patches due to pigment deficiency, use a cover stick first to give a smooth finish.

Powder, if required at all, should have colour and be fluffed on very lightly.

Use blushers to shape and highlight the cheekbones and give warmth to the cheeks. These should be non-greasy and the colours should be deep-red to wine, orange-reds and red-browns. Highlighters high on the cheekbones and around the eye area bring eyes into focus.

Eye-shadows can be varied using deep colours for effect and you will probably find that the powder eye-shadows have more staying power than cream which are inclined to crease. Kohl, and eye pencils accentuate and give depth to the socket of the eye and lipsticks should be bold. Table 13.3 gives suggested colours that could be used.

Table 13.3 Suggested colours for dark skins

Make-up	Light brown	Medium olive brown	Dark brown	Ebony-black
Foundation	Dark golden	Golden, hint of red	Golden and slightly orange	Golden or dark copper
Blusher	Brick red or red brown	Reddish brown	Orange red or sienna	Orange red
Powder	Warm golden	Warm golden	Gold bronze	Copper gold
Eye shadow	Rust or sienna	Sea green	Rust, brown or muted greens	Dark blue or dark green or violet
Shadow under eyebrows	Light beige or salmon	Ivory	Ivory beige or salmon	Ivory or beige
Eyebrow pencil	Chestnut or medium brown	Brown	Medium or very dark brown	Black
Mascara	Black	Black	Black or brown	Black or navy blue
Eyeliner	Black, brown or bronze green	Black or bronze green	Black	Black or navy blue
Lipstick	Red brown or orange brown	Orange red or red brown	Orange brown or redcurrant	Dark chestnut pencil and blueberry shades

Contra-indications

- skin diseases
- skin disorders, e.g. herpes simplex
- eye disorders, e.g. stye, conjunctivitis, eye make-up should not be applied

- pustula acne
- cuts, grazes or black eyes
- recent scar tissue
- not immediately after electrolysis or facial waxing

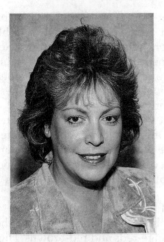

Fig. 13.15 The end result

On completion of make-up

Check the client's face to ensure evenness. Remove headband/cap, comb the hair, remove cape/towel and let her see the end result in the mirror (see Fig. 13.15). It is important that the client approves. It may mean taking away or adding colour to please, but with a happy client, your retail sales could improve!

A simple make-up chart should be made out and given to the client (see Fig. 13.16), and you may also wish to record the cosmetics used on the salon's card for future visits. Return any jewellery and personal possessions to the client, assist with outdoor clothing and accompany her to the reception area where payment can be made.

Return to the cubicle and dispose of all tissues and used orange-sticks; place headband and towels in a laundry basket; clean your pots/jars; clean all used brushes and put them in a clean container or an ultra-violet cabinet. Wipe down your surface area and chair with surgical spirit. Wash your hands.

Self assessment

- what is the purpose of a concealant and describe the difference between a cream and stick
- explain the difference in product content between a cream and liquid foundation
- describe the types of face powder available
- when would you not use a cream eye-shadow?
- what skin type would be suitable for a cream rouge/blusher?

```
┌─────────────────────────────────────────────────────────────────────┐
│                      West End Beauty Clinic                            │
├─────────────────────────────────────────────────────────────────────┤
│ Skin type ........................    Cleanser ......................   Toner/tonic ....................  │
│                                                                        │
│ Moisturiser ........................................    Concealant ........................................  │
│                                                                        │
│ Foundation ........................................    Powder ........................................  │
│                                                                        │
│ Rouge/blusher/highlighter or shader:                                   │
│                                                                        │
│           cream ........................................................  │
│                                                                        │
│           powder ........................................................  │
│                                                                        │
│ Eye shadows: cream ........................................................  │
│                                                                        │
│           powder ........................................................  │
│                                                                        │
│ Eye-liner ........................................    Mascara ........................................  │
│                                                                        │
│ Eyebrow pencil ........................................    Lip pencil ........................................  │
│                                                                        │
│ Lipstick ........................................    Other ........................................  │
└─────────────────────────────────────────────────────────────────────┘
```

Fig. 13.16 Suggested make-up chart

- why are cake mascaras preferred in the salon?
- explain the product content of lipsticks
- what sort of foundation would you use for a client of 55 years of age?
- what is the purpose of rouge/blusher?
- what are the contra-indications to applying eye-shadows?
- your client is blonde with blue eyes, what colour eye-liner and mascara would you use?
- having used mascara, how would you separate the eye lashes?
- your client is 21 years of age with thin lips, what type and colour of lipstick would you suggest?
- how would you apply highlighters to a client with a dark skin?

14 Corrective make-up

Facial and eyebrow shapes, corrective make-up

Basically there are seven shapes of faces: oval, heart, long, diamond, square, round and pear.

The oval face is generally accepted today as the perfect shape and therefore other shapes are highlighted or shadowed to obtain this effect. For make-up and shading purposes note the colour of the hair and its style and the colour of the eyes. Before you decide on the shape of the face, use a crêpe bandage as a headband and wind it around the head at the hairline. Remove all trace of make-up and study carefully from the front and profile angle and note the colour of the skin.

The client's face may fall into one of the above seven categories but with certain exceptions. She may have a low forehead, a protruding or receding chin, eyes set too close together or a long or short nose.

To highlight simply means using lighter shades to bring out the good points and therefore shadowing is the opposite, using deeper shades to minimise imperfections. This can be done quite easily with foundations, contour sticks, blushers, powders and rouges, but to have any effect at all these should be either two or three shades lighter or darker than the original foundation. Expertise and common sense should prevail; no client should leave the salon with a 'doll-like' appearance or so heavily made-up it is obvious. There should be no demarcation of colour; it should harmonise and blend in well.

Taking each type of face it will be seen how improvements can be made.

Oval

As we have said this is perfection. First of all check the eyebrow shaping. Let them follow the natural line of the eyebrow – a gentle curve – but pluck below if they appear too heavy for the face. Your foundation will blend in with the skin tone, but to give warmth apply a triangle of dry rouge or cream, blending it out towards the temples and the level of the earlobes. If the client prefers her cheekbones accentuated, use a darker rouge/blusher to the area under the zygomatic arch towards the ear.

Heart

The aim here is simply to offset the wide forehead and the narrow (or even pointed chin). Check the eyebrows; the arch should be almost

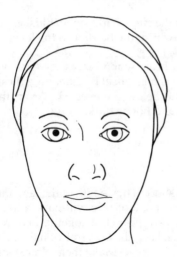

Fig. 14.1 Oval face

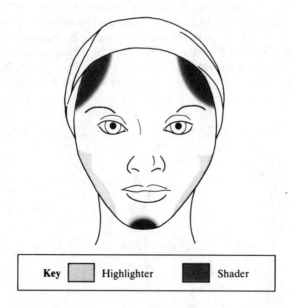

| Key | | Highlighter | | Shader |

Fig. 14.2 Heart-shaped face

centre of the eye and the line ending just beyond the outer corner of the eye. After the original foundation has been applied a darker shade can be used to the sides of the forehead, blending into the hairline and also to the point of the chin. Alternatively, a lighter foundation could be applied beneath the cheekbones down the outer side of the face, along the jawline to either side of the chin, blending in with the original foundation and the darker area of the chin. With rouge/blusher, accentuate the cheekbones and blend it away at the hairline at the level of the eyes and the edge of the zygomatic bone.

Often in the diamond- and heart-shaped faces the eyes will appear quite small. This imperfection can be offset by extending the eye make-up slightly beyond, above and below the eyes. However, the colours should complement the eyes and not be dark.

Long

Obviously you should aim to shorten the length of the face and give the illusion of breadth. Often this shape of face will have a long, narrow nose and this will make the eyes appear close together. To create width between the bridge of the nose, keep the area free of hairs and start the eyebrows at the inner corner of the eye. Make them almost straight but not extending them beyond the outer corner of the eye.

Use two foundations, the lighter shade being used down the sides of the nose to the centre of the cheek area and also around the jawline and into the throat. The darker foundation used elsewhere and down the centre of the nose should blend in well. Apply rouge in a semi-circle from about the top of the ear towards the centre of the cheeks and back towards the level of the earlobe. To keep the balance, when applying eye make-up place the paler shades near the bridge of the nose and the darker shades from the centre to the outer edges of the eyes.

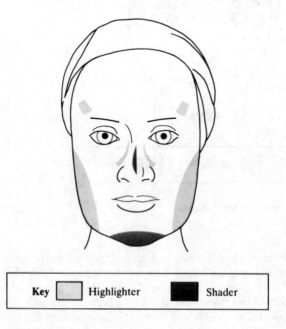

Key ☐ Highlighter ■ Shader

Fig. 14.3 Long face

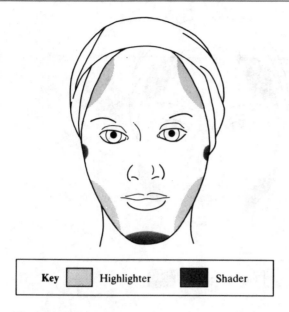

Fig. 14.4 Diamond face

Diamond

A shape similar to the 'heart' with the exception of the narrower forehead. To appear to broaden this area, highlight with a lighter foundation to the sides of the forehead near the hairline. Apply the remaining make-up as for the heart-shaped face.

Square

The aim here is to minimise the squareness of the features. Make sure the eyebrows have a high arch towards the ends and extend the eyebrow beyond the outer corner of the eye. This will soften the squareness of the forehead. Apply the skin-tone foundation all over the face and with a darker foundation start with a thin line just above the ears down the hairline and widen out under the zygomatic arch to end at the jawline near the corners of the lips. This should blend in with the remainder of the foundation used on the face. Rouge is applied from the centre of the cheeks, fading away to the level of the eye at the hairline and the lower border of the zygomatic bone. If the chin is very square, apply a lighter foundation to the central point. It is a very small area and should be carefully blended with the original and darker foundations.

With eye make-up, complement the eyes by making them look wider with the appearance of an upward slant. This can be done by extending the make-up beyond the outer corner of the eye and shading upwards.

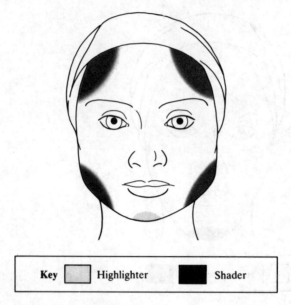

Key ☐ Highlighter ■ Shader

Fig. 14.5 Square face

Round

The aim again is to slim down the face and the application of darker and lighter foundations would be nearly the same as those used for a square face – obviously not to the same extent as there is less to shadow or highlight.

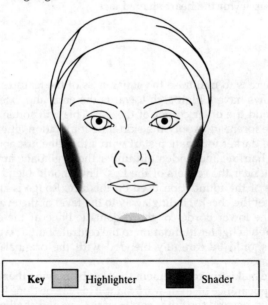

Key ☐ Highlighter ■ Shader

Fig. 14.6 Round face

Pear (or triangular)

This type of face usually has a narrow forehead but the jawline and chin are wide, so the aim here would be to create the illusion of balance by widening the forehead and making the face appear longer and more oval.

If needed, correct the shape of the eyebrows. These should start immediately above the inner corner of the eye and continue towards the end of the cheekbones, arching them slightly towards the ends. Three foundations would be useful here or the use of a cream contour stick (instead of the third foundation). Apply the skin-tone foundation all over the face with the exception of the sides of the forehead near the hairline. Here use a lighter foundation to give the illusion of width. To narrow the jawline, using a darker foundation or contour stick, start a thin line at the temple area, come down over the outer side of the cheeks widening the area of darker foundation, ending near the outer corners of the lips at the jawline. Blend this in well. Rouge can be applied to accentuate the cheekbones.

Use the darker shades of eye shadow in the middle or inner corner of the eyes and the paler shades at the outer corners of the eyes.

The above are very broad outlines. Rarely will you have a client who will exactly represent any of the seven shapes mentioned. These particular shapes rarely apply to the dark-skinned races as their bone structure is quite often different. A prominent jawbone will emphasise a larger mouth or the zygomatics may be more prominent. It is important that you encourage the individual ethnic beauty rather than trying to assert a European image.

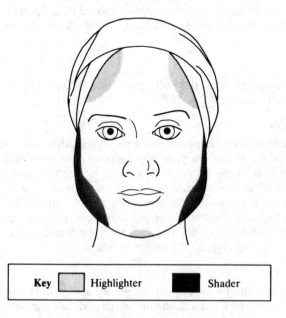

Key		Highlighter		Shader

Fig. 14.7 Pear (or triangular) face

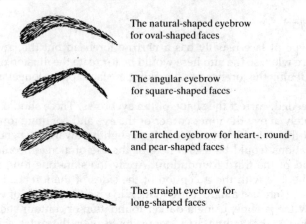

The natural-shaped eyebrow
for oval-shaped faces

The angular eyebrow
for square-shaped faces

The arched eyebrow for heart-, round-
and pear-shaped faces

The straight eyebrow for
long-shaped faces

Fig. 14.8 Eyebrow shapes

Corrective make-up for facial features

Foreheads

A low forehead would appear higher if a lighter than original foundation was applied over the whole area to the eyebrows and the bridge of the nose.

For a high forehead, a darker foundation applied to the upper area of the forehead would appear to bring down the height.

Also the imperfection of a bulging forehead would be lessened if a darker foundation was applied to the area just below the temples, over the eyelids and across the upper part of the nose.

For a narrow forehead the eyebrows should be shaped to form a low arch and for the high forehead a high arch would be more suitable.

Eyes

Eye make-up can often help offset an imperfection. The following are the more obvious (see Fig. 14.9).

Round eyes

For a more almond shape lengthen the eye shadow beyond the outer corner of the eye. Use the paler shades below the brow and the darker shades closest to the lid edge. Ignore the socket line and shadow the colours in an upward slanting effect from the middle of the eye to the outer corner. If an eye-liner is requested, use this only on the top lid and finish just beyond the end of the eye. If it is continued on the lower lid, a rounded effect will result, which defeats the object. When using mascara use a second coat on the upper lashes.

Small eyes

These can be made to appear larger by using pale shades of eye shadow. If two or three colours are requested, use the palest shade on the eyelid and extend it beyond, above and below the eye. A slightly darker shade may be used in the eye-socket area and a paler shade above this, blending them out beyond the corner of the eye. There is an excellent range of blues, greys and beiges available to create this effect. To make the lashes look thicker, apply a light-coloured mascara. Avoid a dark eye-liner.

Bulging or protruding eyes

These can be minimised by the use of a dark eye shadow on the lid and lighter shadows above. Using three shades, take the middle colour and blend it all over the lid into the socket line, slanting it upwards slightly at the end. With the deepest shade start at the inner corner of the eye with a very thin line. At the middle of the eye gradually widen the shadow to the outer corner of the eye. Lighter shadows above the eye socket will appear to bring the area forward and so minimise the protrusion. Mascara may be used for top and bottom lashes.

Close-set eyes

To make these appear wider apart, apply very pale shadow over the lid and above the socket. A darker shadow can then be applied lightly upwards from the middle to outer edge of the eye. Use mascara but only very lightly on the inner corner of the eyes and more than one coat from the middle of the outer corner. If an eye-liner is worn, start this from the middle of the top lashes but avoid dark colours.

Wide-set eyes

This should be the reverse of the above by using the darker shadows on the upper inside of the lid up to the browline. Paler shades can be used over the rest of the lid and above, making sure they blend in well. Eye-liner can be taken into the inner corner of the eye and mascara used on both top and bottom lashes.

Heavy-lidded eyes

A very similar shading to that used for protruding eyes, except that the darker shade can be widened nearer to the inner corner of the eye. As it reaches the outer edge the whole eyelid will be covered with the darker shade. Lighter shades should be used between the socket and the brow line. Mascara can be used, especially if the top lashes can be curled upwards.

Deep sunken eyes

The idea is to create the illusion of bringing them forward. Use very pale shadows at the inner corners of the eyes up to the browline. A very slightly deeper shade can be applied to the outer edge of the lids up towards the temple. Use a light shade of mascara (or matching) to make the lashes appear thicker, but avoid using an eye-liner.

Dark circles and puffy eyes

Dark circles under the eye can be camouflaged with a lighter-shade foundation.

Puffy eyes will need a darker shade of foundation to minimise the puffiness.

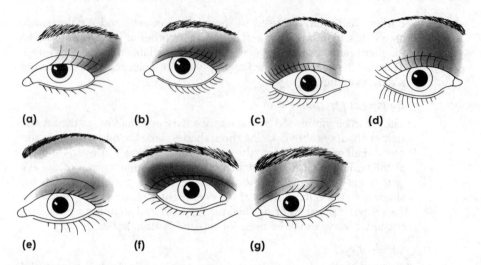

Fig. 14.9 (a) Round eyes (b) Small eyes (c) Protruding eyes (d) Close-set eyes (e) Wide-set eyes (f) Heavy-lidded eyes (g) Deep-set eyes

When both these imperfections are present it requires a great deal of patience. With the client's eyes open, draw a very thin line of the lighter foundation just under the lower lid. Then apply the darker foundation to the puffy area. Then blend one into the other with a clean dry brush. Because of the delicate skin there, be gentle and work towards the nose.

Noses, which come in all shapes and sizes

The large or protruding nose

To make this appear smaller place a darker foundation along the length of the nose. To create fullness in the cheeks – which will also make the nose appear smaller – apply a lighter foundation down the sides of the nose and across the cheeks. Blend in well the dark and the light foundations, being careful not to let the darker foundation slip down the sides of the nose. When using rouge or blusher, avoid placing this too near to the nose.

Broad nose

To slim this type of nose use a darker than original shade of foundation down the sides of the nose and nostrils and shade it into the cheeks. If the nostrils are just flared use a darker foundation there, but be careful with the darker shade; make sure that it does not tone into the laughter lines, otherwise these will be accentuated. Use a lighter shade down the centre from the bridge of the nose.

Short or flat nose

So that this may appear longer, use a lighter foundation down the centre of the nose to the tip, blending in well with the skin-tone colouring.

Boot nose or turned-up nose

Just use a darker shade on the tip and in some cases a lighter foundation along the centre of the nose helps

As common sense would dictate, if a client had a nose that was small for the size of her face it would be obvious to lighten the whole of the nose.

Mouths

Rarely will you have a client with a beautifully even mouth – either the bottom lip is uneven or the top lip is higher one side than the other. Here you will have to judge how to apply the lipstick to complement the shape of the face (see Fig. 14.10).

Uneven top lip

Generally speaking it is better to fill in, i.e. bring the uneven side up to the level of the other side.

Variations of the bottom lip

If the bottom lip is already full, just draw a line across to even the lip, taking the narrower side as a guideline. However, if you consider the lower side to be the correct line, then you would need to fill in again. This simple correction would apply to any imperfection in the lips.

Mouth too oval

The top lip could be made into a very slight cupid's bow.

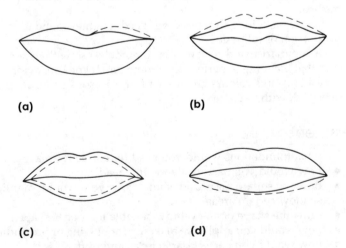

(a)   **(b)**

(c)   **(d)**

Fig. 14.10 (a) Corrective work for uneven lip (b) Corrective work for mouth too oval (c) Corrective work for large lips (d) Corrective work for lips dropping at the corners

Large full lips

These could be slimmed by keeping the lipstick inside the line of the lip with a well-defined clean-cut outline, especially at the corners.

Lips drooping at the corners

Should the lips droop at the corners, build them up with the lipstick to correct this. The whole idea must be of balance and only practice will make this perfection.

Chins

These can sag, recede or protrude. First of all it would be better to highlight the receding chin. Use a lighter than original foundation on the chin area itself and fade it away. A darker foundation just under the chin will also help to give the illusion of prominence.

The sagging or double chin can be minimised if a darker foundation is applied to the area.

The protruding chin will also look less prominent if a darker foundation is applied to the chin area only, but blended in well with the original foundation.

Necks

Clients rarely ask for a foundation for the neck area as it rubs off on to the clothing. However, if they are going out in the evening or wearing a low-cut or off-the-shoulder dress, their necks matter a great deal.

With a proportionate neck the original foundation can be carried down and faded away.

A short thick neck can appear thinner by using a darker foundation at the sides with a narrow strip of the original foundation down the trachea.

Vice versa, a long thin neck will need a lighter foundation to create the illusion of fullness.

To summarise and repeat, it is common sense with expertise to ensure that blending is perfection, and no harsh lines are evident.

Fashions and colours change with the seasons so be careful not to overstock with make-up.

Self assessment

- what foundations would you need for corrective make-up?
- how would you narrow a wide forehead?
- draw a square face and show how you would highlight and shadow certain areas
- draw the shape of an eyebrow suitable for a pear-shaped face
- how would you apply eye make-up for bulging or protruding eyes?
- how would you correct dark circles and puffy eyes?
- draw a diagram showing corrective work for uneven lips
- how would you make a receding chin appear more prominent?

15 Remedial camouflage

This is the art of camouflage, using cosmetics of a special type, to cover blemishes and scars. It must be said at the outset that you will find that this is not a financially rewarding type of treatment as clients will rarely make more than one or two visits. Having shown them how to apply the cosmetics they will return home to apply the techniques expertly themselves.

It should be stressed that anyone undertaking this work must have an understanding and sympathetic nature, a complete knowledge of the skin and of myology (science of muscles), a good eye for colours, considerable practice and above all, patience. People who have facial or even body disfigurements, however small, will tend to be over-sensitive and in some cases psychologically affected by them. Under-standing the individual is very important, as no two cases are the same. Your approach should be to let the client talk! You will often be told something which would not be mentioned to either family or doctor. Listen carefully, gain her or his confidence and treat the client as if he or she were the only person that mattered. Everything that is told to you is, of course, confidential and you must adhere strictly to your Code of Ethics.

You may have a client who is very young, or even a baby, and it is the parent who is emotionally disturbed about the disfigurement. It is very difficult to apply creams to a baby's face that is continually on the move and you will welcome the parent's assistance. The parent will also be there to watch you apply the creams and learn the technique.

However, where young people of either sex are concerned, in the first instance, it is better for the parent to leave the room. Gain the confidence of the young person, make sure he or she realises that you are accepting the blemish as something which can easily be overcome. Children can be very cruel and the child could be developing a complex through being teased. Where a girl is concerned you are halfway there by 'allowing' her to use make-up, but for the boy it is more difficult. He will shy away from make-up as he fears he may be called 'sissy'. He needs the final result to convince him and you could suggest that, after all, he is only using coloured ointments to cover a mark. When you have applied the creams, then is the time to let the parent in to see the result. All the creams should then be removed from the area and ap-plied again, showing or guiding the young person with his or her parent watching. Later, when this is practised and perfected at home it will become as habit-forming as the brushing of teeth.

Your reward is seeing a disfigurement disguised as naturally as poss-ible and know that you have given the client confidence with a completely different attitude towards life in the knowledge that she or he can live with their disfigurement.

Contra-indications

Check for contra-indications. These are:

- over any inflamed or broken skin – which includes cold sores, open spots (pustular acne) or cuts
- over warts
- over painful areas
- over any area which looks infectious
- after surgery – recent scar tissue. This should be left for a minimum of six months. Scar tissue can be recognised easily: it is, when new, red or pink in colour. The skin might have a wrinkled appearance. To the touch it would feel soft or thin and delicate. It could also feel puckered or lumpy especially after plastic surgery.

You may cover moles but if hairs are present these may be cut with sterilised scissors but never removed. Advise the client not to cover them continually, as any change in structure or malignancy might not be noticed. It is always best to let these blemishes breathe freely and be able to cover them for the evening or special occasion.

At this point it should be mentioned that close liaison with the client's doctor, plastic surgeon, surgeon or dermatologist is valuable. You should endeavour to work in conjunction with the medical profession in all your cases. It is not an easy task because of their excessive workload but it is certainly desirable. Often it is possible to be attached to a hospital for this remedial work. If you are working on your own, advise the local doctors and hospitals that you can provide this treatment. It is available under the National Health Service in the UK and the client can obtain the necessary form from his or her doctor.

In view of the few manufacturers making this type of camouflage make-up it will obviously be helpful to mention them by name. At the time of writing, Keromask, Max Factor, Covermark, Coverall, Derma Color, Veil and Boots produce a range of colours and creams which are suitable. The covering creams have an ointment base with a great deal of colouring matter, are non-allergic and some are waterproof. This is something that you must check with the manufacturer. They should last all day, unless they are used on an area which is being constantly rubbed by clothing. If they are being used on the body for sunbathing, swimming etc., advise washing carefully so as not to disturb the creams and pat dry.

Birthmarks

These will be dealt with first as it is much easier to blot out a flat mark with colour. Skin grafts and scars usually leave raised or sunken marks and the texture of the skin is quite different.

There are varying degrees of birthmarks (also known as capillary naevi) ranging from pink to red to purple. They are generally found on one side of the face or neck and are often referred to as 'port-wine' stains or 'strawberry' marks. They are irregular and also vary in size.

To prepare the client with a facial and/or neck naevus, wind a crêpe band around the head at the hairline and tuck in towels to protect her or his clothing. Wash your hands.

Cleanse the face and neck with appropriate cleanser or soap and water and use a tonic or toner to make sure the skin is free from grease and dry thoroughly. If the birthmark is elsewhere on the body, uncover the area, cleanse, tone and dry. Wash your hands again.

Cover the blemished area with a very light – even white – shade of cream to blot out the naevus; the intensity will depend on the colour of the blemish and the pH factor of the skin. Use a spatula to remove the cream from the container and apply with fingers or brushes or both, using a very little at a time and working the cream well into the area. Practise patting, stippling, followed by rocking movements with the pads of the fingers.

Now this is where the art, knowledge of the skin, myology and patience is required to bring the area back to match the remaining skin tone. Use a little of the deeper shade, i.e. deeper than the skin tone, perhaps a brown or red, brush or pat in, following the muscles from origin to insertion or vice versa where possible. The facial muscles are continually moving and the cream will move the various expressions. Keep adding or slightly changing the colours until the desired effect is obtained.

It is worth mentioning here that the fewer colours used the better, as the client will find it easier when applying it herself. You may find, in an attempt to use fewer colours, that it will be necessary to remove all that you have done and start again. It may be found preferable to mix two colours in a small palette with an orange-stick to obtain one colour which may be sufficient. Dab the area with damp cotton wool and pat dry with a tissue. Apply a liberal dusting of finishing powder and leave for ten minutes, then dust off the surplus. Always bear in mind that camouflage must look natural. If the client is an adult male and the naevus extends to the chin area, it will be necessary to use a darker shade for the 'shaving' area to match the other side. Make-up may be applied for the female and a light dusting of translucent powder all over. Freckles can always be painted in, if the client wishes this. Do not use greasy make-up creams on top of camouflage creams as these would tend to slide off; liquid foundations are better. Cover creams can be removed with liquifying cleansing cream or oil plus soap and water. Always take away part or all of the make-up you have applied and let the client apply the cream so that you can advise and guide.

Freckles, moles, varicose and thread veins can also be covered in this way.

To begin with see if you can find a freckle or blemish on your own skin or on a member of the family. Then practise on friends who have blemishes, however small. It is easy enough to blot out a blemish, the art is to match the skin colouring exactly.

Chloasma

These patches may disappear after birth or remain as a permanent blemish. They can also appear during the menopause. The treatment would be as already outlined, using a light cream first and darker shades to bring the patches back to the natural skin tone.

Vitiligo

The preparation of the area is as outlined in naevi, i.e. cleanse, tone and dry. Apply a dark covering first, making sure that it is pressed well into the area. Then use one or more lighter colours to bring it back to the natural skin tone. The rest of the face may be made up. Vitiligo will appear on the hands and although they can be covered satisfactorily, constant immersion in water will disturb the creams, and even the wearing of gloves may do this. Always show the client how to apply the coloured creams, as there may be occasions when her hands are on 'show' and she will feel more confident if the white patches are not evident.

Scars

These are more difficult to disguise and therefore wax (morticians) or theatrical putty is used when they are raised or indented. Often women who have had operations on the stomach want to wear a bikini for their holiday and turn to you for advice. Make sure that the scar is at least six months old and liaise with her doctor. Indentation is easier in as much as you can fill in with wax. Soften the wax by warming and kneading it between the fingers, so that it becomes soft and pliable. Place it into the indentation and with a small palette knife smooth it over and then cover with make-up and powder. Remember that the area must be free of grease. With sunbathing the make-up will have to deepen gradually in colour to continue matching the surrounding skin tone. This method is not very satisfactory on an area with continuous movement – the wax will simply fall out. Softened wax can also be used to fill in large pock marks on the face and an ordinary daytime make-up will cover these.

Raised scars are more noticeable as light will reflect from them, causing a shadow. You should smooth out very small, thin pieces of softened wax either side of the scar or, in some instances, just under the scar. Use ordinary make-up to cover as it could be too small to use a covering cream.

Covering creams may also be used to cover the mottling effect from burns, but again you will need assurance from the client's doctor that the tissues have healed and may be camouflaged.

Plastic surgery

This is used extensively for medical reasons and for cosmetic purposes. Normally the latter is not available under the National Health in the UK but of course there are exceptions. People involved in an accident, or who are born with a hare-lip or cleft palate, or who have a deformity which is causing psychological change in them, can have this type of surgery. If you are working on your own in a salon you will come into contact with women wishing to have cosmetic plastic surgery or post-operative treatment. Your advice should be for the client to contact her own doctor first, who in turn will get in touch with a surgeon recognised by the Association of Plastic Surgeons. When the client sees the surgeon he will have received from her doctor a background report on her health and any medication prescribed. This is important.

Whatever the cosmetic operation, try to liaise with the plastic surgeon. You may be able to assist the pre-surgery treatment, i.e. for the face, removal of comedones, massage or paraffin-wax treatments to soften the tissues. You will need to know what post-surgery treatment may be given and when. The field of cosmetic surgery is expanding and presently includes treatment for the face, eyelids, nose-shaping, chin augmentations and complete facelifts. Remedial camouflage for these types of operations is minimal and often not required. However, surgery to the body, i.e. arms, thighs, abdomen or breasts, usually leaves scars and these can be camouflaged after six months.

Hospital work

Working in a hospital is very different. The work is mainly helping people involved in accidents of all types and size and also in close liaison with the dermatologist when skin diseases or disorders have been cleared up. People are mainly concerned by their facial appearance. Some disfigurements will discourage you at first, but the tissues heal, and the day will come when you can help to conceal the scars. Where skin grafts have been made or prostheses have been added, the texture of the skin varies. It is difficult to explain in theory how you should treat these as every case is different but the end result is to try to bring the area to match the general skin tone.

If you come across a case where the forehead has needed a skin graft, there could be a ridge left and the graft itself could be quite a different colour and texture, depending from where the skin was taken. Use your skills to camouflage the forehead to match in with the rest of the skin colouring. Sometimes you will be defeated in making the perfect match but you will have made a substantial improvement. You could also suggest a hairstyle to the client to at least partially cover the area. If one side of the forehead is damaged and the client is mature, you can show her or him how to use colours to match the furrows and lines on the other side of the brow.

If a prosthesis has been added – for example, a nose – the edges will need to be camouflaged. Occasionally the prosthesis itself can be improved, by taking away the shiny look and matching the colour with the rest of the face. When looking at a disfigured face always find the good points and highlight them; it will help the disfigurement to recede into the background.

There are always many patients to be seen, but never hurry; remember one good result is so much better than three or four mediocre attempts. Your client is full of apprehension and usually very worried; therefore, your entire concentration is needed together with the right kind of approach. If you think a client will not be able to cope after one session, do arrange to see her again.

One final word: the basic theory can be learnt in a day, but the art takes endless practice over months and years. You will never be able to say that you can always give perfection.

Self assessment

- what is your most important asset when performing remedial camouflage?
- give four contra-indications to remedial camouflage
- how would you recognise recent scar tissue?
- what method would you use to cover a port-wine stain?
- how would you remove cover creams?
- how would you deal with raised scars?

16 Eyebrow and eyelash treatments

Eyebrow plucking

Preparation

Prepare the trolley as for a simple cleanse. You will need:

- clean towel
- pair of sharp tweezers or automatic tweezers
- two small strips of towelling
- small bowl of antiseptic lotion
- astringent
- cotton wool
- cream
- small bowl with a solution of boracic acid or an eye lotion
- eyebrow brush

The natural growth of the eyebrow follows the orbital ridge (the bony cavity containing the eyeball) but rarely grows as a clean-cut arch. Hairs appear below the outline required. To make a simple arch, first take a line starting at the corner of the nose through the inner corner of the eye and the eyebrow should commence just above. Then take a line again from the corner of the nose through the outer corner of the eye to above where the eyebrow should terminate. If necessary mark the spot with an eyebrow pencil (see Fig. 16.1).

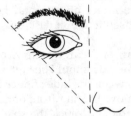

Fig. 16.1 To determine the length of the eyebrow

Thin eyebrows can give a rather hard look; if over-plucked, advise the client to let them grow and brush daily until there is sufficient hair to create a new line. Bushy eyebrows will make a client look older and two or three sessions will be necessary to effect an ideal shape.

Method of plucking

You will require good natural daylight or a magnifying glass. Place the towel over the client's clothing and wash your hands. Cleanse the eyebrows and leave two strips of towelling in hot water. Cotton wool is not

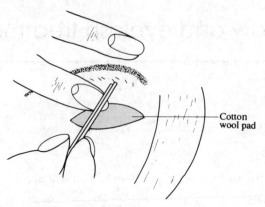

Fig. 16.2 Plucking the eyebrow

advised as it is difficult to ensure that all the hot water has been squeezed out to prevent scalding or making the area very sensitive.

1. Take a little cream (with a spatula) on to your ring fingers and massage in small circles over the eyebrows for a minute or two.
2. Completely remove the cream with damp cotton wool.
3. Squeeze out the hot water from the strips of towelling and place them on the eyebrows. This will help to soften the eyebrow tissue and open the pores.
4. Take two thin pieces of cotton wool, put these in the boracic acid solution, remove and squeeze out the excess and place over the client's eyes.
5. Squeeze out a piece of cotton wool in the antiseptic lotion and place this on the towel on the client's shoulder. Use this to remove the hairs from the tweezers and keep them clean. Wind a small piece of cotton wool around the little finger of the hand holding the tweezers and dip it into the antiseptic lotion. Use this to dab the area being plucked.
6. Throw away the strips of towelling and start by removing the hairs between the brow. In plucking, the skin should be taut and this can be done by stretching the skin between the index finger and thumb or index and middle fingers. Remove the hair from underneath the eyebrows. Brush the hair upwards and pluck the shape required (see Fig. 16.2).

Lift and stretch the skin and pluck each stray hair individually in the direction of the hair growth. Dab the area frequently with the antiseptic cotton wool on the finger.

It is often preferable to do both eyebrows together, a little from each at a time, especially if they are to be reshaped.

7. Halfway through, remove the eye pads and hand the client a mirror to ensure that she is pleased with the progress so far. Plucking above the eyebrows is not advised but the odd stray hair may be removed.

8. When you have finished, brush or comb the hairs into place and check for an even result.
9. Hand a mirror to the client and ensure that she is satisfied with the result.
10. Wipe both eyebrows with antiseptic, use an astringent to close the pores and a little antiseptic cream.

Solutions should be thrown away and bowls wiped clean. The tweezers should be wiped with surgical spirit, rinsed in cold water, dried and placed in a steriliser.

Eyelash and eyebrow tinting

Clients may prefer a tint for the eyebrows and/or eyelashes instead of the everyday use of eyebrow pencil and mascara. The dyes come in liquid form, jelly or cream and you should follow the manufacturer's instructions. There are generally six colours available – black, blue, grey, auburn, light brown and brown and your selection of colour for the client is important.

Table 16.1 Suggested colours for eyelash tinting

Hair colouring	Colour of tint	or	Mixture
Blonde	Brown or grey		Light brown/grey
Grey	Grey		Grey/blue or grey/light brown
Light brown	Brown or grey		Light brown/grey
Auburn	Brown or auburn		Light brown/auburn
Dark brown	Brown		—
Black	Black or brown		Black/brown or blue/black

Take care with the eyebrows: if these are too dark they will give the face a harsh expression. Tinting usually lasts for about five to six weeks.

Preparation

You will need:

- clean towel
- solution of boracic acid or an eye lotion
- bowl of clean water
- small palette or egg cup (non-metallic)
- cotton wool and tissues
- thin damp cotton wool shaped to fit under the eye or use the manufacturer's eye papers
- white non-absorbent lint
- cotton buds (or make these with cotton wool and orange-sticks)
- spatula and small brushes
- Vaseline (petroleum jelly)
- eyelash dyes (tints)
- 10 volume hydrogen peroxide and dropper
- timer or watch

Contra-indications

Check for contra-indications. These are:

- skin infections (i.e. eczema or psoriasis)
- eye disorders or diseases (i.e. styes, conjunctivitis or even redness)
- any cuts or skin abrasions near the eyebrows
- freshly plucked eyebrows
- contact lenses
- nervous or elderly clients who may continually blink

Patch testing

Patch testing is important as most dyes contain toluenediamine, which is a synthetic para-dye and which can cause an allergic reaction. Testing is essential if the tint is to be used for the first time or if a considerable time has elapsed since the last tint. It is a wise precaution to do a simple test whenever possible, preferably a day or two prior to the tint.

For a patch test use very little of the tint and mix with one drop of 10 volume peroxide. Use a cotton bud or brush to mix well and paint a small patch of the tint on the skin behind the ear. Should there be any irritation, wash off the tint immediately and apply an antiseptic cream as a calming agent.

Method of applying eyelash and eyebrow tint

For an eyebrow and lash tint, settle the client comfortably in an almost upright position. If she is lying down, the tint may run backwards into the eyes. Place a clean towel over her clothes. Wash your hands.

1. Cleanse the area well, use a mild toner to remove grease and blot dry. Check for contra-indications.
2. To prevent the tint staining the skin apply, with either a brush or cotton bud, a smear of Vaseline around the eyebrows, on the upper lid and on the skin below the lower lashes.
3. Take the shaped damp cotton-wool pads or papers and place under the lower lashes and ensure that they fit well (see Fig. 16.3).
4. Mix the tint, a small amount, with two drops of the peroxide to a smooth texture, or according to the manufacturer's instructions. A liquid tint is more difficult to apply as it is inclined to run.
5. Request the client to open her eyes and with a small brush carefully stroke down the lower lashes, from the root to the tip of the hair shaft. Repeat for the second eye. The eyes may now be closed and the upper lashes brushed down in the same manner. It may be necessary to open the eyes and brush the tint upward, i.e. under the upper lashes. Cover both eyes with pads of lint. This will keep the tint warm and speed up the action. Dry cotton wool has the same effect but any movement by the client may cause tiny wisps of wool to aggravate the eye. Leave the tint to develop for 5–10 minutes, but check after 5 minutes for colour change. Should the

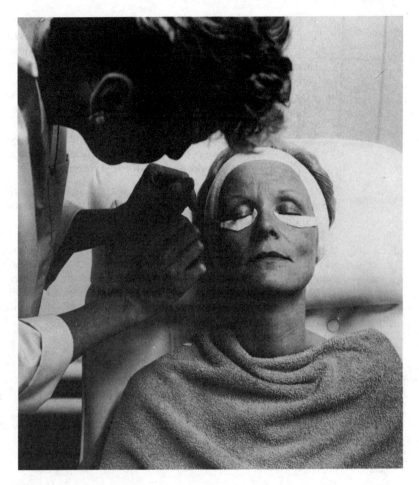

Fig. 16.3 Tinting the eyelashes

client feel any discomfort, remove the tint immediately and bathe the eyes with cold water.

6. For the eyebrows, lightly comb or brush up the brow hairs. Apply the tint with a small brush underneath the hairs, working from the outer corner of the brow towards the procerus. An orange-stick or very small spatula can be used under the brow hairs to support them and to prevent the tint touching the skin. Then reverse the application by stroking down the hairs gently. Repeat for the other brow.

7. By this time a minute will have elapsed which is usually enough time for the tint to develop sufficiently on the eyebrows. Remove the tint from the brow which had the first application, with damp cotton wool using firm strokes until clean, i.e. no tint remaining on the hairs or skin. Repeat for the other eyebrow.

8. Check the lashes again for colour change.

9. When the tint has taken, request the client to keep her eyes closed. Use the lint to remove Vaseline and surplus tint. With a damp cotton-wool pad stroke the lashes down on to the protective paper or cotton wool under the lower lashes until all the tint has been removed. Repeat for the other eye.
10. The client may now open her eyes and for a final check use a small folded piece of damp cotton wool and clean around the rim of the eye and between the upper lashes.
11. Hand the client a mirror to ensure that she is satisfied with the result. To soothe the eyes, pads with a solution of boracic acid may be placed over the eyes and left for five minutes.

Note: If a light colour is requested for the eyebrows and a much darker shade for the lashes, mix the light colour first and complete the brows, then add the darker tint for the lashes.

Remove the towel from the client and if there are no more treatments to be given, return personal possessions, assist with outdoor clothing and accompany the client to the reception area for payment. Return to the cubicle and dispose of all tissues, cotton-wool buds etc., clean the eyelash pot and brushes and wipe down your surfaces with surgical spirit. Complete the client's record card with the colour of the tint and the time it took for the tint to be processed.

Self assessment

- why is it important to give a patch test?
- in which order would you give plucking, eyelash/brow tinting?
- list the contra-indications for an eyelash tint
- should the client feel any discomfort during tinting the eyelashes, what action would you take?

17 Mask therapy

The purpose of masks is to activate circulation temporarily, bring nutrients and oxygen to the epidermis, refine the pores and improve the texture of the skin. There are many masks which are effective if chosen with care. The commercial varieties are popular as they are easy to apply and rarely require mixing. However, they should be used with caution if the constituents are not stated as they may cause an adverse reaction.

Masks are generally divided into two categories, setting and non-setting. Setting masks would appear to be the ideal masks in as much as they immobilise the features and thereby rest the whole cutaneous musculature.

The skill of the therapist is in the choosing of the mask which will give the best result. Make sure the skin is well cleansed before application of the mask ensuring all make-up, oil or cream have been removed. An accurate diagnosis of the skin is all important together with any information gained from the client, i.e. recent skin behaviour, general health and age. Drastic dieting, illness or atmospheric conditions will have an effect on the skin. Masks should not be applied if skin diseases or infections are present, e.g. herpes simplex.

Having examined the skin decide whether it is:

1. dry – requiring general stimulation and a nourishing mask;
2. oily, perhaps with blackheads or pimples – needing desquamation and toning;
3. subject to acne – requiring a cleansing and drying effect;
4. sensitive or delicate with possible thread veins, needing a mask to soothe and stabilise a pH balance;
5. sallow or sluggish, needing to be stimulated, refined and toned;
6. dehydrated, requiring stimulation as with a dry skin and a nourishing mask to improve loss of texture.

Preparation

For all masks you will need:

- crêpe bandage as a headband, head square or cap
- bowl of clean water (if you do not have a washbasin to hand)
- spatulas or tongue depressors
- bowl for mixing mask
- cotton wool in a container (some of which cut into 4 in (10 cm) squares)
- tissues

- disposable paper
- eye pads (in a solution of boracic acid)
- towels
- waste bin at the side of the chair

For particular masks you will also need the following:

Clay masks
- powders
- distilled water, orange flower water, rose water and witch-hazel
- hot/warm towels
- additional ingredients, i.e. honey, cloves, oils, yeast, oatmeal, yoghurt

Manufacturer's masks
- $\frac{3}{4}$ in (2 cm) brushes
- bowl of hot water or double saucepan to heat the mask

Paraffin-wax masks
- container (preferably thermostatically controlled)
- $\frac{3}{4}$ in (2 cm) brush
- creams or essences (optional)

Non-setting masks
- natural preparations, i.e. fruit, yoghurt, etc.

Hot-oil masks
- various oils
- gauze
- infra-red or radiant heat lamp

Setting masks

Clay masks

These contain either china clay (kaolin), Fuller's earth, light magnesium carbonate, powdered calamine and yeast. The content of these masks is detailed in Table 17.1.

The masks are made by mixing the powders with solutions or oils into a smooth creamy paste, i.e.

rose water	mild, toning
orange flower water	stimulating and toning
witch-hazel	lightly stimulating and drying
grapeseed oil	light and soothing
almond oil	slightly stimulating

Table 17.1 Content of clay masks, their action and skin types

Powders	Action	Skin types
Calamine	A very mild soothing effect on the capillaries and help to reduce vascular appearance	Sensitive or delicate skin
Light magnesium carbonate	Mild astringent action which gives a moderate stimulating and toning effect	Dry and normal skins
Kaolin	Quite a strong action. It stimulates vascular and lymphatic flow and has the ability to absorb dirt and grease thereby aiding desquamation	Greasy skin, blackheads or acne
Fuller's earth	Even stronger action and should be used with care. It has the same qualities as kaolin but vascular response is quicker with very definite astringent properties	Greasy skin, blackheads or acne
Sulphur	To be cautiously used as it has a greater desquamating effect. It has a germicidal and drying action and should not be used for general skin textures. It is rarely used as a complete mask. It remains tacky	Applied to actual spots, i.e. acne vulgaris

Tried and tested masks for average skin types

Normal skins
    1 part kaolin
    1 part Fuller's earth

Mix with part distilled water and part rose water or witch-hazel into a smooth paste. Apply and leave for 10–15 minutes. Remove with hot towels.

Dry skins
    1 part kaolin
    1 part light magnesium carbonate

Mix with rose water or orange flower water into a smooth paste, apply and leave for 10–15 minutes. Remove with warm towels.

Oily skins
Fuller's earth mixed with witch-hazel to a smooth paste

Apply and leave for approximately 15 minutes, watch the skin closely for any undue vascular reaction.

   If there are a number of spots this mask can be thinly applied. Make up a small amount of sulphur with witch-hazel and apply to the spots. This latter mix will not dry out. Remove the mask with hot towels.

Sensitive skins
    1 part kaolin
    2 parts light magnesium carbonate
    2 parts calamine powder

Mix with rose water, apply and leave for 5–10 minutes. Before the mask is completely dry remove with warm towels.

Combination skins
Use both: the mask for dry skins over the dry areas – usually the cheeks – and the mask for oily skins for the greasy panel – usually the chin, nose and forehead. Remove with hot towels (see Fig. 17.1).

Sensitive and mature skins
   4 parts light magnesium carbonate
   2 parts calamine

Mix to a smooth paste with grapeseed oil, apply and leave for 5–10 minutes. Remove with warm towels.

For stimulating skins
   3 parts light magnesium carbonate
   1 part Fuller's earth

Mix to a smooth paste with sweet almond oil, apply and leave for approximately ten minutes. Remove with hot towels.

Most skins
Powdered yeast can be used as a good cleansing agent as it softens and improves the appearance of the skin. Use 2 tablespoons of yeast and add a few drops of either rose water (for dry skin) or witch-hazel (for oily skin) to make a smooth creamy paste.

Neck masks
   cleansing $\frac{1}{2}$ teaspoon powdered yeast
                1 teaspoon finely ground oatmeal
                small quantity of yoghurt

Put yeast and oatmeal into a bowl, add a little yoghurt and mix into a paste. Apply to the throat and neck area and leave for 15 minutes. Remove with warm towels.

Discoloration
   2 tablespoons Fuller's earth
   1 teaspoon witch-hazel
   1 pinch of ground cloves
   1 teaspoon honey
   a little milk

Mix the Fuller's earth, cloves and witch-hazel with milk, then add the honey. If it is too thick add a little more milk. Apply to the throat and neck area and leave for 20–25 minutes. Remove with milk or warm water using cotton-wool pads.

   For all mask therapy, it is preferable for the client to remove garments to the shoulder area. Ensure that the client's hair and clothing are well protected with headband, head square or cap, towels and disposable paper and keep the client warm with towels or a blanket.

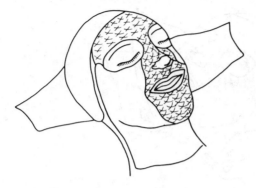

Fig. 17.1 Clay mask (combination)

Application of clay masks

1. Use a spatula or a tongue depressor, which is cheap and can be thrown away after use, to mix the mask in a bowl. Put the powders in first and add the required solution or oil slowly to form a paste. The consistency should not be too thick or runny. The thicker the mask the more difficult it is to remove, which is time-consuming for the therapist and irritating for the client. It is inadvisable to use brushes for clay masks as these are very difficult to clean and sterilise.
2. Warn the client of the effect of the mask where it will feel heavy or cold initially.
3. Apply the mask with the spatula, commencing below the chin (or the base of the neck, if required) with a thin, even film all over the face. Be careful to avoid all apertures (eyes, nostrils and mouth). Practice will ensure evenness and the ability to apply the mask quickly. Should the skin require more than one type of mask, apply them in order of the longest time first with the objective of finally removing the complete mask.
4. Cover the eyes with pads to aid relaxation. These can be dampened with rose water or a commercial eye freshener.
5. Let the mask dry, but not to the extent that it becomes too hard.
6. Remove the mask with hot or warm towels.
7. Apply a toner or an astringent with damp cotton-wool pads all over the face. An electric or aerosol spray with toner may be used instead to stimulate and freshen the skin.
8. Blot with paper tissues.

Peel-off masks

These are commercially available and the therapist should adhere to the manufacturer's instructions or preferably obtain technical and practical advice from a qualified representative.

It may be suggested that a preparation of a cream, oil or phial containing biological elements or essences be applied to a cleansed skin prior to the application of the mask.

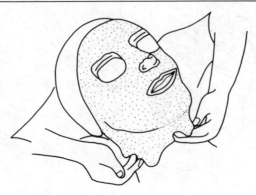

Fig. 17.2 Peel-off mask

These masks are of benefit to dry, mature or dehydrated skins as they solidify on the skin to form a setting type mask, so immobilising the features. The effect of the mask also acts as a compress which assists in isolating the preparation from the atmosphere, therefore allowing some of its properties to be absorbed by the skin.

Some masks will require warming and the jar should be placed in either a basin of hot water or a double saucepan should be used. When the mask is at the right consistency, apply to the face and neck with a spatula or brush, carefully avoiding all apertures and eyebrows. After a few minutes place eye pads on the eyes to refresh and leave the mask for the required time – usually 10–15 minutes.

To remove, peel away from the borders and apertures and the mask should lift off in a complete film. Use damp cotton-wool pads to remove any of the original preparation and tone well in the normal manner (see Fig. 17.2).

Other peel-off masks are in the form of transparent jelly. They usually come in bottles with their own applicator. On a cleansed skin the mask is brushed on, avoiding apertures and eyebrows.

They dry fairly quickly – in about five minutes and give a mildly stimulating and toning effect. The film is thin and can easily be lifted from the face and neck.

Thermal types

The principles mentioned regarding the manufacturer's instructions should be followed. The action of the thermal mask is to promote heat by a chemical reaction caused by the properties contained in the mask. This occurs as the paste hardens and the effect is an improved circulation.

Again an appropriate preparation is suggested prior to the mask application.

The paste should be applied in a fairly thick layer covering the face but avoiding the apertures. Some manufacturers suggest covering the eyes and mouth, but you will soon observe that clients find this too claustrophobic.

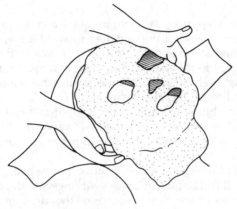

Fig. 17.3 Thermal mask

As with the warm peel-off masks, the thermal types have the same qualities as a compress. Advise the client that a heat effect starts to develop as the paste hardens, but this will gradually disperse. Apply eye pads in the normal manner. Leave the mask to set for the required time, about twenty minutes. Remove the eye pads.

To remove the hardened mask gently loosen it around the edges. Ask the client to smile to loosen the mask around the cheeks and mouth and with an upward movement the mask can be lifted off in one piece. Any residue of the preparation can be removed with damp cotton-wool pads (see Fig. 17.3).

Tone the skin well with an appropriate solution.

These masks are good for dry, mature or dehydrated skins with few contra-indications.

Paraffin-wax masks

For easy reference this mask is included in this section but should not be attempted until electrical equipment has been well studied.

Make sure the skin is cleansed but not over-stimulated. Check for any contra-indications, i.e.

- highly vascular skins
- nervous or tense client
- skin infection
- open cuts or wounds

A semi-reclining position is best for this mask. Protect the client's hairline and the base of the neck area with disposable towels, and protect the eyes with damp cotton wool. It is a simple mask to apply but requires considerable practice.

Here again the use of an appropriate preparation, be it cream or an essence, could be of benefit.

Before commencing the application of the wax ensure that it is at the required temperature (approx 49 °C/120 °F). Test it on the inside of your wrist and check with a patch test that it can be easily tolerated by the client.

Use a small brush (approx $\frac{3}{4}$ in/2 cm) for quick and neat application. Wipe the brush gently against the container to avoid drips; commence at the base of the neck and apply a firm layer of wax to the neck and throat areas. Proceed to the cheeks, chin, nose and forehead, carefully avoiding apertures, eyebrows and hairline. Ensure that the edges of the mask are even and firm – this aids removal.

Initially, heat will build up within the mask but as it sets it will also cool. The length of time the mask is left on will vary from 10 to 20 minutes, depending on the client's tolerance to heat and reaction to the wax.

After the required time has elapsed, remove the eye pads. To remove the wax, which will still be pliable, place your fingers under the edge of the mask at the base of the neck and all around the edges up to the forehead. Lift the mask upwards from the neck and face. If the wax has been applied evenly and firmly, wax fragments will not be left behind.

Remove the disposable papers and use paper tissues to blot any preparation left on the skin. Use damp cotton-wool pads or an astringent to tone the skin.

Benefits

It is useful for seborrhoeic conditions or uneven textured skin as it is a deep cleansing treatment. Natural perspiration is induced, allowing the skin to excrete impurities and toxic waste.

The heat promotes intercellular activity and increased circulation, thereby benefiting dry, mature and dehydrated skins. The skin will appear softer and finer in texture, and the colour and tone will be improved.

It should be emphasised that with all setting masks the therapist remains with the client. It is not only reassuring for the client, who will then be able to relax, but the therapist will be able to attend to any needs, i.e. keeping the client warm or cool or removing the mask early if it is uncomfortable. To obtain maximum results and to allow the skin time to restore its pH balance, make-up should be avoided with the exception of the eyes and lips.

Non-setting masks

Although these masks form a film over the skin which often becomes firm and dry, they do not immobilise the features. These masks are made with natural or biological ingredients or essential oils.

Natural preparations

These include fruit, vegetables, milk, eggs, honey, nuts, oatmeal and oil. They can be prepared in the salon but should be used the same day as they can go rancid if left.

As a very general guide these ingredients can be mixed to good effect.

oatmeal	cleansing, calming and refining
avocado	rich in oils for a dry skin
cucumber	astringent and cooling
honey	rejuvenating, stimulating for sluggish skins
egg white	temporary tightening effect on wrinkled skin
lemon juice	a bleaching effect

The following are a few basic recipes for various skin types. Always ensure that the face is well cleansed and use eye pads to relax and refresh the eyes.

Normal skin

1 banana
1 tablespoon honey
1 beaten egg

Mash the banana and mix with the honey and egg. It may be necessary to sieve the ingredients to form a smooth paste and apply with a spatula. Leave for 15–20 minutes and remove with warm towels. Apply appropriate toner.

Dry skin

1 egg yolk
few drops of cider vinegar

Mix with a little almond oil. This is better applied with a brush. Take the usual precautions to avoid soiling the client's clothing and tuck tissues in the band around the hairline. Leave 15–20 minutes and remove with warm damp cotton-wool pads. Apply rose water as a toner.

Sensitive skins

Mix almond meal (obtainable at health stores) with milk to a paste. Apply with a spatula and leave for 20 minutes. It will be quite dry so remove with hot towels. Use cotton-wool pads which have been placed in warm milk to sponge the face. Tone with rose water and apply appropriate moisturiser.

Dehydrated or mature skins

1 egg yolk
6 drops of olive oil
3 drops benzoin or peppermint oil

Mix and apply with a brush. Leave for 20 minutes and remove with warm towels.

Note: If your recipe includes an egg, it will often become sticky. Put almond or olive oil on to cotton-wool pads for easier removal.

Greasy skins

Cut a double-thickness gauze and make holes for the eyes, nostrils and mouth. Crush and pummel strawberries and place between the gauze. Apply to the face and leave for 15 minutes. Remove the mask and any residue with an astringent.

There are many masks of this type featured in magazines and books. They are all worth trying, preferably on friends or relatives before using them in the salon!

Biological preparations

These are also based on natural ingredients such as flower, plant or herbal extracts and essential oils. These are usually supplied by skin-care houses in creams, gels or emulsions and are used to stimulate circulation, balance and regenerate the skin.

Hot-oil masks

There are two methods of applying hot-oil masks. Various oils may be used, i.e. olive, wheatgerm grapeseed, jasmine or sweet almond.

1. The oil should be heated and be as hot as the client can tolerate. It can be tested on the inside of the wrist of the therapist. Cut several shapes of gauze for the face and neck and place these into the oil. Place dampened cotton-wool pads on the eyes. Take out the gauze, sliding along the edge of the bowl or container to avoid dripping on to the client and apply to the neck and face. Replace with fresh pieces of gauze and oil for 15–20 minutes. The eye pads may now be removed. To aid absorption the excess oil left on the face and neck may be used for gentle massage. Remove residue with paper tissues and blot carefully then use an appropriate toner. Check the skin first before applying a moisturiser as this may not be necessary. Excellent mask for dry, crêpey and dehydrated skins.
2. This method requires a thorough knowledge of infra-red or radiant-heat lamps before attempting its use. There are a few contra-indications to be noted.

    *   highly strung or nervous clients;
    *   advanced vascular or hypersensitive skins;
    *   surface damage or capillaries – the treatment needs to be restricted.

Advise the client that the skin will be stimulated and make-up should be avoided until the tissues have had time to settle down.

Again warm oil is used. Cut the gauze to fit the face and neck, making holes for the eyes, nostrils and mouth but making sure the tip of the nose is covered. Fold the gauze and place in the warm oil. Cover the eyes and any areas restricted, i.e. broken (or thread) veins with dry cotton wool. Unfold the gauze and place on the face and neck closely fitting the contours. The lamp may now be placed over the face. Its distance will vary accordingly to the sensitivity of the skin and the client's tolerance of heat from $1\frac{1}{2}$ to 3 ft (0.45–0.9 m). As with all electrical treatments the client must not be left unattended. The therapist should check the skin's reaction regularly to observe that a gentle perspiration is induced, that there is a softening of the skin and that the colour is not excessive. This will determine the time for the lamp which will range from 8 to 15 minutes. As the lamp produces a rise in skin temperature

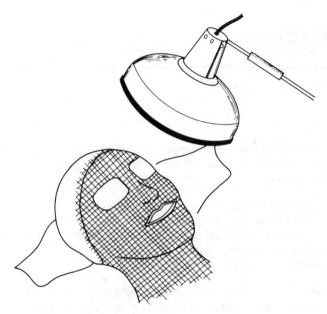

Fig. 17.4 Hot-oil mask with lamp

heat penetration will increase vascular flow, activate the sebaceous glands and have a calming effect on the sensory nerve endings (see Fig. 17.4).

Switch off the lamp and turn it away from the client. Remove the gauze from the neck upwards and the cotton-wool pads. Again the residue of oil may be used for gentle effleurage. Tone and refresh the skin. It is rarely necessary to use a moisturiser immediately.

This mask helps to combat the ageing process by promoting cellular function. It is useful for young skins drying prematurely due to excessive temporary climatic conditions, and invaluable for dehydrated or mature skins.

Self assessment

- what type of clay mask would you use for a sensitive skin? and list the ingredients and solutions to be used
- how would you treat spots on an oily skin?
- give reasons why you should not leave the client while the clay mask is setting
- using natural products make up a mask suitable for a greasy skin
- list contra-indications for a hot-oil mask
- what are the benefits of a paraffin-wax mask?

18 Massage

The most important requirement for any massage is a thorough knowledge of anatomy and an understanding of skin conditions. The purpose of massage is to:

1. **cleanse the skin**, by improving venous, arterial and lymphatic circulation and increasing sweat and sebum secretion;
2. **improve muscle tone**, by increasing blood supply; muscles are nourished and stimulated;
3. **soothe and refresh nerve endings**.

Your hands are the tools – they should be strong and flexible. Hand-mobility exercises and practice will ensure an even rhythm, alternating pressure and a full range of movements. Practise the following exercises several times daily until your hands are loose and mobile.

Exercises for the hands

1. (a) In a prayer position, palms and fingers together.
   (b) Press the hands and lift the elbows.
   (c) Press the hands away from the body downwards and then upwards.
   (d) Press the hands over the radio-carpal joint to the left and then to the right.

2. (a) Bend the fingers over the palm then stretch one finger out at a time.
   (b) Clench the fist and stretch all the fingers out.
   (c) Roll the thumbs around – first one way then the other.

3. (a) Bend the elbows close to your sides and rotate the hands and wrists slowly and rhythmically in both directions.
   (b) Shake the wrists together and then alternately.

4. To obtain a light touch, practise drumming with the fingers on a hard surface. Work from the little finger to your index and then reverse the sequence.

In all your exercises, music will help to practise rhythm and speed. Sensitivity can be practised by feeling the shapes of different objects with the eyes closed. To progress, feel over limbs and the face. The sense of touch is all-important as it will determine the pressure to be used in any given area.

Classification of movements

Massage is generally divided into five main groups of movement, i.e. effleurage, petrissage, frictions, tapotement and vibrations.

Effleurage

All stroking movements fall into this category. The palmar surface of one or both hands is laid flat on the part to be treated and with pressure applied over the skin in the direction of the venous or lymph flow. The hands must mould themselves to the contour of the body or face over which they are moving. Any degree of pressure may be applied from the lightest touch to deep pressure, dependent upon the underlying structures. The hands should follow each other in slow and rhythmical movements without jerkiness or breaking contact with the skin. The cushion of the fingertip may be used but not the tips of the fingers as they cannot control the degree of pressure and the free edge of the nail could scratch the skin (see Figs 19.1–3).

The effects of effleurage are:

- venous circulation is improved;
- arterial circulation is aided by removal of congestion in the veins;
- lymphatic circulation is also improved with oxygen being brought to the area by the blood, and carbon dioxide and waste products being carried away;
- aids desquamation through an increase in sweat and sebum secretions;
- aids relaxation as the underlying muscles are nourished by an increase in blood supply and the fibres are loosened.

Petrissage

All pressure movements come under this heading and can be sub-divided as follows.

Picking-up

The muscles are grasped and lifted away from the bone, released, and the movement repeated with the other hand. The release must be sudden to be effective. The whole muscle is worked in this manner from origin to insertion, e.g. gastrocnemius (a leg muscle). When the movement is completed the hands slide back to the origin of the muscle to begin again.

Kneading

On the body this is a single-handed movement whereby the heel of the hand is pressed on to the part and moved in small circles, not sliding the part but moving the tissues with it. Again the whole muscle is worked from origin to insertion, e.g. tibialis anterior (leg muscle).

For the face or neck area digital kneading is performed using gentle pressure. Knuckling can also be used for this area where your fingers are lightly curled into the palm of the hand and the dorsal aspect of the phalanges used to make small circles, kneading and lifting the tissues upwards, e.g. sterno mastoid (see Figs 19.5(a) and 19.8).

Scissoring

When classed as a petrissage movement the index and middle fingers of both hands are separated to make a 'V' shape. As this is normally performed on the forehead, the hands are horizontal and pressure can be applied where there is a flat surface of bone. The fingers are placed inside each other and they apply gentle pressure in small circles, lifting the tissues and working on the lines of the forehead from one side to the other (see Fig. 19.13).

If a friction action is required the middle and ring fingers can make quick criss-cross movements across the forehead still maintaining the scissor action.

Pincement

This type of massage is useful for fatty tissue. It is performed by lifting the superficial fascia between the fingers and thumb and gentle squeezing or rolling with light but firm pressure. Care should be taken to ensure the skin is not pinched. There are others including squeezing and wringing which are mainly used over large areas of the body (see Fig. 19.21).

The effects of petrissage

- compressions and relaxation of muscles causes the blood vessels and lymphatic vessels to be filled and emptied;
- circulation and removal of waste products is increased;
- eliminates fatigue;
- increases basal layer activity giving a more refined skin texture;
- muscle tone is improved.

Frictions

These are small circular or to-and-fro movements produced with the first two fingers or thumb. The skin must move with the fingers (see Fig. 19.4(b)).

The effects of friction are:

- breaks down fat and fibrous thickenings;
- removes oedema, i.e. swelling due to effusion of fluid into the tissues;
- stimulates circulation and glandular activity.

Tapotement

This includes all percussion movements, which should be performed lightly and briskly to stimulate the tissues. These are tapping, hacking, beating, pounding and clapping; the last three are generally performed on the body.

Tapping

This is performed with the palmar surface of the fingers and, dependent on the area to be covered, two to four fingers gently tap rhythmically and in rapid succession (see Fig. 19.7(a), tapping along the mandible). Two or three fingers may be used to slap gentle as in Fig. 19.7(b).

Hacking

This employs a twist of the wrist using edges of the outer three fingers, loosely held to flick against the part being treated. It should not be performed over bony areas nor during a relaxing massage.

The effects of tapotement

- causes muscle fibres to contract, thus strengthening the muscles;
- due to an increased blood supply there is warmth which will promote sebum secretions;
- stimulates the nerve endings in the skin which can improve elasticity and have a toning effect.

Vibrations

These are given to a nerve; the pads (or cushions) of the fingers are placed on the nerve and the muscles of the operator's arm contracted and relaxed rapidly so that a fine trembling is produced. This is static vibration. When the vibrating fingers are run along the course of a nerve it is known as running vibrations (see Fig. 19.6(b).

The effects of vibrations are:

- stimulates the nerves;
- relieves pain and fatigue;
- loosens scar tissue and stretches adhesions;
- promotes relaxation and avoids capillary damage;
- useful for fine, sensitive skins.

Contra-indications for a manual facial massage

Contra-indications or conditions which would preclude you from giving a facial massage are:

- sepsis;
- skin infections or diseases;
- over recent fractures;
- inflammation, bites or stings;
- sinus disorders or asthmatic conditions (except with care).

The use of hand-held vibrators

Percussion vibrator

Percussion vibrators (see Fig. 34.3) produce vibrations of low penetration. They have a range of applicator heads and a variable intensity control to allow application on both soft and muscular tissue. They are very useful for dry or dehydrated skins needing general stimulation, for mature skins requiring regeneration and for general relaxation. The skin is cleansed and talcum powder or cream applied and the applicator chosen – normally the soft head for the face and neck.

For the direct method, place the applicator head on the client's neck and commence stroking up the platysma, then follow the facial contours, again with upward strokes or lifting circles. All these strokes should be applied smoothly and, as only one hand is required to operate the vibrator, the free hand should maintain personal contact. This method can also be used on the trapezius to relax the muscle and prevent stiffness and tension developing.

For the indirect method, which is for use over bony areas or areas where there is a lack of firm subcutaneous tissue, the vibrator head is placed on the back of the therapist's fingers.

Audio-sonic vibrator

Audio-sonic vibrators produce sound waves in surface body tissue to encourage circulation of the blood and lymph and relieve tension. In the main, the applicator heads are made of hard plastic; a smooth disc-shaped head, about an inch in diameter which is used for general work and a small rounded ball-shaped head which is used for concentration in small areas, i.e. between muscle fibres or around joints. On the head of the vibrator is a control knob, which controls the current to the motor and by turning this the level of intensity is increased or decreased. The frequency is 50–100 Hz. The depth of penetration beneath the skin is up to about 2 in (5 cm) in soft tissue and therefore it cannot be recommended over bony areas. Beneath the head of the vibrator lies a plate into which the applicator head is attached and in the handle of the vibrator is the on/off switch.

As for the percussion vibrator, the skin is cleansed and talcum powder or cream is applied.

The audio-sonic vibrator has limited use on the face, but by using the indirect method, it can be used to stimulate either delicate or sensitive skins, or mature skins with loose skin tissue.

Using the direct method fibrositis nodules in the trapezius muscle can often be broken down by stroking along the length of the muscle, from insertion to origin. This can be followed by increasing the level of intensity and using circular movements over the same muscle (see Fig. 18.1). Care must be taken when altering the frequency to ensure the correct depth of vibration. Migraine-type headaches can be relieved by stroking the upper fibres of the trapezius to the occiput, using a mild frequency.

The effects of hand-held vibrators:

- increases local skin temperature
- no chemical formation on the surface of the skin
- improves blood and lymph flow
- relieves tension in muscle fibres.

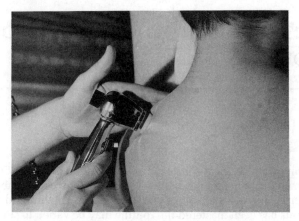

Fig. 18.1 Audio-sonic over the trapezius muscle

Contra-indications to hand-held vibrators

These are the same as for manual facial massage but should also include:

- over bony areas
- sinus disorders
- asthmatic conditions.

There are varied skin conditions and the massage must relate to these. Highly vascular areas, i.e. zygomatics, should be avoided but a suitable massage may be given to the rest of the area. Ageing skin which is loose will not benefit from further stretching but vibrations, tapping and very light finger stroking will increase blood supply and improve appearance.

Self assessment

- what is the purpose of massage?
- give three hand mobility exercises
- what are the effects of petrissage and friction?
- state the contra-indications for manual massage of the face
- your client has loose crêpey skin, what facial massage would you perform?
- what are the effects of hand-held vibrators?

19 Massage of the head, neck and shoulders

It is important to learn a basic massage routine incorporating all the movements mentioned in Chapter 18. This will give invaluable experience in evaluating skin types and developing rhythm and pressure. Once this has been mastered the routine may be varied to suit the individual, taking into account general health and temperament.

Preparation

You should have ready, prior to the arrival of your client:

- roll pillow
- sheet or towels
- towels to cover or blanket to keep client warm
- headband or crêpe bandage
- headsquare or cap
- cotton wool cut into 4 in (10 cm) squares (dampened with water)
- tissues
- spatulas
- cleansers, toners and tonics
- massage cream
- waste-bin at the side of the chair

To prepare your client, assist with the removal of outer clothing, blouse or shirt and have salon chair or couch at an angle of 45 degrees. Wrap the client up neatly with sheet/towels and blanket to maintain warmth and place a towel across the chest and under the arms to avoid soiling linen and clothing. A roll pillow may be placed under the knees for further comfort. If there are bra straps these may be taken down towards the elbows. All jewellery and earrings should be removed. Cover the client's hair with a cap or headsquare, use a crêpe bandage or hairband and draw this back from the hairline.

Wash your hands.

Sequence of massage

Apply cleanser to eyes and then lips as outlined in Chapter 12 and wipe clean with damp cotton-wool pads. Cleanse the neck and face well and wipe off all cleanser with damp cotton-wool pads and repeat if necessary.

Take sufficient massage cream with a spatula on to the palms of your hands.

1. Commencing at the left clavicle with effleurage movements, lift the platysma muscle from origin to insertion, first with the left hand followed by the right hand. (This movement is similar to the cleansing movement Fig. 12.5(a).) The hands follow each other across the sternum, avoiding the trachea to the right clavicle. Effleurage is repeated back to the left clavicle. Rhythm and rate of movement is slow at approximately 7 ins (18 cm) per second (see Fig. 19.1).

2. Again with alternate hands repeat six effleurage movements from the left clavicle along the sterno-mastoid up to the mandible so that the fingers are pointing towards the chin and pull firmly back (see Fig. 19.2). Leave the right hand at the right ramus while the left hand continues lifting up the masseter, zygomatics, then sweeping across the frontalis in a horizontal position (see Fig. 19.3). To finish the movement reverse the hands.

3. Both hands will be at their respective mastoid processes. Slide the left hand down the sterno-mastoid over the clavicle and swing the palm and fingers over the deltoid. Keeping the thumb forward, lift the trapezius muscle towards the last cervical vertebrae. Repeat six times. Slide the left hand to the left mastoid process and with the right hand repeat the movements over the right deltoid and finish at the right mastoid process.

4. Slide both hands down to the clavicle, point the fingers together in a horizontal position and swing the hands towards the deltoid. Place the thumb at the back – on the trapezius – and give thumb

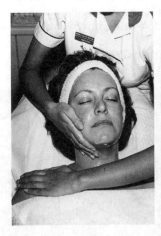

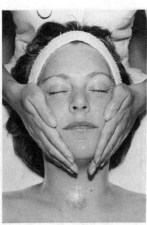

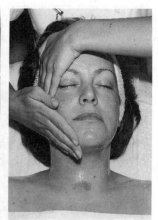

Fig. 19.1 Effleurage from the right clavicle across the sternum to the mandible

Fig. 19.2 Fingers pointing to the chin – pull back firmly

Fig. 19.3 Lifting masseter and zygomaticus

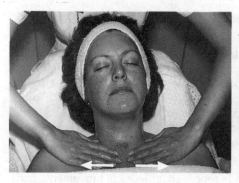
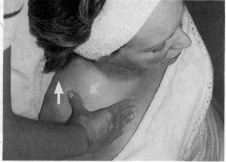

Fig. 19.4 (a) Horizontal hands sweeping towards deltoid (b) Thumb frictions on trapezius

frictions (i.e. circling lifting movements) into the trapezius. Move towards the third cervical vertebrae, ensuring that there is minimum pressure from the hands which are on the sternomastoid/platysma. Slide the hands into the insertion of the trapezius and repeat the thumb frictions three times as indicated (see Fig. 19.4(a) (b)).

5. Slide both hands down to clavicle and place in a horizontal position. Use knuckling movements along the pectoral muscles to the axillae (see Fig. 19.5(a)). Use thumbs to give friction movements over the acromion process followed by three palmar strokes down the deltoid. Keeping the thumbs forward, swing the fingers to the back and firmly lift the trapezius muscle to the third cervical vertebrae (see Fig. 19.5(b)). Repeat three times.

6. Again slide both hands to the chest in a horizontal position. This is a swimming movement, whereby you stroke towards the axillae, around the deltoid (see Fig. 19.6(a)) and lifting along the trapezius to the occiput. Give vibrations at the end of each movement (see Fig. 19.6(b)). Repeat six times.

The following three movements should only be performed when

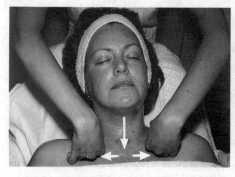
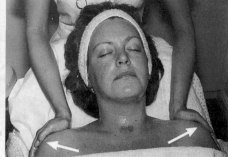

Fig. 19.5 (a) Knuckling movements towards axillae (b) Movement to lift the trapezius muscle

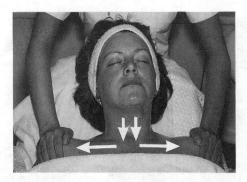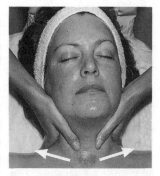

Fig. 19.6 (a) Swimming movement around the deltoid (b) Vibrations at the occiput

there is fatty tissue present and care should be taken to avoid slapping or tapping the mandible itself. It should not be performed on sensitive skin.

7. Slide the hands down and place the fingertips beneath the centre of the mandible. With the middle and ring fingers of both hands use firm but light slapping, lifting movements on the tissues beneath the mandible moving towards the right ramus. Reverse to the left ramus and back to the centre. This is a stimulating movement given very quickly – approximately seventy slaps altogether. Move the fingers to the right side of the face and lift the masseter and buccinator, continue under the mandible and then lift these muscles on the left side of the face as indicated (see Figs. 19.7(a) and (b)).

8. Slide the middle and ring fingers of both hands under the mandible at the centre and tap quickly and firmly beneath, moving towards

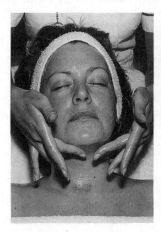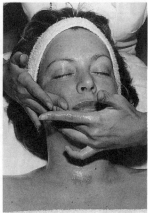

Fig. 19.7 (a) Light slapping beneath the mandible (b) Light slapping lifting masseter and buccinator

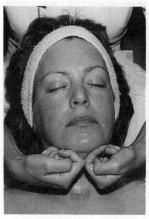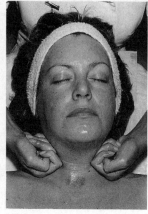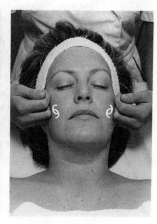

Fig. 19.8 (a) Knuckling beneath the mandible (b) Kneading the platysma (c) Kneading the mentalis, depressors, masseters and buccinators

the right ramus, reverse to the left ramus and back to the centre (see Fig. 19.8(a)).

9. Form the hands into loose fists and place both knuckles at clavicle. Using each knuckle in rotation making lifting, circular movements on the sterno-mastoid and trapezius towards the mastoid processes. Sweep the knuckles beneath the mandible and from the centre carefully knead the platysma and finally bring the knuckles on to the mentalis, depressors, masseter and buccinators. Repeat this movement three times, being careful to avoid the mandible and trachea as indicated (see Figs. 19.8(b) and (c)).

10. Slide hands again to beneath the centre of the mandible and with the middle and ring fingers of both hands stimulate lymphatic activity with small petrissage movements. Exert a little pressure and

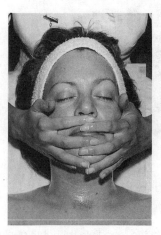

Fig. 19.9 Throat brace

release, moving along to the ramus of the mandible. Slide the hands back to the centre and repeat three times.

11. To relax the area stimulated, use effleurage by forming the hands into a 'V' shape with the fingers interlocked over and below the mandible. As you pull the hands and fingers apart, lift the platysma and sterno-mastoid muscles back to the mastoid process. This is sometimes referred to as a throat brace. Slide the hands back to the centre and repeat six times as indicated (see Fig. 19.9).

    From this movement onwards one or both hands should be in contact with the skin.

12. Leave the right hand at the right mastoid and slide the palm of the left hand across the base of the throat to the left sterno-mastoid (see Fig. 19.10(a)). Leave the left hand there and take the right hand and lift the zygomatic muscles and turn the hand horizontally across the frontalis avoiding the corrugator (see Figs. 19.10(b) and (c)). Repeat this movement for the other side of the face.

13. Slide the hands down to rest lightly beneath the centre of the mandible. Using the thumbs only, make opposing circular movements along the right side of the face lifting the muscles. Reverse the thumb movements to lift the muscles again on the left side of the face and return to the centre of the chin, taking care that the thumb circles lift the tissues and that you do not circle downwards.

    Now let the thumbs swing apart and pointing upwards, lift the buccinator six times (see Fig. 19.11). Finally slide index and ring fingers up the laughter lines, sides of the nose, on to the forehead and finish at the temples.

14. Slide the hands to place each index finger in a horizontal position on the upper orbicularis oris, the middle finger on the lower part of this muscle and palms supporting the lower facial muscles (as in

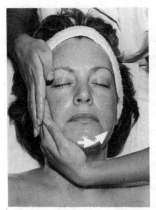 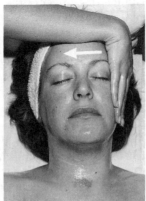 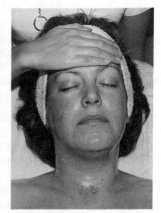

Fig. 19.10 (a) Right hand at mastoid and left hand sliding over throat to left sterno-mastoid (b) Lifting the zygomatic muscles (c) Taking the hand across the frontalis

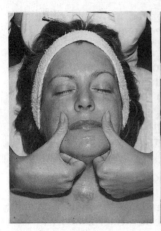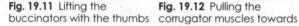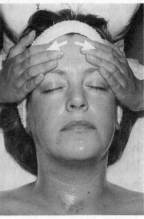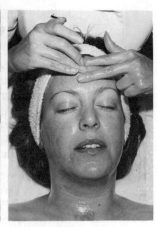

Fig. 19.11 Lifting the buccinators with the thumbs

Fig. 19.12 Pulling the corrugator muscles towards the temporalis

Fig. 19.13 Circling movements over the frontalis

the throat brace Fig. 19.9). Being careful not to touch the mouth, pull the hands apart and turn them so that the fingers are pointing downwards. Bring the hands up until the palms are on the frontalis. Carefully avoiding nose and eyes, lift the frontalis and turn the hands into a horizontal position; as the fingertips touch, pull the corrugator muscles towards the temporalis (see Fig. 19.12). Point the fingers downwards and slide lightly down the face to repeat the movement six times as indicated.

15. Slide the middle and ring fingers of both hands to the centre frontalis and make quick criss-cross movements across to the right temple, reverse to the left temple and finish at the centre.

16. Leaving the left hand in a horizontal position, part the index fingers so that you have a 'V' shape or that resembling an open pair of scissors. With the ring finger of the right hand make slow, circling movements over the frontalis, moving down to the left temporalis. Without losing contact with the skin, make the right hand into the 'scissor' hand and use the left, ring finger, repeating the movement to the right temporalis. Reverse the hands again to the centre as indicated (see Fig. 19.13).

17. Follow these two movements with deep stroking, lifting the frontalis. Leave the right hand horizontally on the forehead. Start by placing the left index finger (horizontally) beneath the centre of the brow. The right hand strokes up the frontalis followed by the left index finger and the remaining fingers of the hand towards the hairline. As soon as the distal finger of the left hand has reached the upper fibres of the orbicularis oculi, follow with the right fingers. Repeat this movement slowly and smoothly across to the right temporalis – approximately 15–18 strokes (see Fig. 19.14).

With the thumbs resting on the forehead, use the ring fingers to

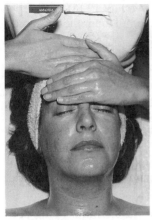 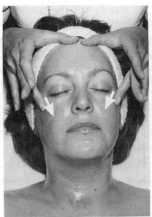 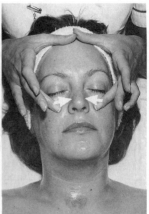

Fig. 19.14 Stroking the frontalis

Fig. 19.15 Half-moon lifts at the crow's feet area

Fig. 19.16 Stroking the ring fingers under the eyes

make eight light half-moon lifts at the outer edge of the orbicularis oculi, i.e. 'crows feet' area (see Fig. 19.15).

This is followed by eight strokes with the ring fingers under the eyes (see Fig. 19.16). Even though the touch is as light as a feather, it is important to work towards the nose to avoid the slightest drag of the delicate skin beneath the eyes. Repeat eight half-moon lifts. Repeat the deep stroking and lifting of the frontalis from the right to left temporalis (as Fig. 19.14).

18. Turn the hands so that the fingers at the centre of the forehead are pointing downward and slide the ring fingers along the eyebrows to the right and left temples (see Fig. 19.17). Lightly swing the ring fingers along the infra-orbital ridges (i.e. ridges beneath the orbits (as Fig. 19.16) up the sides of the nose. With the addition of the

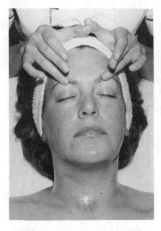 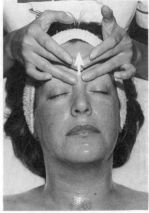

Fig. 19.17 Stroking the ring fingers along the eyebrows

Fig. 19.18 Lifting the procerus

middle finger, firmly lift the procerus (see Fig. 19.18) and upper fibres of the orbicularis oculi before completing the sweeping movement at the temples. Repeat twice.

With ring fingers at the temples, use feather touch to slide under the eye towards the nose and under the eyebrow to the temples. Repeat three times.

19. With the fingers pointing towards the chin, the palms of the hands supporting the frontalis, thumbs crossed and with their base, followed by the palms, lift the frontalis. When the base of the thumbs reach the hairline, turn the hands to a horizontal position and maintain pressure as they stroke across the forehead to the temples. Repeat the movement five times more as indicated (see Fig. 19.19).

20. From the temples, slide hands down to the sternum. Using both hands and a lifting movement, stroke up the platysma, over the mandible to lift the masseter. By this time the heels of your hands will be free of the nose and eyes and can be placed on the frontalis. As you lift this muscle, index and middle fingers stroke up the sides of the nose on to the frontalis (see Fig. 19.20). Continue to stroke up the hairline and repeat the movement three more times.

21. Repeat step 20 until the fingers stroke up the nose. With the ring fingers make a circle – along the eyebrows, beneath the eyes, below the eyebrows, finishing with light pressure at the temples.

Using damp cotton-wool pads remove all traces of massage cream, check behind the ears. At this stage mask therapy may be applied. If this is not a requirement complete the treatment by using an appropriate toner/tonic and if needed – a moisturiser.

This sequence of a basic routine combines all the petrissage/tapotement movements at the beginning of the massage, followed

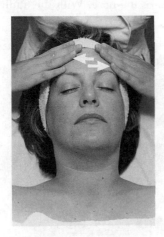

Fig. 19.19 Hands in horizontal position maintaining pressure to the temples

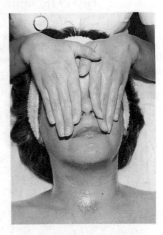

Fig. 19.20 Fingers stroking up the nose with palms of hands on frontalis

by soothing relaxing movements. Some clients are irritated by a sequence which changes to and from petrissage to effleurage. Just as they are beginning to relax completely, an operator may start tapotement movements again, which will negate the relaxation.

However, if a facial massage needs to be specific in its requirements, to be stimulating or increase desquamation, improve cellular function where pores are blocked or comedones have formed, obviously more petrissage and tapotement may be needed. Try to ensure that these are given linked with effleurage and finish the massage for at least five minutes with soothing, relaxing movements.

Additional movements

The following are a few movements which can be incorporated into a stimulating massage.

The jacquet or pincement movement

This is where the tissues are picked up between the tips of the thumb and index finger using rapid rotatory movement and released quickly. This movement can be used on fatty tissue areas, i.e. neck, chin and cheeks, to increase lymphatic and vascular flow. Always commence at the lower area first, working towards the temples and follow with effleurage (see Fig. 19.21).

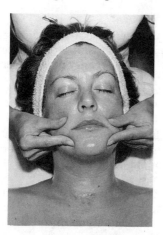

Fig. 19.21 Jacquet method

Digital tapping

Already mentioned for use beneath the mandible, it can also be used as a petrissage movement using three or four fingertips in rapid succession; place the little fingers at the corners of the mouth and apply tapping movements along the naso-labial furrow, or digital tapping over the same area with all finger tips and continue over the zygomatics.

Tapping needs considerable practice to ensure rhythm and rapid, even pressure.

Frictions for the chin, nose and forehead

For the chin, place the fingers loosely beneath the mandible and use the pads of the thumbs to make small circular movements over the entire chin area. For the nose, use the index finger, as the pad of this is usually smaller than the pad of the thumb and can make smaller and deeper circles aiding desquamation. Use one finger at a time, which will enable the client to breathe! From the tip of the nose along the nasalis, use the index fingers to make criss-cross movements.

Vibrations

For tense clients, these help to soothe nerve endings. They are made by contracting and relaxing your arms very quickly to produce a fine trembling action. In the basic routine they are given at the end of movement 6 at the occiput (see p. 190). Horizontal vibrations can also be given in a zig-zag movement across the frontalis. Rest the left hand at the left temporalis and with the right hand make vibrations across the forehead, reverse hands and vibrate back to the left temporalis. Vibrations to the procerus, corrugator and upper fibres of the orbicularis oculi will also help to combat fatigue and headaches.

Contra-indications

These are given at the end of Chapter 18 but facial massage can be given if the client has an asthmatic or sinus disorder, diabetes or has excessively loose skin *providing* your movements are chosen and performed with great care.

On completion of massage

Remove headband, towels and blanket from client and comb hair into place. If there are no more treatments to be given, return personal possessions, assist with outdoor clothing and accompany the client to the reception area.

Return to the cubicle and dispose of all tissues, cotton wool etc., place towels in the laundry basket, tidy the couch and blanket and ensure your jar/pot is clean, closed and ready to use for the next client.

Self assessment

- how would you prepare your client for a basic facial massage?
- what type of massage would you use for tense clients?
- describe the movements used to relax the trapezius
- describe 'knuckling' movements and give diagrams showing where they would be used
- describe the movements you would give to a client with a sinus disorder.

20 Lymphatic drainage of the face and neck

Lymph

The purpose of the lymph has been mentioned in Chapter 5 but further knowledge is required before attempting lymph drainage.

The lymphatics resemble veins in structure but with the following exceptions

- lymphatics have thinner walls;
- lymphatics contain more valves;
- lymphatics have lymph nodes located at certain intervals along their course.

It has been said that the close network of lymph vessels is interrupted by one-way valves which keep the lymph moving in the right direction.

The nodes, which are oval-shaped or bean-shaped, vary in size, some as small as a pin-head and others as large as a lima bean. They consist of a thin connective tissue sheath of white fibrous tissue with some yellow elastic fibres containing cells similar to white blood cells (lymphocytes). The functions of the nodes are:

1. to filter lymph and bacteria along with any foreign materials such as dirt particles; and
2. to manufacture new lymphocytes which are carried away in the lymph to the bloodstream.

Lymph nodes become swollen if invaded by bacteria from a septic area, e.g. lymph nodes at the back of the neck become swollen and tender if there is an infection in the scalp area above the node.

As will be seen in Fig. 20.1 the node is made up of

1. marginal or cortical sinuses which are irregular spaces within the node through which the lymph flows; and
2. trabaculae which are the supporting structures for the sinuses.

Hilium are depressions for the lymph vessels to enter and exit. The **afferent vessels** which enter the hilium at different parts of the periphery bring lymph to the node and the purified lymph vessels leaving the node at the hilium are known as **efferent vessels**.

There are approximately 600 lymph nodes throughout the body, of which 200 are in the neck area.

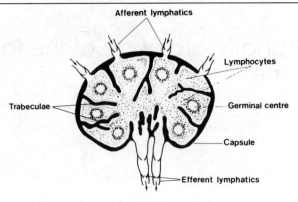

Fig. 20.1 Section through a lymph node

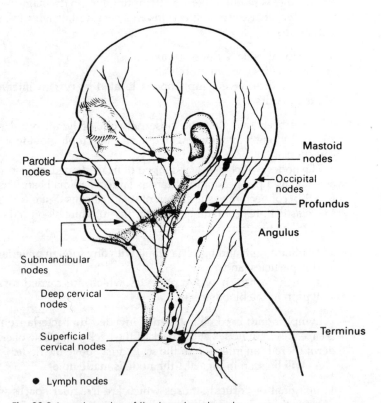

Fig. 20.2 Lymph nodes of the head and neck

The right side of the head, neck and right arm drain into the right lymphatic duct and then into the right subclavian vein. The left side of the head and neck, the left arm, the lower limbs and abdomen drain into the left subclavian vein. The lymph is thus returned to the bloodstream.

There are six main groups of nodes in the head, parotid, mastoid (or *retro-auricular), occipital, submandibular (including sub-mental), profundus or upper deep cervical and superficial cervical (see Fig. 20.2).

Massage movements

As the lymphatic system carries away the waste products of metabolism, the use of this specialised pressure-and-release type of massage may increase the flow of lymph and so speed the removal of waste products.

The following are simple massage movements for the face and neck and should not be confused with the more advanced techniques used for lymphatic drainage of the body.

The hands must be touch-sensitive and supple to feel, by palpitation, the condition of the lymph nodes. The wrists should be flexible. The pressure used is dependent on the tissues but generally soft tissue requires light pressure. The movements are rhythmical and slow.

It is important to practise the stationary circular movement as this is used extensively. The pads of the fingers or thumbs are placed flat on the skin (the number of fingers/thumbs used depends on the area). Pressure is applied in small tight circles, about five in all and then released. Move the fingers along the direction you are working before applying the pressure and release again. The direction of pressure is determined by the lymph drainage. Very little cream or oil should be used as the fingers may slip rather than move lightly. Each movement can be linked with expanding spirals or effleurage.

Massage sequence

The client is prepared as for the basic facial massage. For the neck, stand in front of the client.

1. From the sternum, use the thumbs to make six outward effleurage strokes and the last stroke should be along the clavicle (see Fig. 20.3). Repeat four times more.

2. Slide the fingers up to the medial upper deep cervical nodes, often named as the profundus; make stationary circles as you work your way down to the medial lower deep cervical nodes, also known as the terminus.

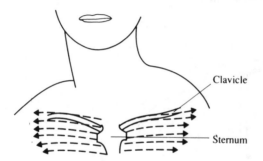

Fig. 20.3

3. Make three thumb effleurage movements from the profundus to the terminus (see Fig. 20.4).

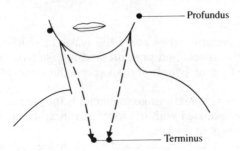

Fig. 20.4

4. Slide hands to the occiput and make stationary circles from the cervical vertebrae to the terminus followed by three effleurage strokes (see Fig. 20.5).

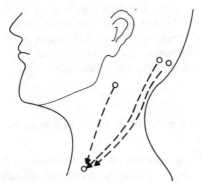

Fig. 20.5

5. Slide hands to the centre of the mandible and make stationary circles to the terminus (see Fig. 20.6). Repeat three times being careful to avoid the trachea.

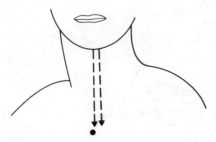

Fig. 20.6

6. Slide hands back to the acromion process and make stationary circles along the edge of the trapezius and finish at the terminus (see Fig. 20.7).

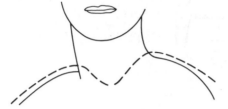

Fig. 20.7

7. Slide hands back to the acromion process and make stationary circles along the top of the clavicle to the terminus. Follow this movement with effleurage.

    With one hand resting on the client, move to stand behind the head of the couch.
8. Place both hands on the lower triangularis and with fingers make stationary circles along the submandibular nodes to the profundus and continue down to the terminus (see Fig. 20.8). Slide hands back to the tip of the chin and repeat three times more.

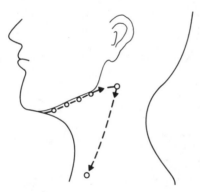

Fig. 20.8

9. Effleurage with parallel strokes over the upper and lower lip, stroke up the sides of the nose and across the frontalis (see Fig 20.9).
10. Slide hands to the orbicularis oris and make stationary circles from the middle of the lip to the angulus and with the index finger drain (light continuous pressure) all the way down to the terminus (see Fig. 20.10).
11. Slide hands to the nasalis and make stationary circles laterally from the bridge of the nose to the zygomatics. Cover the entire nasalis

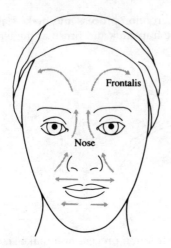

Fig. 20.9

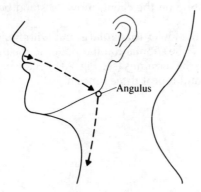

Fig. 20.10

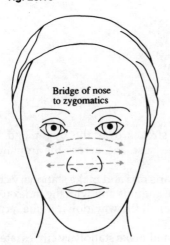

Fig. 20.11

from the tip to the root of the nose carefully, avoiding the orbicularis oculi. It is better to do this alternatively to the left and right zygomatics to enable the client to breathe freely (see Fig. 20.11).

12. Make stationary circles from below the orbicularis oculi along the nasolabial furrow, past the corners of the orbicularis oris to the mentalis.

13. Slide the hands up the procerus and begin very light pressure all round the orbicularis oculi and with both index fingers lift the procerus (see Fig. 20.12). Repeat the movement three times.

14. Take the eyebrows between thumb and index finger and press lightly and then make stationary circles over the eyebrows.

15. From the middle of the frontalis make stationary circles to the temporalis three or four times (see Fig. 20.13).

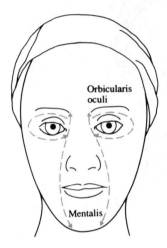

Fig. 20.12

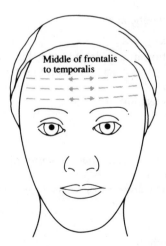

Fig. 20.13

16. Slide hands back to the temporalis and make stationary circles to the profundus. Make 5 or 6 circles here before continuing the circles down to the terminus.
17. Slide hands back to the corrugator and drain with the balls of the thumbs to the temporalis three times.
18. Using index fingers drain from the corrugator to the angulus three times.
19. Effleurage across the frontalis around the orbicularis oculi, from the nasalis over the zygomatics down to the orbicularis oris and finally to terminus (see Fig. 20.14).

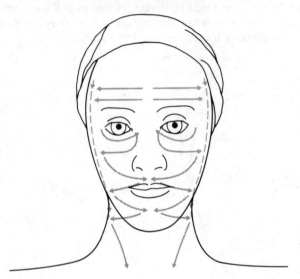

Fig. 20.14

Lymph drainage is especially beneficial for:

● superficial lines and wrinkles;
● poor local circulation resulting in dry/dehydrated skin conditions;
● skin congestion, blocked pores, acne vulgaris, seborrhea and keloids;
● general relaxation, nervous tension or fatigue.

Contra-indications

For the face and neck area there are few, mainly acute inflammation, naevi or skin diseases and asthma.

Common sense will dictate the amount of pressure to be used, but observe the following cautions:

● avoid broken capillaries;
● do not stretch crêpey loose skin;
● do use a medicated cream if acne is present;

- do not treat a client suffering from asthma – stimulating the para-sympathetic nervous system could spark off an asthma attack.

Self assessment

- explain the difference between veins and lymphatics
- what is the purpose of lymph nodes?
- explain the following:

  hilium
  efferent vessels
  afferent vessels

- how does lymph leave the head and neck to be returned to the bloodstream?
- explain the most important massage movement used during lymphatic massage
- draw a diagram, show the positions of the profundus and terminus
- what are the benefits of lymphatic massage?
- list the contra-indications to lymphatic massage.

21 Electro-physics

The study of electricity involves some knowledge of the structure of the substances from which all things, including living organisms, are made.

Elements

These are the simplest substances as they are the building blocks for all substances. There are 92 different occurring elements, e.g. carbon, oxygen, hydrogen, nitrogen, sulphur, phosphorous, fluorine, chlorine and all the metals. Elements cannot be split into any simpler substances by chemical action but may join together chemically to form new and more complex substances called compounds.

Compounds

These have a fixed composition but an enormous number of different compounds can be produced from the 92 elements. Examples of compounds are sugar (a compound containing carbon, hydrogen and oxygen atoms), common salt (sodium and chlorine atoms) and water (containing atoms of hydrogen and oxygen).

Atoms

An atom is the smallest part of an element and all atoms are made up of two different types of electrically charged particles. Positively charged particles, called protons, lie in the nucleus of the atom while negatively charged particles, called electrons, move around the nucleus in paths called orbits (see Fig. 21.1).

The atoms of each element have different numbers of circulating electrons, but each atom is electrically neutral because the number of negatively charged orbital electrons is balanced by an equal number of positively charged protons in the nucleus. Electrons are lighter than protons and are more easily removed. This is demonstrated by the production of **static electricity** (frictional electricity). For example, electrons may be rubbed off the hair by brushing dry hair vigorously and these collect on the brush giving it a negative charge and leaving the hair positively charged. Since like charges repel each other and opposite charges attract each other, the hairs fly apart but are attracted to the brush so that the hair will not lie flat. Similarly, a man-made polymer, i.e. nylon overall, will cling to the body and crackling and sparking occurs when it is removed. Again it is because it has acquired an electric

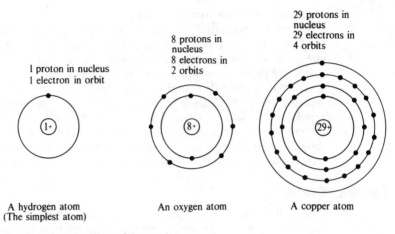

1 proton in nucleus
1 electron in orbit

8 protons in
nucleus
8 electrons in
2 orbits

29 protons in
nucleus
29 electrons in
4 orbits

A hydrogen atom
(The simplest atom)

An oxygen atom

A copper atom

Fig. 21.1 Construction of three atoms

charge by friction. The charges are eventually lost by leaking away to earth.

If electrons can be made to move from atom to atom through a substance, the drift or flow of the electrons is called an **electric current**. The ease with which electrons will pass through various substances differs.

Conductors

These are materials which allow the free flow of electrons and will allow an electric current to pass through them. Most metals, silver, copper and aluminium have atoms which provide free electrons and will conduct electricity. To a lesser extent the human body is a conductor of electricity.

Insulators

These are substances which do not provide free electrons and therefore do not conduct electricity, namely rubber, nylon, dry air, glass and most plastics. You will appreciate why electric wires are made of copper as a good conductor and then covered with a plastic coating as an insulator to make an electrical flex efficient and safe.

Production of electric current

An electric current may be produced by a chemical reaction (i.e. a battery) or by magnetic forces (i.e. a mains generator) and these create an electrical pressure which is known as an electromotive force (EMF). They act like a pump to drive electricity through the wiring. When a continuous closed pathway is provided for electrons to flow from the source (battery or generator) to an appliance and back to the source, it is called a circuit. Switches are used to complete or break the circuit which in turn starts or stops the flow of electricity.

Batteries produce **direct current** (DC) (i.e. current in which electrons flow in one direction) by chemical action taking place in the battery.

Mains electricity is produced at power stations where mechanical energy is converted into electrical energy by rotating a coil of wire between the poles of a magnet. An **alternating current** (AC) is produced where the electron flow periodically changes direction (100 times per second), i.e. it completes 50 alterations per second (forwards and backwards) and is said to have a **frequence** (or frequency) of 50 cycles per second or 50 hertz (Hz). An alternative current may be converted to a direct current if required by the use of a **rectifier** or semi-conductor, which allows electrons to flow through in one direction only.

Electrical units

Electrical pressure (EMF) produced by either a battery or generator is known as the voltage and is measured in units called **volts**. A volt meter may be included in a circuit to measure voltage. For example a battery produces a low voltage.

- for a torch 1.5 volts DC
- for a car 12 volts DC

whereas a domestic mains supply produces 240 volts AC. In mains circuits a transformer may be used to alter voltage, i.e. a step-up transformer to increase voltage and a step-down transformer to give a reduction in voltage.

The size (or intensity) of a current flowing in a circuit

This is measured in units called amperes (amps A). An ammeter (or sometimes a milliammeter) may be included in an appliance to record amperage. A milliampere (mA) is 1000th of an ampere.

The size of the current (amps) flowing through a conductor depends on

1. the voltage
2. the resistance of the wiring

(i.e. the ease or difficulty with which the current will pass). This in turn depends on the type of metal used and its length and thickness; for instance, the thinner or the longer the wire the greater the resistance. Flexes are usually made of copper which has a low resistance and the current flows freely. There is always some heating wherever an electric current flows but this is intensified for some equipment used in the salon where heating elements are required. Heating occurs in wires made of materials such as tungsten in a lamp bulb, which becomes hot and gives out light as well as heat. To obtain considerable heat, i.e. heating elements, thin nichrome (mixture of nickel and chromium) wires are used. They have a high resistance as the current flows with difficulty. Resistance is measured in ohms and a device included in a circuit to provide resistance to a current and control electron flow is called a **resistor** (or a resistance). You may have equipment with a switch that can be turned to high, medium or low. This means that in a low position the electric current must pass through two resistances and in the medium position it will pass through one resistance. A *rheostat* is a variable resistance and is used to control current flow.

The relationship between these quantities is expressed as Ohm's Law which states that the amount of steady current through a conductor is directly proportional to the voltage across the materials. For example:

$$\text{intensity of current} = \frac{\text{electrical pressure (EMF)}}{\text{resistance}}$$

$$\text{or amps} = \frac{\text{volts}}{\text{ohms}}$$

or very simply it takes the pressure of 1 volt to push a current of 1 ampere through a resistance of 1 ohm. The most important variation for beauty therapists is that at constant voltage, the current intensity varies inversely with resistance, i.e.

- Increasing resistance reduces current.
- Decreasing resistance increases current.

For this purpose the rheostat is used.

The power of the appliance

This is measured in watts (W) and is the rate at which the appliance uses electrical energy. A high-powered light bulb of, say, 250 watts will give a bright light, consume a great deal of electricity and therefore cost more to run compared to a low-powered light bulb of only 15 watts, which in turn gives a dimmer light using less electricity. The power of the appliance will depend on the voltage and current flow.

power = voltage × intensity of current
Watts = volts × amps (W = V × A)

Electricity meters are situated at the point of entry of the mains supply to a building and they measure the total electricity used in kilowatt hours (kWh), that is, power in kilowatts multiplied by time in hours. One kilowatt hour is recorded by the meter as 1 unit of electricity. The cost of electricity is therefore given for the use of 1000 watts (1 kW) for an hour using one unit of electricity. As an example a simple sunbed using 20 tubes would use 2 kW per hour consuming 2 units of electricity. The cost to run the sunbed would be 2 × the price of the unit, e.g. 2 × 6 p = 12 p per hour.

Mains electricity

This is supplied from power-generating stations by overhead cables to a local distribution centre and then to individual premises by underground cables. These supply cables, containing live and neutral (or return) wires, first lead into the Electricity Boards' sealed fuse box (which may only be opened by the Boards' engineers) then through the meter to the consumer unit which contains the mains switch and fuses, together with an earthed terminal.

In older installations individual plugs were wired separately to the fuse box. In modern electricity installations various circuits from the consumer unit radiate for power and lighting. Power sockets depend on a ring main circuit where a cable runs around the salon in a closed loop and sockets can be wired at any point (see Fig. 21.2).

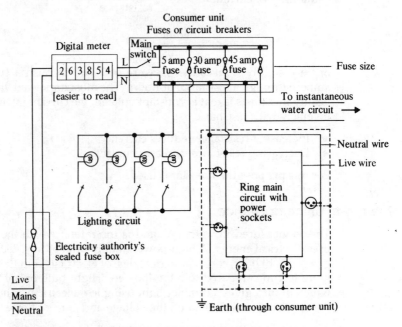

Fig. 21.2 Modern installation with ring main circuit

Safety devices in mains circuits

The chief dangers with mains electricity are electric shocks, electrical burns and fires due to electrical faults.

Electric shock is experienced if a person's body completes a mains circuit by either

1. touching both live and neutral wires, e.g. while replacing a light bulb without switching off; or
2. touching both a live wire and a tap or simply touching a plug with wet hands. Impure water being a good conductor has the same effect as touching a live wire; or
3. touching a live wire, or a live unearthed metal, and the earth. This can happen if the earthing wire is not connected to an appliance whereby a person can complete the circuit through the ground. It can also happen that, if a live wire is touched, a person will conduct the current to earth.

Fires are usually started by improper use of electrical equipment. All electrical appliances must be correctly fused and earthed in accordance with the British Standards Institution's recommended practice. Generally speaking wires (or conductors) carrying the ring main circuits are usually enclosed in conduits (metal or plastic tubing) behind or below salon walls and only the switches and socket outlets are visible. The thickness of the wire varies in different circuits and if the wire carries a greater current than that for which it was intended it will become **overloaded**, e.g. using an adaptor with too many plugs in one socket. It will become hot and start a fire. An overheated plug will emit a 'fishy' odour as it melts, but overloading should cause the circuit fuse to melt which will cut off the current so avoiding a fire.

Loss of insulation can lead to a **short circuit** where live and neutral wires touch. This can happen when alterations are taking place and nails are driven into walls or floors. It can also happen if the plug is pulled out of the socket by the flex so dislodging the wires inside the plug.

Insulation

One important use of insulation is to prevent an electric shock. Non-conductors such as plastic or rubber are used for the outer covers of switches, plugs and sockets. Metal-cased pieces of equipment may have extra insulation fitted to prevent live wires touching the metal case. As poor insulation can lead to a short circuit, cracked or broken plugs or switches should be replaced immediately.

Fuses

The purpose of a fuse is to protect the wiring or appliance. The fuse wire (or cartridge) itself is the weakest part of a circuit and will not carry as much current as the wiring it protects. It acts as a safety device, cutting off the power long before heat builds up to the point where insulation could melt or a fire could start.

Circuit fuses

These are the main fuses in the consumer unit adjacent to the electricity meter. Each circuit fuse has a rating (in amps) which must not exceed the current-capacity of the wire it protects. A circuit that provides outlets for lighting has a fine fuse wire with a current rating of 5 A, whereas a ring circuit providing a number of socket outlets to beauty-therapy equipment would require a thicker fuse wire with a current rating of 30 A. The more powerful the appliance, the higher rating of the fuse, i.e. an instantaneous water heater would require a fuse wire with a current rating of 45 A.

There are two types of circuit fuse. The rewirable type and the cartridge fuse. The former is usually found in older types of fuse boxes. To replace a blown circuit fuse disconnect all appliances and switch off the main switch. Locate the blown fuse by checking each holder. If the fuse is a cartridge type, discard the blown fuse and replace with a new one of exactly the same size.

Fuse-box cartridge fuses are coded by size and colour i.e.

white are for   5 A
blue   15 A
yellow   20 A
red   30 A
green   45 A

These consist of a fuse wire inside a small glass or ceramic tube with a metal cap at each end. It is impossible to fit the wrong size of cartridge into a holder due to the variance in size, i.e. the higher the current rating the larger the cartridge.

If it is a rewirable type remove the old fuse wire. Wind the new fuse wire of the same rating around one screw and tighten. Take the wire across the bridge and twist it clockwise around the second screw being careful not to stretch the wire when tightening the screw. Cut off any surplus wire and replace the fuse holder.

Should a fuse blow in quick succession the circuit or equipment must be examined by an electrician. Never attempt to replace a fuse with a higher amperage wire or cartridge.

As an alternative to the use of a main fuse, trip switches or **circuit breakers** may be fitted and these are designed to turn themselves off automatically when there is a fault or when the circuit becomes overloaded. Switch off some of the appliances or find the faulty appliance on the circuit. Reset the circuit breaker, usually by pushing a button or flipping a switch.

The consumer unit may also be fitted with an **earth-leak** circuit breaker. If some current flows via the earth instead of by the correct route, i.e. through the neutral wire, this breaker immediately disconnects the power supply.

Plug fuses

A plug fuse is a cartridge-type fuse designed to protect the flex to which it is attached and its appliance. The size of the fuse depends on the voltage rating of the appliance and although the cartridges appear the same physical size there are three current ratings.

- 3 A fuse for appliances up to 700 watts
- 5 A fuse for appliances with loading between 700 and 1000 watts
- 13 A fuse for appliances with loading between 1000 and 3000 watts

When replacing a plug fuse check that it has the correct size fuse and this can be easily calculated. Check the wattage plate which is normally positioned at the side or back of the equipment. For appliances made abroad the voltage may vary and you would need to consult an electrician for advice. The plate usually shows how much power the appliance uses, in watts (W) or kilowatts (kW). Divide the figure in watts by 240 and the result is the minimum size of fuse necessary in amps. The fuse size must be rated at just a little more than the normal appliance current. For instance, an appliance using 1.5 kW (1500 watts) i.e. 1500 watts divided by 240 volts) would require a 6.5 amp fuse but in practice a 13 amp fuse would be used. Other appliances may have the voltage and amperage marked. A facial steamer may have a plate marked '240 V 3.5 A', therefore a 5 amp fuse would be required.

The earth wire

This is an addition to the live and neutral wires, providing a path of low resistance between the metal case of the appliance and the ground. It represents less resistance than the human body and acts as a safety device to prevent electric shock by carrying away electric current harmlessly into the earth. It must run continuously from the outside of an appliance with metal casing through the flex, through the plug and socket, along the circuit cable, through the consumer unit into the ground. An earth wire is not always necessary if the outer casing of an appliance is either plastic or has extra insulation fitted inside to ensure that live wires cannot touch the metal case. Such appliance are marked with a square within a square (see Fig. 21.3).

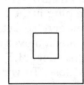

Fig. 21.3 Symbol for double insulation

Correct wiring of a plug

The plug attached to the flex from an appliance must be suitable for the socket in the wall. The flex has three cores coated with plastic insulation and are coloured (see Fig. 21.4 and Table 21.1) so that it is easy to connect the correct wire to the terminals in the plug. These are as in Table 21.1, together with the colours used for appliances purchased prior to 1970.

The wiring of a plug is important to all beauty therapists as wrong

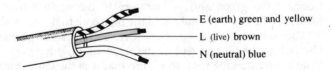

E (earth) green and yellow
L (live) brown
N (neutral) blue

Fig. 21.4 Three-core flex

Table 21.1 Colours of wires in three-core cables

Present colour	Connected to terminal marked	Colour (pre-1970)
brown	Live (L)	red
blue	Neutral (N)	black
green and yellow	Earth (E or $\doteq$)	green

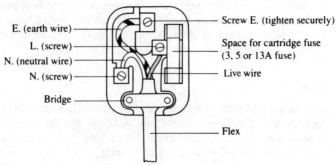

E. (earth wire)
L. (screw)
N. (neutral wire)
N. (screw)
Bridge

Screw E. (tighten securely)
Space for cartridge fuse (3, 5 or 13A fuse)
Live wire
Flex

Fig. 21.5 Wiring of a mains plug

connections in a plug are dangerous. Connecting an earth wire to a live terminal would make the metal parts of an appliance 'live' and crossing over the live and neutral connections would mean that the switch would not cut off the live wire and the appliance would still be 'live'. Most beauty therapy equipment must contain an earth wire, therefore a 3-pin plug is required. The earth pin on the plug is the longest and will make contact with the socket first. Most modern sockets are **shuttered** and when the earth pin is put into the socket it moves the shutter to open the holes for the neutral and live pins (see Fig. 21.5). When the plug is withdrawn from the socket the holes close. To wire the plug keep a screwdriver and a knife or cutters to hand.

1. Cut back the outer covering about 1 in (2.5 cm) to expose three coloured plastic cores, so that when the plug is complete only the outer covering is visible from outside giving protection to the coloured cores.
2. Cut the plastic cores to the length required. Usually the earth and neutral cores should be a little longer than the live core. Cut the plastic core about 0.5 in (1.25 cm) to give sufficient bare wire to make the connection.
3. If necessary twist the strands of the bare wires and trim the ends.
4. Usually there is a bridge across the plug; loosen one screw and remove the other and press in the outer covering of the flex.
5. Connect the green and yellow core to the earth terminal E, the brown to the live terminal L and the blue core to the neutral terminal N. There should be no slack bare wires and the screws must be tight.
6. Go back to the bridge, replace the screw and tighten both screws.
7. Check the cartridge fuse, to ensure that it is the correct size for the appliance and press the fuse in place.
8. Screw down the top of the plug.

General precautions

To prevent accidents occurring in the salon and to minimise the risks of starting a fire or suffering an electric shock the following precautions should be taken:

1. Water and electricity must be kept apart. It should not be possible to reach a plug socket or an electrical appliance at the same time as a source of water because the current can flow between live and neutral wires by passing through the live wire, the water, the human body and the earth. Extra care must be taken when using certain appliances, e.g. steam baths, saunas, facial steamers and electrical foot baths. Never touch electrical equipment with wet hands.
2. To prevent anyone tripping over trailing flexes, ensure that these are carefully coiled out of the way. Do not make a definite 'bend' in a flex as this could produce a weak spot and eventually fray or break and cause a short circuit.
3. Check regularly and replace worn insulation, i.e. cracked or broken plugs and switches or frayed flexes.
4. If you have more than one appliance on a socket, check the total load by adding up the current that each appliance uses. Overloading can cause overheating and a possible fire.
5. Ensure that plugs are firmly pushed into sockets and always use the appropriate plug fuse for the appliance.
6. Finally, make a *regular* check on plugs, flexes and equipment.

Self assessment

- explain the difference between elements and compounds
- what is a conductor and an insulator?
- how is an electrical current produced?
- what is the meaning of EMF?
- explain Ohm's Law
- explain the chief dangers of mains electricity and say how you would avoid accidents
- explain the purpose of

    insulation
    fuses, both circuit and plug

- draw a diagram showing the correct way to wire a mains plug.

22 Electrical therapy

Use of high-frequency current

High frequency (HF) is a rapidly alternating current in excess of 500,000 Hz (hertz) which oscillates (or alternates) so rapidly that when applied to the skin there is no stimulation of nerves or muscles but heat is produced in the tissues. (This may be compared with the low frequency of normal mains current of only 50 Hz.)

The units themselves vary slightly with each manufacturer but generally contain an intensity control, an applicator holder, glass electrodes of varying shapes (i.e. an arc, roll, rake, flattened dome and rod) and a saturator which is either a glass electrode attached to the holder or a metal rod (see Fig. 22.1).

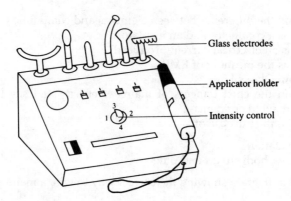

Fig. 22.1 High-frequency unit

There are two methods of application, direct and indirect.

Direct high-frequency method

The current is supplied through a glass electrode. This is hollow and the air inside is partially vacuumed to allow the current to flow through. When the machine is operating, a crackling sound will be heard and a blue/violet colour will be seen. This may be disturbing to the client, therefore it should be explained prior to the treatment.

The **benefits** are:

- a stimulating effect on the skin, producing a mild erythema;
- aids desquamation;

- aids elimination of waste products by increasing lymph action and glandular activity;
- no harmful effects on nerves or muscles;
- germicidal effect, which is due to the ozone formation if sparking is allowed to take place;
- helps to clear pimples or spots in an oily skin;
- alleviates pain from chilblains.

Method of application

Remove all jewellery. Prepare the client comfortably, cleanse, tone and blot the skin dry.

For the electrode to move slowly over the facial contours, apply a very light dusting of talcum powder. To ensure that it is light, place a little in the palms of your hands, shake off the surplus and gently slide the hands over the client's face. This will also absorb any natural secretions occurring during the treatment.

Choose the electrode required. For the face this is usually a flattened dome and place this firmly in the applicator holder.

Switch on the machine and check that the intensity control is at zero.

Test the electrode on your arm first by increasing the intensity and then returning the intensity control to zero. The client will be able to observe the light and noise from the electrode and be reassured.

Place the electrode on the client's face, increase the intensity until the client can feel a mild tingling sensation. There are many schools of thought as to where to begin treatment. Some prefer to start on the forehead as this normally bony area requires less intensity; others prefer to start on the face or neck area to allow the client to become accustomed to the treatment. Whichever method is chosen, ensure smooth and even circular movements with a definite pattern covering the face and neck. The pressure and the intensity of the current should be consistent with the degree of subcutaneous tissue and the skin's sensitivity to allow for maximum client comfort (see Fig. 22.2).

To help to dry pimples or spots these may be 'sparked', which is made by creating an air gap between the electrode and the skin. Raise the electrode about 0.25 in (6 mm) from the skin for a second. This must

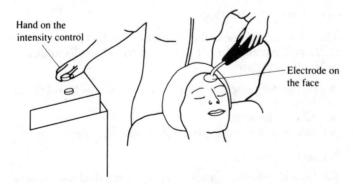

Hand on the intensity control

Electrode on the face

Fig. 22.2 Direct high-frequency, with dome

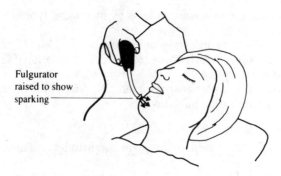

Fulgurator
raised to show
sparking

Fig. 22.3 Direct high frequency

be done with care as the surrounding skin may also dry and could start flaking. You may meet the word 'fulguration' which merely means 'treatment by electric sparks'. A fulgurator is a glass rod, the end of which resembles a large needle with a small aperture at the top. It may be necessary to insert this type of glass electrode into the holder to spark spots or pimples. Certainly it is far more precise for the odd blemish. Sparking near the eyes or lips should be avoided (see Fig. 22.3).

Apart from sparking, the electrode must remain in contact with the skin at all times. Application times will vary from 3–5 minutes for a dry, dehydrated skin to 10–15 minutes for an oily or blemished skin.

Turn the intensity control to zero, switch off the machine and remove the electrode from the face.

The remains of the talcum powder should be removed with damp cotton wool and patted dry with tissues. The skin is best left devoid of make-up (except eye shadow and lipstick).

If deeper penetration is required, for aching muscles and joints, the electrode is moved over the part at a small distance from the skin. Two thicknesses of towelling can be laid on the skin and the electrode passed over this. This means that the sparks have to jump a greater distance and therefore penetrate deeper.

Indirect high-frequency method

This involves the use of the saturator, which is the electrode held by the client and where your hands replace the glass electrodes.

The **benefits** are:

- stimulating effect as lymphatic and venous blood circulation is improved;
- relieves tension;
- aids dry or mature crêpey skins and dry acne.

Method of application

Remove all jewellery, make the client comfortable, cleanse, tone and blot the skin dry.

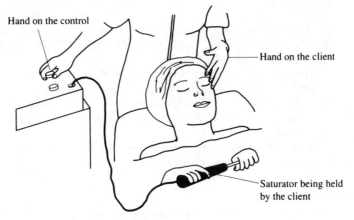

Hand on the control

Hand on the client

Saturator being held
by the client

Fig. 22.4 Indirect high frequency

Be careful to avoid touching metal (i.e. arms of chairs).

Cream or a lubricant (i.e. glycerine) for a relaxing effect or talcum powder for a stimulating action should be applied to the face and neck to allow your hands to move smoothly over the entire area.

Give the saturator to the client to hold with both hands throughout the treatment.

Explain to the client that a pleasant tingling sensation will be felt.

Ensure that the machine is within easy reach and check that the switch is off and that the intensity control is at zero.

Place your hand on the client's forehead, as this is the most sensitive area and with the other hand switch on the machine and turn the intensity control slowly until either you or the client feel the vibrations. Talking to the client will enable you not only to dispel nervousness of the treatment but also to judge the client's tolerance level (see Fig. 22.4).

Commence massage slowly with one hand and as soon as the intensity has been regulated, the other hand can leave the machine and the two hands start a facial massage. Depending upon the skin type and

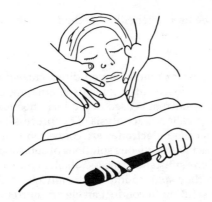

Fig. 22.5 Indirect high-frequency massage

the result required, use the pads of the fingers for a light stimulating effect, or the fingers and hands for a deep relaxing effect. Should you wish to increase/decrease the intensity, ensure that one hand is left on the client's skin before adjusting the machine. Client's reactions must be watched closely (see Fig. 22.5).

When the massage has been completed, with one hand turn the intensity control to zero, switch off the machine and remove your hand from the client's face. Take the saturator from the client.

Use damp cotton wool to remove cream/lubricant or talc and wash your hands.

The length of the massage will vary from five to ten minutes and can be given twice a week for about six weeks.

Contra-indications

For both methods these are mainly the same, i.e.

- any heart condition or high blood pressure
- skin infections
- oedema
- bruises, cuts and abrasions
- metal pins, braces or excessive number of metal fillings in the teeth
- new scar tissue
- headaches or migraine
- medical conditions, i.e. epilepsy
- asthmatics
- severe sinus infection
- nervous clients or others who have a fear of electrical currents
- later stages of pregnancy

While an acne condition persists, only acne cream should be used on the face. Direct HF is suitable for pustular acne and indirect HF for dry acne. Liaison with the client's doctor is advisable when giving treatments for this disturbing condition.

For thread veins massage lightly over the area for about three minutes using either method.

After high-frequency treatment has been completed wash and sterilise all equipment.

Suitable masks may be used after either method of high frequency.

Use of galvanic current

Galvanic current is a constant uninterrupted direct current (DC) produced either by battery or by rectifying mains alternating current. In beauty therapy a galvanic current is used to produce chemical changes in the skin by a process called **electrolysis**. This process takes place when metal conductors called **electrodes** are connected to a source of DC and also make contact with aqueous solutions of substances known as **electrolytes**. These are substances (acids, alkalis and salts) which **ionise** in water, that is, they split up into electrically charged particles or **ions** and enable the solution to conduct an electric current.

One of the most important electrolytes in the human body is sodium chloride. In water, sodium chloride produces positively charged sodium ions (Na+) and negatively charged chloride ions (Cl−). The water itself ionises very slightly to produce positively charged hydrogen ions (H+) and negatively charged hydroxyl ions (OH−) (see Fig. 22.6). Ions carrying a positive charge are called **cations** and those carrying a negative charge are called **anions**.

Sodium ions are key regulators of the water balance of the body and are necessary for the normal function of muscles and nerves. Both sodium and chloride ions are present in body-tissue fluid. Thus the electrolysis of sodium chloride can be used to illustrate the changes which may take place during galvanic treatment of the skin.

If two electrodes are immersed in a solution of sodium chloride and are connected to a source of DC, the movement of ions in the electrolyte completes the circuit. The positive ions move towards the negative electrode, namely the **cathode** and the negative ions move towards the positive electrode, the **anode**.

When ions are neutralised at the electrode, chemical changes take place.

At the cathode (−ve electrode) or negative pole, sodium hydroxide (caustic soda) is produced in the electrolyte as the positive sodium (Na+) ions receive a negative charge and the neutralised hydrogen (H+) ions form hydrogen gas which is released as bubbles. The hydroxyl (OH−) ions increase and the solution round the cathode becomes alkaline.

At the anode (+ve electrode) or positive pole, chloride (Cl−) ions and hydroxyl (OH−) ions are neutralised and chlorine is formed, some of which reacts with water to form hydrochloric and hypochlorus acid in the electrolyte. The solution round the anode becomes acid due to the increased concentration of hydrogen (H+) ions.

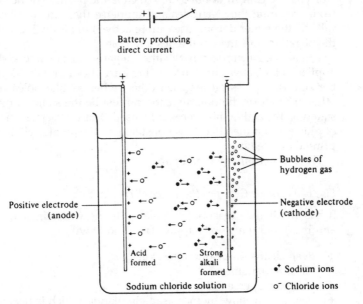

Fig. 22.6 Electrolysis of sodium chloride solution

Galvanic units vary slightly with each manufacturer but will incorporate:

- a pilot light (which advises you that the machine is switched on)
- an intensity control
- a polarity changer
- an indicator or mA meter (determining amperage used and shows the level of skin resistance)
- outlets for lead connections marked (+) positive and (−) negative

Most galvanic machines have fixed polarities, the red lead is for the positive electrode connection and the black lead for the negative electrode connection. However, the colour of the leads may change in different parts of the world and you should check carefully before using the machine. They usually operate from AC mains so the machine will have a transformer to reduce the voltage of the AC, a rectifier to change the current from AC to DC and a capacitor to iron out any irregularities in the DC.

The equipment will have a *passive* (i.e. non-working) or indifferent electrode which can be held by the client or strapped on to the client (see method of application). The indifferent electrode comes in the form of either a metal rod or a small metal plate which must be covered with damp viscose sponge. The *active* (i.e. working) or differential electrode can be found as metal ball rollers, or metal rollers, tweezers or a rod with a round flattened head. If tweezers or a flat applicator head is used, these must also be covered with lint or viscose sponge. The electrodes are connected by leads to the machine. The client completes the circuit between the two electrodes.

If you are ever in doubt as to which is the positive or negative electrode, separate the electrodes and immerse them in water containing salt. As the water decomposes, more active bubbles will accumulate at the negative pole than at the positive pole.

The active electrode can be either negative or positive and this also applies to the active substances being introduced into the skin, remember opposite poles attract each other, whereas like poles repel each other. Therefore, the polarity chosen must be the same as the polarity stated on the active substances to be used. These are usually in the form of phials and if the polarity is not stated on the phial itself, it should be printed on the box.

The action of the two poles are:

Use of a cathode (−ve) as the active electrode

It has an alkaline reaction, stimulates the nerve endings, opens pores and increased the blood supply. Therefore it will:

- deep cleanse and soften the skin
- aid desquamation
- help to disperse milia
- help sebum flow by increased circulation which is beneficial for a dry skin

- improve dehydrated skin by drawing fluids to it or by iontophoresis to help the skin retain moisture content
- benefits mature skin as the tissue fluid can be drawn to the area and so help plump out crêpey or ageing skin.

Use of an anode (+ve) as the active electrode

It has an acid reaction and is therefore germicidal, soothes nerve endings, decreases blood supply and firms the tissues. Therefore it will:

- improve facial contours and help to revive tired and exhausted skins
- assist in the removal of spots and pimples
- helps to tighten open pores
- helps to reduce high colour and rosacea conditions and prevent inflammation.

These poles can be reversed and generally speaking so are the benefits.

Changing the polarity of the electrodes

If the polarity of the electrodes is changed, the chemical effects of the current are reversed. Often it is necessary to reverse the polarity of the electrodes at the end of a treatment to restore the pH balance of the skin. If a reversal of polarity is required, always reduce the intensity control to zero before changing over. The negative electrode should not be used over skin with broken capillaries or a pustular condition.

Treatments using galvanic units include:

Desincrustation, which is a deep cleansing action normally applied to the face to remove impurities and waste matter and the products used are soap-based. It is the chemical reaction on the fatty acid of the sebum trapped in the skin, blockages or enlarged pores which softens the sebum making it easier to remove by either comedone extraction or by normal cleansing methods, and,

Iontophoresis introduces ions of a chosen solution into the skin and its purpose is to moisturise, stimulate, regenerate, firm or just calm and heal the skin.

(a) Cataphoreses is the name given to a process where a solution contains +ions (i.e. cations moving towards the cathode) and the active electrode is positive so that the ions are repelled into the skin and the passive (−ve) electrode is held by the client (see Fig. 22.7(a)).

(b) Anaphoresis is the opposite where it is required to move −ve ions (i.e. anions moving towards the anode) into the skin and a solution containing these ions is placed under the negative electrode (see Fig. 22.7(b)).

A skin-care house will always suggest the types of ampoules to be used for varying skin types.

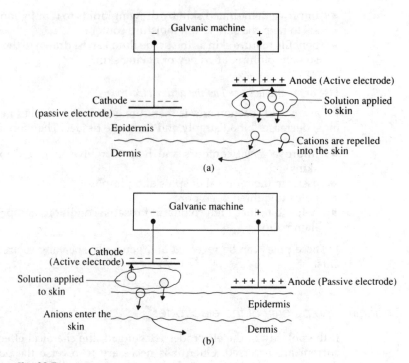

Fig. 22.7

Method of application for desincrustation

1. Settle the client comfortably, i.e. warm and well wrapped up – especially the feet! Ensure that all jewellery is removed (perhaps with the exception of a wedding ring) and that he or she is not able to touch any metal objects (i.e. metal arms of chairs).
2. Cleanse the skin thoroughly and steam the face if required. A clean skin will ensure that the current will not be impeded. However, if there is the odd small lesion or spot, this should be smeared with vaseline (petroleum jelly) to insulate it against the current and prevent an unpleasant sensation with the risk of a burn.
3. For the face, the positive electrode is usually in the form of a rod or bar and is given to the client to hold. If a metal electrode is used, this must be covered with a thick layer of damp viscose sponge or layers of lint and placed on a fleshy part of the shoulders or arms. This is held in place by either a rubber band or velcro strap. This method may be preferred due to the fact that clients do not always hold the rod firmly and the efficiency and flow of the current can be affected. The negative electrode (active electrode) is either tweezers (see Fig. 22.8) or a roller.

    For the tweezer method:

4. Insert cotton wool or lint between the prongs and wrap around the

tweezer, ensuring that it is covered well and connect this electrode to the negative pole.

5. Place the desincrustation fluid (or electrolyte) into a clean bowl. Dip the padded tweezers into the solution and squeeze out any excess liquid. Apply the fluid (or the contents of a phial) to the face and neck, taking care to avoid any seepage towards the eyes.

6. Check the machine: the indicator must be in the 'off' position, the intensity control at zero and the polarity checked. Switch on the machine.

7. Place the covered tweezers on the chin, and very slowly turn up the intensity control. Watch the progress of the mA needle. Advise the client that a slight prickling sensation may be felt, or even a degree of warmth in the area. The client may experience a slight metallic taste in the mouth which could be from one or two fillings in the teeth or due to changes in the saliva.

8. As you gradually increase the intensity ask the client to describe the feeling and when a sensation is felt, turn down the intensity very slightly. In most cases 1.5 mA is sufficient. As a guide use 0.5–1.0 mA for a fine but clogged skin and up to 1.5 mA for an oily skin.

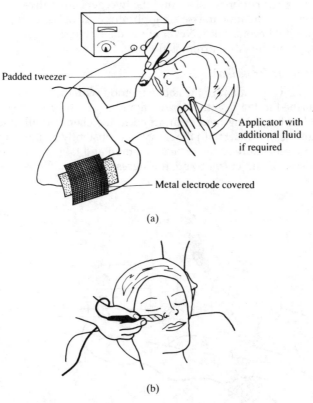

Padded tweezer

Applicator with additional fluid if required

Metal electrode covered

(a)

(b)

Fig. 22.8 (a) Tweezer electrode method (b) Using the tweezer method on a blocked area

9. For the face and neck a maximum of 4–6 minutes should be suffi-cient for a general deep cleanse but allow 8–10 minutes for an oily skin with adjustments in timing for a combination skin. You will probably need to reduce the intensity over bony areas, i.e. cheek-bones, temples and forehead. Always watch both your client's re-action and the mA needle, which should remain nearly stationary.

10. Roll back and forth on the mentalis, move up on to the right side of the face using stroking or rolling movements, over the masseter and zygomatics and across to the middle of the frontalis. Proceed down the nose (nasalis), the upper lip (orbicularis oris) mentalis and right-hand side of the neck (platysma). Avoiding the trachea, complete the left-hand side of the neck and face in the same man-ner.

11. Turn the current down slowly, i.e. returning the intensity control to zero before removing the electrode from the client. Switch off the machine. Alternatively the intensity control can be returned to zero to change polarity (i.e. to positive) if you consider it necessary to neutralise the effects of the negative pole before switching off the machine.

12. Remove the positive electrode from the client.

Note: The cotton wool around the tweezers must always remain moist during the treatment. Use an applicator or dropper to apply additional fluid if it becomes dry. Never allow the electrode to break contact with the skin while the current is flowing.

For the roller method

This is very similar to the above method with the roller electrode being attached to the negative terminal and again the positive electrode (i.e. rod or bar) being held or attached to the client. At all times the roller must be in contact with the skin, kept constantly on the move, using the same procedure as the tweezer method and taking into account the in-tensity of the current and the necessary precautions (see Fig. 22.9).

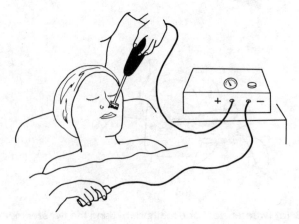

Fig. 22.9 Roller-electrode method

After the treatment desincrustation products must be thoroughly removed from the skin.

Contra-indications for galvanic desincrustation

- skin infection or irritation
- vascular and/or hypersensitive skin
- sinusitis
- epileptics
- asthmatics
- very nervous clients
- pacemakers
- excessive fillings in the teeth
- metal pins or plates in the head

Method of application by iontophoresis

This often follows desincrustation to introduce substances into the skin and the client is prepared using the same procedure as for galvanic desincrustation. Although solutions vary with each manufacturer, the glass containers (phials or ampoules) are clearly marked with the polarity either on the product or its box.

Nourishing ampoules are generally cation-active, being introduced from the anode (+ pole) and requiring a positive charge. Therefore the client will hold the −ve electrode and the covered tweezers or roller will be the +ve electrode and the polarity is chosen accordingly.

1. Break the neck of the glass ampoule and apply the solution to the face and neck evenly with your fingers. Any area of the face and neck not requiring the treatment should be moistened with water.
2. Check the polarity of the ampoule and select the polarity on the machine (i.e. negative ampoule requires negative polarity and viceversa). Some ampoules require both negative and positive polarity and this will be clearly stated by the manufacturer's instructions. Always return the intensity to zero before changing polarity.
3. The damp-covered tweezers or moist roller is placed on the face and using circular or rolling movement cover the face and neck, checking the mA intensity during the entire treatment. You will require a very low level of intensity and it is important not to exceed more than three minutes in any small area of the face. Always ensure the skin is moist.
4. Turn the intensity control to zero before removing the tweezers or rollers.
5. The whole treatment will require about ten minutes to allow full penetration of the substances. Do not rinse off the ampoule, leave it to be gradually absorbed into the skin and bloodstream and to be finally excreted from the body over a few days.
6. After the treatment has been completed protect the skin with a moisturising agent. Clients should be advised not to use make-up (other than lipstick and eye make-up) or shave for six to eight hours after this deep cleansing facial. Also advise against the use of a sun-bed,

unless the face is covered, for the same length of time. Facial waxing and electrolysis treatments should likewise be avoided.

If for any reason the circuit is broken between the client and the active electrode, the intensity control must be returned to zero and the intensity brought up again slowly. Galvanic current itself will not cause a burn but if there is a concentration of alkali or acid formed, a chemical burn may occur. This is recognised by the area appearing grey in colour or a series of grey spots. Should this happen wash the affected area with plenty of cold water and cover with a dry dressing. It must be emphasised that tweezers, rollers, etc., should be in continual motion, i.e. if allowed to dwell in one place for any length of time it is easy to cause this type of burn. If the client feels a burning sensation return the intensity control slowly to zero and examine the skin. It may be necessary to discontinue the treatment to avoid a burn or the client may have an allergic reaction to the cosmetic gels being used.

This type of facial may be given once a week for normal/greasy skins and once a fortnight for dry/dehydrated skins.

Contra-indications for iontophoresis

- skin infection or irritation
- vascular and/or hypersensitive skin
- sinusitis
- epileptics
- asthmatics
- clients of a nervous disposition
- pacemakers
- excessive fillings in the teeth
- metal pins or plates in the head.

Combined galvanic and high-frequency treatments

Units are available providing sources of both currents, so giving an efficient method of cleansing the skin by galvanic desincrustation together with the germicidal and toning effects of the high-frequency current. These 'modular' units usually have two roller electrodes with a double lead attachment and a third lead acting as indifferent electrode. It is important to follow the manufacturer's instructions carefully, especially with regard to the electrical routine and application of the treatment products. The units supply DC at a safe low voltage level between 10 and 20 volts and the current transmitted by the galvanic electrodes at the skin level is less than one milliampere, plus the supply of AC for the high frequency.

General method used

1. Ensure that all jewellery is removed and that the skin is cleansed thoroughly and dried.
2. Some manufacturers will supply a conductive lotion which is applied using fingertips. Ensure that scrunched tissues are placed either side of the neck to catch any surplus lotion.

3. A film of specially formulated galvanic gel is spread evenly over the neck and face by gentle use of a spatula.
4. The indifferent electrode is either attached to the client on the arm or if in the form of a bar, the client is requested to hold the electrode firmly (in the hand opposite the wedding ring, if worn).
5. Switch on the galvanic current and remember to reassure the client that the electrical current is so light that he/she is unlikely to feel the current. Most units have a timer and this can be set for five to eight minutes, depending on the condition of the skin.
6. Select the galvanic setting on the intensity control. Usually two rollers (both +ve) are used, and these are placed on the sterno-cleido mastoid muscles. Commence the treatment with rhythmical rolling movements, each side of the face, working over the muscles, i.e. platysmae, mentalis, masseters, zygomatics and frontalis, ensuring that the rollers remain in contact with the skin but do not touch each other (see Fig. 22.10).
7. Change from rollers to the single electrode applicator, usually in the form of a ball, dome or fork. This is for areas inaccessible to the rollers, where blackheads can gather or where a concentrated application is beneficial. Re-apply the gel where appropriate, usually to the creases around the nose, nose to mouth lines and between the eyes. Again set the timer for approximately seven minutes and commence the treatment at the frontalis, covering the procerus, nasalis, orbicularis oris and the lateral orbicularis oculi (see Fig. 22.11).
8. Switch off the galvanic current and remove the indifferent electrode from the client. Examine the skin under a magnifying glass and, without removing the gel, gently remove the dead surface of the skin with a sterile probe, using circular movements. Blackheads may be removed at this stage with a comedo extractor, but pressure must not be applied as this may result in scarring (see Fig. 22.12).

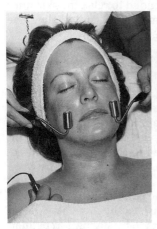 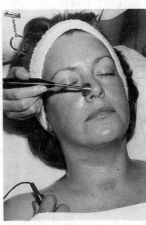 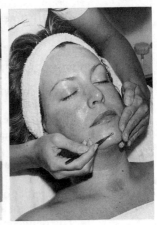

Fig. 22.10 Use of roller electrodes

Fig. 22.11 Use of small single electrodes

Fig. 22.12 Use of comedo extractor

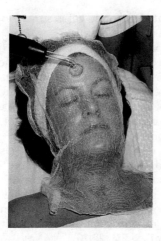

Fig. 22.13 Direct high frequency; face covered with gauze

9. Gently remove excess gel with tissues and apply (by careful use of a spatula) a special emulsion or cream over the face and neck on top of the remaining gel. The two products combine and a chemical change occurs whereby oxygen is produced on the surface of the skin.
10. Cover the face and neck with a piece of dry gauze. If a client is claustrophobic, small holes may be cut in the gauze. Plug in the high-frequency electrode, attach the glass bulb and set the timer to seven minutes. (Take all necessary precautions as previously mentioned.) Adjust the current accordingly and glide the electrode over the face and neck. Always check with the client that the level of the current is comfortable (see Fig. 22.13).
11. Remove all traces of gel/emulsion with damp cotton wool or sponges. A product is usually recommended to relax the skin after the treatment followed by an appropriate mask and cooling eye pads.

Use of faradic current

A faradic current is an interrupted direct current producing groups of short pulses of current separated by intervals when no current flows. Figure 22.14 shows a typical example of a faradic current, each vertical line representing one pulse of current. If applied to the skin through an electrode, each group of pulses may be used to cause muscle contraction, the interval between the groups allowing a period of rest between contractions.

The circuit governing the pulses allows the periods of current flow to be varied from about 0.1 to 1 millisecond (ms). At the same time the intervals between the pulses are also short, thereby giving a repetition rate of 50/100 pulses per second. Due to the short period of time the current flows during each pulse, there is no chemical effect such as

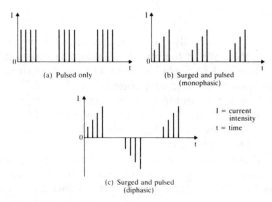

Fig. 22.14 Faradic stimulation patterns

takes place with galvanic current. However, as muscles tend to react less and less to a succession of identical pulses, faradic current is modified to give a series of pulses which increase in size to form a surge, again followed by a period of rest before the surge is repeated. Various forms of surged pulses are shown in Fig. 22.14.

All nervous and muscular activity is caused by minute electrical currents originating in the brain passing along nerves causing muscles to contract, i.e. motor nerves of the cerebrospinal system. A surged faradic type current will produce a similar effect; contracting muscles without the participation of the client, resembling natural muscular exercises.

There are many **benefits** derived from the use of the faradic current:

- toning up the muscles of the face, sagging contours will be improved and sluggish skin will appear more taut;
- the effects of ageing are delayed due to the improved blood circulation and increased cellular function;
- arches of the feet can be improved and oedema around the ankles can be reduced.

Units vary with manufacturers and, before any purchase is made, insist on a demonstration and investigate the machine yourself. With the concept of computerised machines it is necessary to familiarise yourself thoroughly with the unit.

The methods available to obtain the benefits are mainly the use of a button- or disc-handled electrode on the motor points or the use of facial electrodes.

An in-depth knowledge of anatomy is needed for a good, comfortable treatment. Preparation of the client for facial faradism is the same as for all electrical treatments – a thorough cleansing of the skin, followed by toning the area with a tonic or toner and drying with paper tissue.

For a faradic facial it is preferable for the client either to sit upright or to be in a semi-reclining position for you to observe the facial contours and the muscle tone. Therefore, to note contractions and operate the machine efficiently, you should sit facing the client.

Motor-point method

The motor point is normally the point at which the nerve enters the muscle or is in the belly of the muscle. A diagram showing the motor points of the face and neck is given, but as faces may differ the exact location of the point may also vary slightly (see Fig. 22.15).

As with galvanism the indifferent (passive) electrode should be well covered with damp lint or viscose sponge material and placed between the scapulae on the lower cervical vertebrae. If the passive electrode is hand-held, give this to the client.

Cover the active button electrode with damp lint previously soaked in a 1 per cent solution. This will help conductivity, especially if the epidermis is dry or if there is fatty tissue present which can act as an insulator.

Check the machine, test the current, then ensure that the intensity control is at zero. Explain to the client that the initial reaction will be a prickling sensation before a contraction is felt.

Commence at the neck and place the active button electrode on to the motor point in the sternocleidomastoid muscle. Slowly turn up the intensity until a contraction is seen or felt. If the client should advise you that the feeling is uncomfortable or the contraction is not smooth, return the potentiometer to zero as inevitably it will mean that you have missed the exact position of the motor point. Move the electrode to a different placing and start again. When the desired effect has been obtained 6–8 contractions will suffice before moving on to the next motor point at the platysma (see Fig. 22.16).

Work gently and carefully all over one side of the face and as you reach the temporalis, orbicularis occuli, frontalis and corrugator, turn down the intensity as the tissues here are much finer. Work down the other side of the face and neck, regulating the intensity.

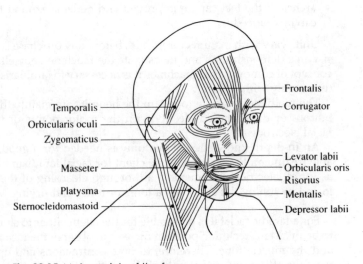

Fig. 22.15 Motor points of the face

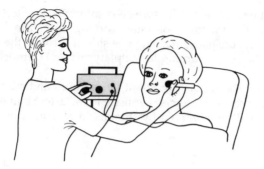

Fig. 22.16 Faradic, use of button electrode

Visible contractions are obviously the most satisfying for an operator, but the client may feel these positively with a subliminal current. A constant rapport with the client will ensure a smooth effective treatment. It is important not to distort the face or produce unnatural movements; the entire treatment is meant to uplift the tissues by improving muscle tone. The intensity control must be seen and be within easy reach of the operator to enable continual adjustment of the current.

Facial electrode method

These electrodes contain both the active and passive electrodes within the head and are therefore larger than a button electrode. This is a more comfortable application but care must be taken as this electrode will exercise more muscles at one time (see Fig. 22.17).

As before, cover the electrode with lint previously soaked in a salt solution. Test the current then reduce the intensity to zero.

Place the electrode on the sternocleidomastoid. Increase the intensity of the current slowly until the client can feel the prickling sensation and

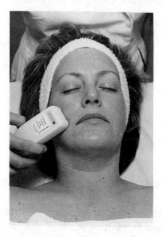

Fig. 22.17 Use of Faradic facial electrodes

slight contraction. Providing the surge is comfortable the electrode may be stroked up the muscle. Continue working with firm but gentle movements along the platysma, over one side of the face, the forehead, other side of the face, returning to the platysma and sternocleidomastoid muscle.

The treatment should last for about ten minutes and may be given once a week. Never over-exercise a muscle to the extent that it becomes fatigued. This will be observed by tremors or slowing down of contractions.

Contra-indications

- high blood pressure
- vascular complexions and very sensitive skins
- sinus congestion
- migraine
- care should be taken if the client has metal in the mouth, i.e. numerous fillings or bridge work, to ensure that contractions do not cause discomfort
- highly strung nervous clients

Self assessment

- what are the benefits of

    (a) direct high-frequency, and
    (b) indirect high-frequency?

- explain the purpose of fulguration
- give a list of the contra-indications for high-frequency
- for what purpose is a galvanic current used in beauty therapy?
- explain cations and anions
- explain

    (a) the benefits of a negatively charged cathode as the active electrode, and
    (b) the benefits of a positively charged anode as the active electrode

- explain the purpose of

    (a) desincrustation, and
    (b) iontophoresis

- give the contra-indications for both

    (a) desincrustation, and
    (b) iontophoresis

- what action would you take if grey spots appeared during a galvanic treatment?
- what benefits are derived from the use of a faradic current?
- draw a diagram giving the main motor points of the face
- what are the contra-indications for facial faradic treatment?

23 Electrical brush-cleansing and massage

Brush-cleansing

This is another form of deep-cleansing especially useful for sallow or discoloured skins. The equipment can be free-standing or combined in a facial stacking unit. The control panel usually has an on/off switch, a regulator controlling the speed of the brush, a switch denoting which direction the brush is rotating (clockwise or anti-clockwise) and a socket for the brush holder. Inside the unit there is a variable-speed motor which rotates and vibrates the brushes. Usually there are three or four different brush sizes with varying bristle composition (see Fig. 23.1).

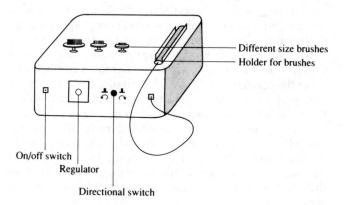

Fig. 23.1 Brush-cleansing machine

The *benefits* are:

- general deep cleanse
- aids desquamation
- improved vascular circulation
- improves sallow complexion by increasing skin temperature and colour.

Method for brush-cleansing

1. Prepare the client as for a facial massage and cover the eyes with damp cotton wool.

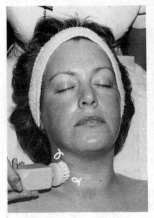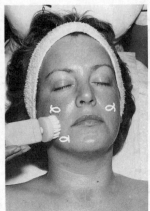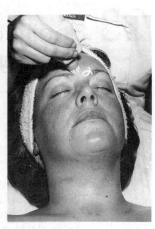

Fig. 23.2 Brush cleansing

2. Apply a water-based preparation over the face and neck. You can make your own preparation by mixing 50 per cent mineral oil, 15 per cent beeswax, 1 per cent borax and 34 per cent distilled water.
3. Push the selected brush, slightly damp, into the brush holder and place on the sternocleidomastoid. Turn on the regulator to the required speed and *stroke* up the muscle. Let the brush rotate without any pressure, otherwise the speed will drop and you will soon spoil the bristles. Change the rotation of the brush after two or three strokes and repeat before moving on to the other side of the neck.
4. Carefully brush-cleanse as above under the mandible before coming on to the triangularis. To avoid changing the size of the brush you may prefer to continue up to the zygomatics, frontalis etc., but you must check the speed especially over bony areas (Fig. 23.2).
5. Use a smaller brush for the orbicularis oculi, procerus, nasalis, orbicularis oris and mentalis, increasing and decreasing the speed of the brush to suit the various skin conditions.
6. The entire cleanse should take about eight minutes to complete and the residue of the cleansing product can be removed with damp sponges.
7. Clean the bristles of the brushes well and ensure that all particles of the cleansing product or make-up are removed before sterilisation.

Contra-indications

- fine textured or highly sensitive skins
- acute acne or inflamed areas
- over dilated capillaries
- skin infections or disease

Brush-massage

This is a stimulating form of massage to improve skin texture and is good for sallow, discoloured, scarred or pigmented skins.

Method for brush-massage

1. The preparation of the client is the same as for a brush-cleanse.
2. Apply cream or talc, according to the skin type, to the face and neck.
3. Select the brush required and, if using cream, ensure that the bristles are fairly firm. The sequence of the strokes is the same as that used for the brush-cleanse, but more time and strokes are required over each area. Again the speed of the brush must be reduced over sensitive or bony areas. The massage should take about twenty minutes to complete.
4. Remove the cream or talc and examine the skin. A suitable mask may be applied, taking into account that this massage has a greater stimulating effect, promoting a quicker vascular response than manual techniques and that erythema may be present.
5. Clean the bristles of the brush thoroughly in a mild detergent before sterilisation.

Contra-indications

- fine textured or crêpey skins
- sensitive skins
- pustular acne or inflamed areas
- skin infections or disease
- dilated capillaries
- mature skins where there is a distention of surface tissue.

Self assessment

- what are the benefits of brush cleansing?
- how would you prepare a client for brush cleansing?
- how would you prepare your own water-based preparation for brush cleansing?
- which brush would you use for cleansing the orbicularis oculi?
- give contra-indications for a brush cleanse
- what is the purpose of a brush massage?
- when would you avoid giving a facial brush massage?

24 Use of steamers, vaporisers, aerosols and hot towels

Use of steamers

The purpose of a steamer unit is to apply a warm vapour to the face, neck, shoulders and back. There are numerous models available, and some have the addition of a high-pressure mercury vapour lamp (HPMV) to produce ozone or it may be designed with a glass container for lotions to be atomised.

The benefits of vaporisation are:

- slight perspiration is induced which helps the skin to rid itself of impurities
- pores are opened, effecting a deep cleanse
- circulation is increased
- the stratum corneum is softened and comedones can be expressed more easily
- sebaceous glands are stimulated.

With the addition of the HPMV lamp emitting ultra-violet radiation, some of the oxygen of the air will convert into ozone which helps to destroy bacteria, promotes healing and sterilises the skin.

The machine whether hand-held or free-standing will comprise a container for the water, a small electric immersion heater, a tube with an outlet nozzle, pilot lights, switch mechanisms, air vents for machines combining steam and ozone, a small HPMV lamp and a switch for ozone steaming.

It should be mentioned here that when switching on the ozone control, there is a distinct smell, and a slight noise from the head. The steam vapour changes into a bluish-white cloud. Newer models are now fitted with safety features which guard against over-heating and the container running dry. They also have an adjustable steam force to ensure client comfort.

Method of application

1. Ensure that the container has sufficient water. Distilled water is preferred to prevent the deposition of scale and also tap water will often contain some chemicals which may cause spitting.
2. Plug in the appliance. Ensure that the nozzle is directed away from the client and turn on the vapour switch to permit the water to heat.
3. Prepare the client as for a facial treatment and cleanse the skin.

4. Place the client in a semi-upright position to ensure an even distribution of the vapour. Again, talking to the client and explaining the treatment will alleviate any anxiety. During treatment never leave the room or cubicle (see Fig. 24.1).
5. Cover the eyes and any area of sensitivity with *dry* cotton wool.
6. Check that the water has heated and that the steam is flowing well. Turn the nozzle towards the client, and position it so that it will evenly bathe the forehead, face or jaw and neck area.
7. You will find that it will be necessary to reposition the nozzle end of the machine to complete the treatment from the forehead to the base of the neck. The switch to ozone vapour if required is made once the steaming has begun and at a time you consider to be beneficial.
8. The following are guidelines for the approximate application time with suggested distances between the nozzle end and the skin.

Normal skins to maintain texture – at a distance of 12 in (30 cm):

5 mins on jaw and neck area
5 mins on full face
5 mins on forehead.

Sensitive skins (any small area of thread veins cover with dry cotton wool) – at a distance of 14 in (35 cm):

5 mins on jaw and neck area
5 mins on full face
5 mins on forehead.

Pale, faded or dry skins – at a distance of 10 in (26 cm) to stimulate sebaceous glands and increase blood circulation:

7 mins on jaw and neck area
7 mins on full face
7 mins on forehead.

Mature or dehydrated skins at a distance of 15 in (38 cm) for a regenerating effect and increased cellular function:

3 mins on jaw and neck area
2 mins on full face
2 mins on forehead.

Greasy skins at a distance of 10 in (26 cm) to heal and disinfect the skin:

7 mins on jaw and neck area
7 mins on full face
7 mins on forehead.

If comedones are present these can be gently expressed more easily after the treatment has been completed. Ozone steaming may be used on the back to help disinfect the skin to promote the healing of blemished areas.

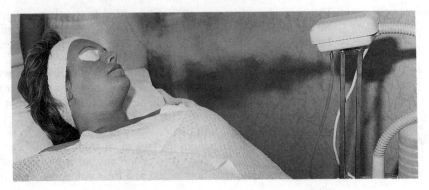

Fig. 24.1 Use of facial steamer

9. If you have used ozone steaming turn off the switch and leave the vapour steaming for two minutes before turning it off.
10. Turn off the machine, place away from the client, remove the plug and wind up the flex carefully.
11. The skin should be gently wiped with damp cotton wool. If no further treatment is required apply a skin toner to close the pores.
12. After the client has left ensure that the container is refilled with distilled water.

Contra-indications

- very sensitive skins
- acne rosacea
- Skin irritations, cuts or abrasions
- inflammation
- infection
- sunburn
- extremely vascular skins

Ozone steaming is restricted in some overseas countries. This is probably due to the fact that the USA Food and Drug Administration research findings discovered ozone to be a contributory factor in lung cancer. However, it is doubted that the small amount inhaled during a treatment given, even weekly, would subscribe towards this disease.

Vaporisers

These are usually hand-held appliances often combined with other small facial equipment giving pressure spray toning. A variety of toning and astringent lotions can be prepared for varying skin conditions.

The fine spray is directed on to the face and neck at a distance of approximately 9–12 in (22–30 cm). In order to complete the vacuum inside the container the index finger should be placed over the air outlet. Any surplus moisture forming can be removed with a sponge held in the other hand. For client comfort small eyepads can be used to prevent droplets of moisture forming in the inner eye.

There are large vaporisers available, whose spray jets produce a continuous stream of water. These are useful for the removal of setting-type masks. The client should sit upright, be protected with towels and hold a cuvette or plastic bowl under the chin. The client's eyes must be kept closed as the mask is sprayed off and, by directing the water in a downward movement, both mask fragments and excess water will be collected in the cuvette.

Aerosol sprays

These are commercially available and normally contain natural mineral water. By pressing down the cap at the top, the valve is opened and a fine mist is produced under pressure. This method is often used after exposure to the sun to refresh, moisturise and cool the skin. These sprays are not permitted in certain countries as they contravene environmental laws and these may also affect the UK in the future.

Hot towels

Hot towels have really been superseded by the facial steamer. However, if the latter is a low priority on your equipment-purchasing list the following will serve the purpose, giving the same effect.

You will need hot water close by – as hot as your hands can bear – and two or more towels.

1. Prepare the client as for a facial and cleanse the skin well.
2. Place damp cotton-wool pads over the eyes and sensitive areas.
3. Soak the towels in hot water and wring dry. Fold the towels lengthwise quickly and neatly – test on the inside of your arm first before placing on the face of your client.
4. Place the towels diagonally from the forehead across the zygomatics, across the jaw and neck, leaving the nostrils and mouth free (see Fig. 23.1).
5. The towels will have cooled on the face in about two to three minutes and will need to be removed. Therefore, to replace with fresh

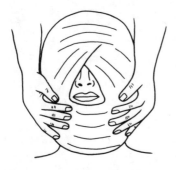

Fig. 24.2 Use of hot towels

hot towels quickly, keep spares in hot water and repeat the process for about ten minutes.

Self assessment

- what are the benefits of vaporisation?
- give suggested application times and distances when using a facial steamer for:

  (a) dehydrated skins
  (b) greasy skins.

25 Use of facial vacuum units

Vacuum (or suction) massage is an electrical method for lymphatic drainage. Units vary with each manufacturer but most will have large perspex or plastic cups for the body and small cups or ventouses for the face and neck which have round, oval, narrow or very small apertures (see Fig. 25.1). The control panel on the unit has an on/off switch, a pilot light and a vacuum gauge which registers the amount of pressure being exerted by the machine. There is also a regulating knob or switch controlling the intensity of the vacuum and a small hole which receives a flexible plastic tube. The selected ventouse is attached to the other end of this tube. The unit itself contains an electrically driven pump which draws the air from the ventouse and, when the latter is placed on the skin, the suction created by the partial vacuum pushes the tissue into the ventouse.

The **benefits** are:

- increased blood and lymph flow;
- increased elimination of waste products, i.e. removal of skin blockages, e.g. comedones, oily matter and dead keratinised cells;
- general deep cleanse;
- stimulates dry or dehydrated skin conditions.

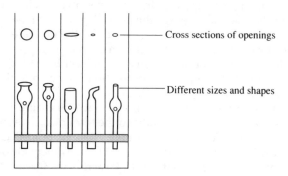

Fig. 25.1 Facial vacuum cups or ventouses

Method of application

1. Prepare the client as for facial massage and cleanse the skin well. Steaming will open the pores and soften the skin, preparing it for this treatment. It is also effective after galvanic desincrustation.
2. Put a drop of oil in the palm of your hand. Spread it over the hands

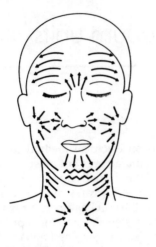

Fig. 25.2 Facial vacuum strokes

and then apply to the face and neck, giving it a very light coating of oil – just enough to allow the ventouse to glide over the skin. Wash your hands.

3. Choose the size of the ventouse required for the neck and test the strength of the suction on the back of your hand. The rise of the skin in the ventouse should not exceed 20 per cent, otherwise there is a risk of bruising, capillary dilation or distention of the skin. The ventouse must glide and not drag or pull the tissues. For lymphatic drainage the stroke may be followed immediately with a hand stroke. For the pattern of facial vacuum strokes see Figure 25.2.

4. As with manual lymphatic drainage you may prefer to stand in front of the client to massage the neck. Stroke down the profundus to the terminus (see Fig. 20.4). Cover the entire neck area, avoiding the trachea, and observe the skin reaction. If the purpose is to stimulate the area, the strokes may be quicker but still rhythmical.

5. Stroke under the mandible from the tip of the chin to the profundus and from there to the terminus.

6. Select appropriate ventouses for the face. Standing behind the client stroke from the temporalis to the terminus, covering the entire cheek area. Avoid any sensitive areas or dilated capillaries. Check the intensity at all times. Repeat for the other side of the face.

7. From the centre of the frontalis stroke across the forehead over the temporalis and through to the terminus. Cover the entire forehead and repeat for the other side of the face.

8. For the sides of the face, stroke from the sides of the nose to the angulus.

9. To treat the nose, chin, labial lines and eye area choose a smaller ventouse. Stroke down the labial lines to the nodes beneath the mandible.

10. For the chin, zig-zag lines are excellent when there is skin congestion and blackheads are present.

11. For the nose, the smallest aperture can be used with quick, short strokes to produce more concentrated suction pressure. The procerus should be stroked upwards towards the frontalis and corrugator.
12. While the oil is still on the face, give effleurage movements away from the face towards the terminus. This will counteract the acceleration of blood to the face by this treatment, which can, on occasions, give rise to headaches.
13. This treatment may also be given for the shoulders. The client will need to sit slightly forward and the strokes will start from the occiput over the trapezius to the acromion process covering the entire area. From the front of the client the strokes may be taken from the trapezius over the acromion along the top of the clavicle to the terminus. This will generally relax any tension in the area. Always remember to lower the intensity of the pressure over bony or delicate skin areas.
14. Remove the oil with damp cotton wool and continue with further treatment, i.e. a mask.
15. Ensure that cups etc. are well cleaned with diluted Savlon (or any similar antiseptic) and placed in a steriliser. If at any time cups/ventouses crack or chip these must be thrown away.

The length of the treatment will vary according to the purpose. A deep cleanse can be completed in 6 minutes whereas lymphatic drainage massage will take twice as long, i.e. 12–15 minutes.

Contra-indications

- thin or sensitive skin
- dilated capillaries
- pustular acne
- over or near scar tissue
- inflammation other than chilblains

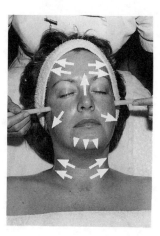

Fig. 25.3 Automatic intermittent suction

- delicate under-eye tissue
- crêpey or ageing skin.

Units are also available which have an automatic intermittent suction which provides a gentle tapping or patting action on the skin. These usually have two tubes with their ventouses. These are placed simultaneously on either side of the neck or face, and lymphatic drainage massage is applied (see Fig. 25.3).

Self assessment

- what are the benefits of vacuum suction?
- what ventouses would you use for the neck and chin areas?
- give a list of the contra-indications to the use of vacuum suction on the face.

26 Anatomy of the arm and hand

Bones of the arm and hand

The upper arm

This contains one bone, the **humerus**. It has a shaft (or diaphysis) and two extremities (or epiphyses). The upper extremity has a head; an anatomical neck; two tuberosities (i.e. elevations or protuberances) called the greater and the lesser; and intertubercular groove and surgical neck.

The head articulates with the glenoid cavity of the scapula to form a ball and socket joint.

The anatomical neck directly joins the head.

The greater tuberosity occupies the lateral part of the humerus and the lesser tuberosity occupies the anterior part of the humerus and they are the projections for adjacent muscles.

The shaft flattens as it approaches the lower extremity which is formed of two condyles (i.e. rounded eminences at the articular end of a bone, external and internal). The former, which is called the **trochlea**, articulates with the ulna and the latter, called the **capitulum**, articulates with the radius (see Fig. 26.1).

The lower arm

This has two bones, ulna and radius. The **ulna**, which is the larger (on the little finger side of the arm), has a shaft and two extremities. The upper extremity is strong and thick and enters into the elbow joint. The olecranon process, commonly known as the 'funny bone', projects up the back and fits into the olecranon fossa of the humerus. The latter prevents the backwards bending of the forearm which explains why it is a hinge joint. The projection on the anterior surface of the proximal end of the ulna is called the coronoid process. The trochlea of the humerus fits snugly between the olecranon and coronoid processes.

The shaft narrows to the carpal (wrist) area and the lower extremity is small with two eminences. The head joins the radius forming the inferior radioulna joint. The styloid process projects downwards from the back of the lower extremity.

The **radius** or outer bone (on the thumb side) of the lower arm has a shaft and two extremities. The upper extremity has a small head which

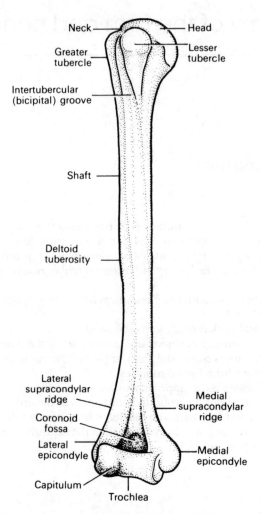

Neck

Head

Greater tubercle

Lesser tubercle

Intertubercular (bicipital) groove

Shaft

Deltoid tuberosity

Lateral supracondylar ridge

Medial supracondylar ridge

Coronoid fossa

Lateral epicondyle

Medial epicondyle

Capitulum

Trochlea

Fig. 26.1 The right humerus (anterior view)

articulates with the capitulum of the humerus and the sides of the head articulate with the radial notch of the ulna.

The shaft flattens and widens to the lower extremity and articulates with the scaphoid and lunate carpal bones and with the head of the ulna (see Fig. 26.2)

The wrist or carpus

This has eight carpal bones in two rows:

First row   scaphoid   boat shaped
               semi-luna (or lunate)   crescent shaped
               triquetrum
               pisiform

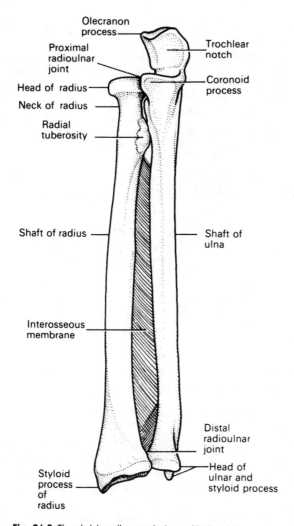

Fig. 26.2 The right radius and ulna with the interosseous membrane (Anterior view)

Second row   trapezium
trapezoid
capitate
hamate

The palm of the hand or metacarpus

This has five metacarpal bones. Each has a shaft and two extremities – carpal and distal, i.e. to the wrist and to the fingers (see Fig. 26.3).

Fingers or digits

These have 14 bones in all, 3 in each finger and 2 in the thumb.

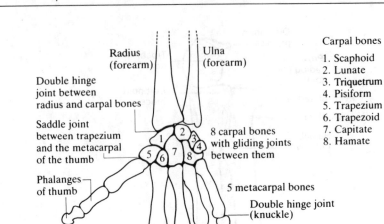

Carpal bones
1. Scaphoid
2. Lunate
3. Triquetrum
4. Pisiform
5. Trapezium
6. Trapezoid
7. Capitate
8. Hamate

Radius (forearm)

Ulna (forearm)

Double hinge joint between radius and carpal bones

Saddle joint between trapezium and the metacarpal of the thumb

8 carpal bones with gliding joints between them

Phalanges of thumb

5 metacarpal bones

Double hinge joint (knuckle)

Phalanges with hinge-joints between them

Fig. 26.3

Muscles of the arm and hand

Further anatomical terms are used to assist in the identification and use of muscles.

Abduct is to move away from the mid-line, e.g. the deltoid muscle is an abductor in as much as it lifts (or abducts) the upper arm.

Adduct is the opposite to abduct and it means to move towards the mid-line, e.g. the pectoralis major is used to move the arm across the chest.

Pronators turn the hand inward so that the palm faces down, e.g. pronator teres.

Supinators turn the hand outward so that the palm faces upward, e.g. brachioradialis.

Flexors bend the wrist and draw the fingers towards the forearm, e.g. flexor carpi radialis.

Extensors straighten the wrist, hand and fingers in a straight line, e.g. extensor carpi ulnaris.

The muscles of the arm are detailed in Table 26.1 together with Fig. 26.4.

The muscles of the hand, detailed in Table 26.2 and Figs 26.5 and 26.6, are generally divided into three groups:

1. the thenar eminence;
2. the hypothenar eminence; and
3. the adductor pollicis and palmar and interosseous muscles.

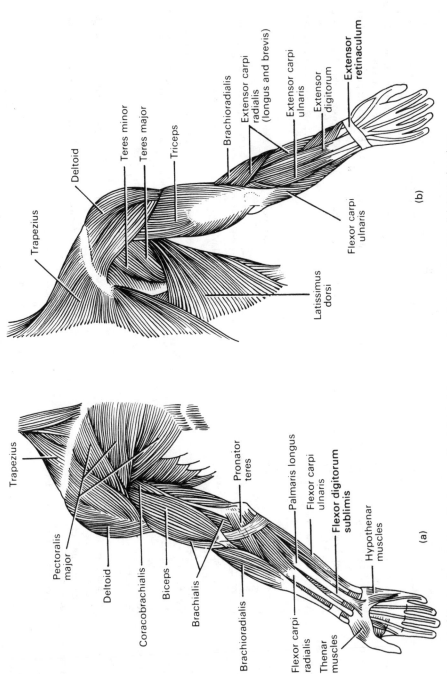

Trapezius

Deltoid

Teres minor

Teres major

Triceps

Brachioradialis

Extensor carpi radialis (longus and brevis)

Extensor carpi ulnaris

Extensor digitorum

Extensor retinaculum

Latissimus dorsi

Flexor carpi ulnaris

(b)

Trapezius

Pectoralis major

Deltoid

Coracobrachialis

Biceps

Brachialis

Brachioradialis

Flexor carpi radialis

Thenar muscles

Pronator teres

Palmaris longus

Flexor carpi ulnaris

Flexor digitorum sublimis

Hypothenar muscles

(a)

Fig. 26.4 The main muscles which move the joints of the upper limb (a) Anterior view (b) Posterior view

Table 26.1 Main muscles of the arm

Name	Location	Origin	Insertion	Action
Deltoid	Shoulder	Clavicle and acromion process of scapula	Lateral side of the humerus	Abducts upper arm. Assists in flexion and extension of upper arm
Pectoralis major	Across the chest to the arm	Medial half of clavicle, sternum and costal cartilages of true ribs	Humerus (greater tubercle)	Flexes upper arm and adducts upper arm anteriorly
Latissimus dorsi	Below the shoulder to the pelvis	Vertebrae and ilium crest (part of the pelvis)	Humerus (intertubercular groove)	Extends upper arm. Adducts upper arm posteriorly
Triceps brachii	Posterior and anterior upper arm	Scapula and humerus	Olecranon of the ulna	Extensor of the lower arm, extends arm forward
Biceps brachii	Anterior upper arm	Scapula	Radius	Supinates forearm and hand
Brachialis	Lower part of anterior upper arm	Humerus	Ulna	Flexes pronated forearm
Brachioradialis	Anterior aspect of lower arm	Humerus	Radius (styloid process)	Flexes forearm and hand
Pronator teres	Anterior aspect of lower arm	Humerus	Radius	Pronates and flexes forearm
Palmaris longus	Anterior aspect of lower arm	Humerus	Fascia of palm	Flexes hand
Flexor carpi radialis	Anterior aspect of lower arm	Humerus	Base of second metacarpal	Flexes forearm and hand
Flexor carpi ulnaris	Anterior aspect of lower arm	Humerus and ulna	Pisiform bone and 3, 4, 5, metacarpals	Flexes and adducts hand
Flexor digitorum sublimis	Anterior aspect above the wrist	Ulna and radius	Terminates in long tendons passing through the palm of the hand to the fingers	
Extensor carpi ulnaris	Posterior aspect of lower arm	Humerus and ulna	Base of fifth metacarpal	Extends and adducts hand
Extensor carpi radialis longus	Posterior aspect of lower arm	Humerus	Base of second metacarpal	Extends and adducts hand
Extensor carpi radialis brevis	Posterior aspect of lower arm	Humerus	Base of second and third metacarpals	Extends hand
Extensor retinaculum	Wrist		Strong fibrous band	

Table 26.2 Muscles of the hand

Name	Location	Origin	Action
Thenar eminence	Thumb		
Abductor pollicis brevis		Flexor retinaculum	Draws the thumb forward to the palm of the hand and rotates it medially
Opponens pollicis		Tubercle of the trapezium	Flexes the metacarpal bone of the thumb
Flexor pollicis brevis		Flexor retinaculum and tubercle of the trapezium	Flexes the proximal phalanx of the thumb
Hypothenar eminence	Thumb		
Opponens digiti minimi		Tubercle of trapezium and flexor retinaculum	Opposes thumb
Flexor digiti minimi brevis		Hook of hamate bone	Flexes little finger
Abductor digiti minimi		Pisiform bone and tendon of flexor carpi ulnaris	Abducts little finger
Abductor pollicis		Two heads: oblique: 2nd metacarpal, capitate and trapezoid; transverse: 3rd metacarpal	Adducts thumb
Dorsal interossei	Back of hand	2 heads from adjacent sides of metacarpal bones	Abduct, flex proximal and extend middle and distal phalanges
Palmar interossei	Palm of hand	Sides of the 1st, 2nd, 4th and 5th metacarpal bones	Adduct, flex proximal and extend middle and distal phalanges
Lumbricals	Hand, linking one tendon to another	Tendons of deep flexor muscle of the fingers	Flex proximal and extend middle and distal phalanges

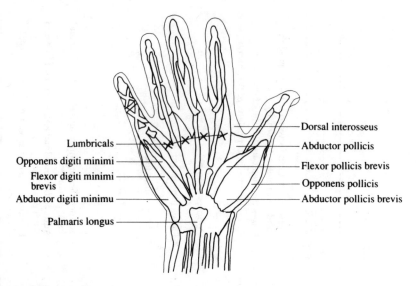

Fig. 26.5 Muscles of the palmar surface of the hand

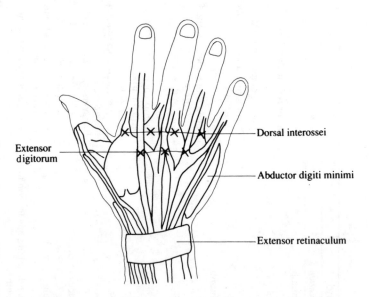

Fig. 26.6 Muscles of the dorsal surface of the hand

Circulatory system of the arm and hand

The main arteries are shown in Fig. 26.7 and are:

- brachial
- radial

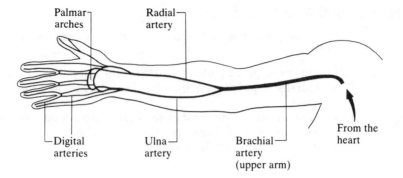

Fig. 26.7 Main arteries of the arm and hand

- ulna
- palmar arch deep and superficial
- digital

The main veins are shown in Fig. 26.8 and are:

- cephalic
- basilic
- median basilic
- median

The main veins in the hand are:

- palmar venous plexus
- palmar digital veins

(Dorsal metacarpal and digital veins are not shown on Fig. 26.8)

The lymph nodes are:

- axillary
- supratrochlear

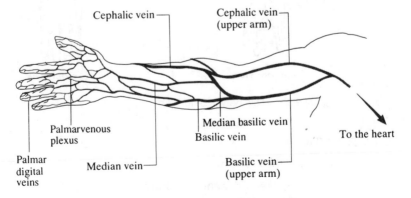

Fig. 26.8 Main veins of the arm and hand

Nerves of the arm and hand

The principal nerves are sensory-motor. They are shown in Fig. 26.9 and are:

- **ulnaris**, supplying ulna side of the arm and palm of the hand;
- **radialis**, supplying the thumb side of the arm and the back of the hand;
- **median**, supplying most of the flexor muscles on the front of the forearm, the thumb and the skin of the palm;
- **digital**, which supplies the phalanges.

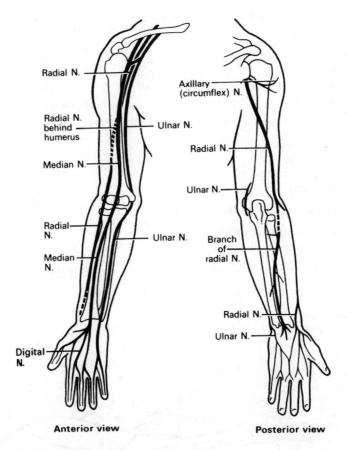

Fig. 26.9 The main nerves of the arm

Self assessment

- name the bones of:

    (a) the upper and lower arm
    (b) the wrist

- give the origin, insertion and action of the following muscles:

    (a) deltoid
    (b) latissimus dorsi
    (c) brachialis
    (d) palmaris longus

- name the main arteries from the heart to the hands
- which nerves supply:

    (a) the ulna side of the arm and palm of the hand
    (b) the phalanges.

27 Nails (structure and growth)

Structure of the nail

The technical term for the nail is 'onyx'. Like hair, nails are appendages of the skin, which develop from an embryo state as a jelly-like substance to the hard keratin of an adult nail by about the twentieth week of foetal life.

Nails are protective translucent plates covering the tips of the digits. These plates are composed of horny epidermal cells. The most important constituent is keratin, which is a protein containing an amount of sulphur and very small quantities of calcium, arsenic, phosphorous and trace metals.

Nails consist of three parts.

1. The **nail plate** (or body) which rests on the nail bed and extends from the nail root to the free edge. It does not contain nerves or blood vessels.
2. The **nail root** is at the base of the nail underneath the skin originating from the matrix.
3. The **free edge** is that part of the nail plate which extends over the finger/toe tip and is grey/white in colour. There is a dividing line which separates the pink portion overlying the nail bed from the free edge.

There are structures adjoining the nail and these are:

4. The **nail bed** which lies immediately below the nail plate. The soft tissue is arranged in ridges instead of papillae as in the skin. It is supplied with blood vessels and nerves.
5. The **matrix** is that part of the nail bed which extends beneath the nail root. It is the most important and the most sensitive part of the nail and contains nerves, lymph and blood vessels.

   A bad manicure/pedicure, with digging or poking or using a nail brush on this area can dent or damage the matrix. As nails grow these dents will also grow out but will break off at the free edge.
6. The **lunula** (or half-moon) is the intermediate stage between the matrix and the nail plate. Its pale colour is due to the lessened blood supply. It is often prominent, which means that the matrix lies very near to the cuticle and therefore very sensitive as it is soft. If the lunula is not so well defined, the matrix will lie well back and therefore the nail-hardening process will be nearer to the cuticle and less likely to be damaged by exterior pressure.
7. The **cuticle** is the natural fold of overlapping epidermis. It should

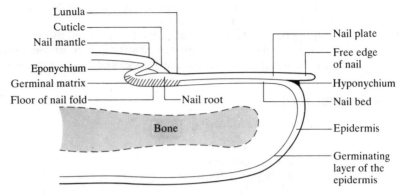

Fig. 27.1 Section through the end of a finger to show structural relations of the nail

be in the form of a fine rim surrounding the lunula, which should be even and unattached to the nail plate.

8. The **eponychium** is the extension of the cuticle at the base of the nail plate. It is also known as the nail fold or scarf skin.
9. The **perionychium** is the portion of the cuticle surrounding the entire nail border.
10. The **hyponychium** is the portion of the epidermis upon which the nail plate rests and under the free edge.
11. The **nail grooves** are furrows which reach up to the finger/toe tip. As the nail plate grows it moves along these grooves.
12. The **nail walls** are simply the folds of skin overlapping the sides of the nail plate (see Fig. 27.1).

Growth of the nail

Nail growth begins at the matrix and normally takes about six months to grow from there to the free edge. The germinative zone of the nail bed consists of two parts. The part between the root of the nail and the lunula is concerned with the growth of the nail, the epidermal cells gradually being hardened by keratinisation and converted into the nail substance. The part beneath the rest of the nail plate is thinner and provides a surface over which the growing nail can glide (nail grooves).

As already mentioned the matrix and the nail bed are well supplied by blood vessels which bring nutrients and oxygen to the growing nail. There are also numerous sensitive nerves which explain why pain is experienced when a nail is injured by pressure or when a nail is torn below the free edge.

The average rate of growth for an adult nail is about 0.0195 in (0.5 mm) a week. As ultra-violet rays stimulate cell division, nails grow faster in summer than in winter. The nail on the middle finger appears to grow the fastest and the thumbnail the slowest. Children's nails will grow more quickly than adults and elderly people's nails grow more slowly due to the lessening supply of keratin. Toenails grow slowly but they are usually thicker and harder.

If the nail bed is injured after the loss of a nail this usually results in a badly formed nail. To encourage strong nails advise a sensible diet, adequate rest and avoiding hard knocks or bruising to the nail.

Self assessment

- describe the following:

    (a) lunula
    (b) nail grooves
    (c) hyponychium
    (d) cuticle

- what is the average rate of growth for an adult nail?
- why do nails grow faster in summer?
- what part of the nail contains nerves, lymph and blood vessels?
- what can happen when the nail bed is injured?

28 Nails (irregularities or disorders and diseases)

Irregularities or disorders

These come within the scope of the beauty therapist, but when infection, soreness or irritation is present, the client should be referred to a doctor.

A normal healthy nail is firm, flexible and slightly pink. The surface should be smooth without any hollows or wavy ridges.

Fragilitas unguium (brittle nails)

This condition is often caused by an inadequate diet but there are other contributory factors and these could include continual use of nail polish, hard chalky water, frequent immersion of the hands in hot water, detergents and disinfectants, anaemia, rheumatism, illness e.g. hypothyrodism, or a nail infection, occupational hazards or a genetic factor. Burns can injure the nail and can, in severe cases, destroy the matrix. Too much exposure to X-rays may also injure the nail, making it brittle.

For treatment, clip the nails short and square and with the fine side of the emery board gently file the entire surface and edge of the nail plate. It will look dull but the application of a paste polish and buffing the nail will increase the circulation to the nail area and will also give a shine to the nail. If the free edge is long enough a nail hardener may be applied to the tip.

Your advice to the client would obviously call for a balanced diet with fresh fruit and vegetables, dairy produce, vitamins and protein. Also advise the use of rubber gloves for wet work and cotton gloves for dry work. Rubber gloves should not be worn for any length of time as they cause the hands to perspire and the skin loses its natural oils (see Fig. 28.1).

Longitudinal ridges

These are usually caused by an illness, faulty circulation or rheumatism. The ridges run from the lunula to the free edge.

The nail plate becomes dry and brittle and, if not cared for, may open up and expose the nail bed. Again smoothing down the ridges with the fine side of the emery board, using paste polish or a base coat and a nail polish containing nylon fibres will protect the nail plate. There are products on the market, ridge fillers, which will help to fill in ridges.

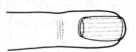

Fig. 28.1 Fragilitas unguium   **Fig. 28.2** Longitudinal ridges

Read the manufacturer's instructions as these can be applied before or after the base coat. However, should the nail bed be exposed, cover it with a very narrow strip of adhesive to prevent infection. In an older person you will find fine longitudinal lines but this is only a sign of age (see Fig. 28.2).

Transverse ridges (Beau's lines)

These run horizontally across the nail plate. They are usually the result of an illness, i.e. measles or pneumonia when a temporary interference with the formation of nail keratin can occur. A ridge will occur in the matrix and will show as the nail grows. A bad manicure/pedicure can also result in transverse ridges, i.e. damage to the cuticle affecting the matrix. When chilblains occur the swelling can press into the matrix and again a transverse ridge will appear on the nail plate. If these ridges are seen close to the cuticle do not attempt to push back the cuticle; just apply cuticle cream to the area with a cotton bud. In the unlikely event that the transverse ridge opens up use a narrow piece of adhesive (see Fig. 28.3).

Leukonychia

These are white spots which appear on the nail plate and are usually caused by an external injury to the matrix, or a nervous disorder. There is a separation in the nail cells allowing air to permeate the cells. They will grow out but treat the nail gently as the nail plate will be fragile.

Advice to the client would be to protect the nails whenever possible, using rubber or cotton gloves (see Fig. 28.4).

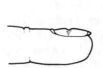

Fig. 28.3 Beau's line   **Fig. 28.4** Leukonychia

Onychophagia

This is the technical name for nail biting which varies in degrees from person to person. A client may have bitten the nail down below the free edge and the surrounding tissue looks red and ragged. Another client may have bitten so low as to lose half the nail, the shape of the finger tip is bulbous and the cuticle has been bitten back and left ragged and inflamed. This is nearly always caused by nervous tension or worry and gradually becomes a bad habit.

There are commercially available bitter-tasting paints for the nails which will deter some clients, but they do not treat the cause. Your immediate task is to clip away hanging pieces of nail or skin and clear the cuticles. Gaining the confidence of the client is important and try to see her at least once a week. Suggest the use of wearing gloves when possible, especially when studying, reading or watching television.

Unfortunately, nail biting is often an unconscious habit, but if you can get the client to leave one nail alone to see the improvement, progress can often be made with other nails.

Onychauxis (hypertrophy)

This is an over-growth of the nail, usually in thickness rather than in length. It is often caused by an internal disturbance or a nervous disorder. If there is any infection a manicure/pedicure should not be undertaken.

Onychotrophia

As the name would imply an atrophy or wasting away of the nail. It becomes smaller and can shed entirely. The causes are various from an injury to the matrix, nervous disorders to illness, i.e. tuberculosis or diabetes.

The nail must be treated very gently and the client should seek medical advice and wear gloves to protect the nail plate (see Fig. 28.5).

Pterygium

This is the forward growth of the cuticle which adheres to the base of the nail plate. Advise the client to use cuticle cream every night and gently to push back the growth. When giving a manicure/pedicure try to lift the cuticle and gently push it back. Unless you are very experi-

Fig. 28.5
Onychotrophia

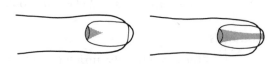

(a)   **(b)**
Fig. 28.6 Pterygium (a) early stage (b) later stage

Fig. 28.7 Onychorrhexis

enced and know how to cut the cuticle this should not be attempted. Simply cutting all round the cuticles will thicken them and leave hangnails. A warm oil treatment (described in Chapter 29) should help to improve the condition (see Fig. 28.6).

Onychorrhexis

This is a term describing split or brittle nails, which are often caused by an external injury or by glandular disturbances. However, they can be caused by excessive use of cuticle solvents and nail polish remover. It is therefore important that you use these nail cosmetics with care if several manicures are being given every day. Any split should be treated as for transverse ridges (see p. 264 and Fig. 28.7).

Hangnails (agnails)

This is where the cuticle is split or where there is splitting of narrow strips of nail along the nail groove. The former is usually due to the dryness of the cuticle and the latter often caused by a careless manicure/pedicure. A warm oil treatment will help to soften the cuticle and then clip away any part of the skin or cuticle which is likely to catch in clothing etc. and tear.

Warn the client about possible infection and advise nail care, especially at night.

Eggshell nails

These can appear quite healthy, but cannot stand up to daily wear and tear because they are so thin. They usually peel off leaving no free edge. This condition can be caused by internal disorders and, in liaison with the client's doctor, advice should be given for a nutritional diet. Poor circulation may result in weak nails, digestive disturbances and vitamin deficiencies may impair their growth. The nails can be helped by using cuticle massage cream, suitable gloves, avoiding external injury and immersion in water. Cuticle removers, nail polish and false nails (or extensions) should be avoided until the condition improves.

Blue nails

These are mainly attributed to poor blood circulation and possibly a heart condition. As a beauty therapist there is little you can do and a plain manicure/pedicure may be given.

Bruised nail

This usually results from an external injury and bleeding in the nail bed. The dried blood adheres to the nail and makes the nail plate appear discoloured but as the nail grows this too will grow out with it. A plain manicure may be given but avoid any pressure and treat the nail gently.

Nail diseases

Onychosis is the technical term applied to any nail disease. Although it is not within your field to treat, it is important that you should be able to recognise a disease and advice the client to see a doctor immediately. *Never* give a manicure/pedicure.

Onychomycosis

This is ringworm (or tinea unguium) of the nails. It is a fungal infection which invades the free edge and spreads to the root. People who do a great deal of gardening without wearing gloves may get this infectious disease (see Fig. 28.8). It is recognisable by:

1. whitish patches that can be scraped off the nail;
2. long yellow streaks within the nail plate;
3. the infected part of the nail is thick, spongy and discoloured;

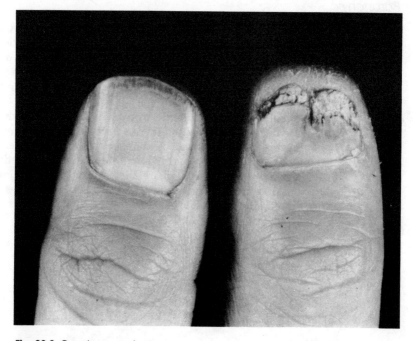

Fig. 28.8 Onychomycosis

4. if the deepest layers of the nail are invaded, the infected layers peel off to expose the diseased part of the nail bed.

Tinea

This is a ringworm of the hands caused by a fungus. It is a highly contagious disease and is recognised by red circular patches or rings over the hands and is often very irritating. Like onychomycosis, the cause is usually due to external damage through coming into contact with infection through animals, gardening and even nursing. It is a persistent and virulent type of fungus which can attack the nail plate and matrix.

Athlete's foot (Tinea pedis)

This is a fungus infection of the skin of the foot. It can be seen between the toes as thick white skin or as watery blisters. It can appear on the soles of the feet and spread to the nail walls and infect the nailbed.

Onychitis

This is inflammation of the matrix of a nail.

Paronchyia

Most infections of the nails originate in the folds of tissue around them and inflammation of this area is called paronychia. An infection may be caused by staphylococci, streptococci or other bacteria or a yeastlike fungus gaining an entrance through a hangnail or a break in the skin. It causes a painful swelling around the nail with red, shiny skin and often there is a pus formation present.

If this condition is not treated, paronychia may spread to the nail bed and cause further inflammation there which is known as onychia.

Paronychia is often caused by damage to the cuticle, i.e. biting or picking at the cuticle or a bad manicure/pedicure. Occupational hazards play an important role where clients' hands are continually immersed in water, detergents or chemicals. Illness, i.e. diabetes, may also cause this condition (see Fig. 28.9).

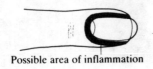

Possible area of inflammation

Fig. 28.9 Paronychia

Onychia

An extension of paronychia is the inflammation of the nail bed where bacteria grow under the nail. The nail may change colour and in extreme cases onychia may cause the nail to separate from the nail bed.

Psoriasis

This is recognised by minute pittings or holes scattered over the nail plate affecting one or more nails. Silvery scales may also form on the nail fold, the nail bed or under the free edge (see Fig. 28.10).

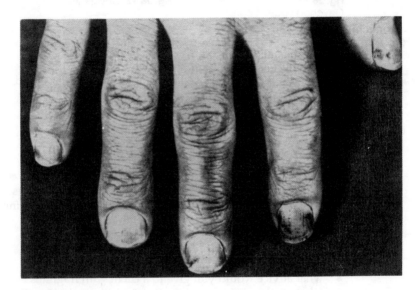

Fig. 28.10 Psoriasis

Eczema

As this disease can be found on the terminal phalanges it will often involve the nail fold. The nails are often pitted and ridged and when the cuticle becomes infected the whole area is vulnerable to inflammation. It is recognised by its smell and weeping condition under the nail plate.

Onychocryptosis

The technical name for ingrown nails where the nail grows into the sides of the flesh of the digit. This may be caused by filing too deep into the corners of the nail or by failing to correct hangnails. Do not attempt to correct an ingrown nail in the toes; always refer the client to a chiropodist.

Onychogryposis

This is an abnormal elongation and twisting of the nails, giving a claw-like appearance (see Fig. 28.11).

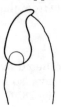

Fig. 28.11
Onychogryposis

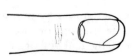

Fig. 28.12 Onycholysis

Onycholysis

This denotes a loosening or separation of a nail from its bed without shedding. It is usually caused by an internal disorder or a disease (see Fig. 28.12).

Onychopyma

This is a term used to denote a swelling of the nails.

It is very important if you have come into contact with any disease, or have any doubts of a disease, to wash your hands and use surgical spirit all over the hands, not only to prevent you from catching the disease but to prevent any cross-infection to another client.

Self assessment

- what advice would you give to a client with fragilitas unguium?
- what is the difference between longitudinal ridges and Beau's lines?
- describe the condition of

    (a) onychophagia
    (b) pterygium
    (c) agnails

- how is onychomycosis recognised?
- how would you recognise tinea and tinea pedis?
- what is onychia?

29 Manicure (including nail cosmetics) and massage of the arms and hands

Purpose of a manicure

Well-manicured nails are vital to a groomed appearance and regular attentive care is necessary to keep the nail shape and cuticles in trim. The procedure files the nails to an acceptable length, frees the cuticle and nail wall from the nail plate, thereby avoiding the risk of hangnails.

Nail cosmetics

The following are the main products used on the nails.

Nail polish removers

The purpose of these is to remove polish quickly and efficiently without excessive dehydrating effects on the nail plate and skin.

Liquid types of polish remover contain solvents (i.e. amyl acetate, ethyl acetate or butyl acetate) with the addition of glycerol or lanolin to counteract any drying effect of the solvents. Acetone is rarely used now as it does seem to degrease the nail plate and skin.

Cream polish removers are O/W emulsions containing oil (i.e. mineral oil or castor oil in the oil phase) and about 60 per cent of the solvents are therefore less degreasing than liquid removers.

Cuticle cream

There are available milks or creams but the latter are more popular as they contain a larger proportion of oil and act as an emollient to soften the cuticle skin. The constituents of the cream usually include beeswax, borax, liquid paraffin and petroleum jelly.

Cuticle remover

The purpose of this nail cosmetic is to loosen and release the cuticle when it encroaches too far over the nail plate. It generally consists of 2 per cent potassium hydroxide, 20 per cent glycerol or lanolin and 78 per cent distilled water. As the potassium hydroxide is a caustic alkali it will soften the keratin and therefore tend to dry the nail and surrounding skin tissue. It also acts as a nail bleach removing discoloration, i.e. nicotine stains.

Buffing paste or powder

The paste is usually composed of a derivative of jeweller's paste and the buffing powder contains talc or kaolin and stannic acid. The friction caused during the buffing increases blood circulation in the nail bed. Buffing also helps to minimise ridges and makes for a much smoother nail base for the application of nail polish.

Nail white pencil

The pencil is composed of a soap base containing a white pigment, i.e. titanium dioxide. The pencil is wetted first and used to whiten the underneath part of the free edge of the nail. It is very useful for a client who prefers to wear a colourless polish or only wishes the nails to be buffed.

Nail bleaches

These may also be used for whitening under the free edge but in the main they are useful to remove nicotine and vegetable stains on the nail plate and surrounding skin. These can be used as a product, i.e. cream or paste containing titanium dioxide, talc, oils, petroleum jelly and zinc peroxide, or by the simple use of half a lemon or lemon juice. Either method is very drying to the nail plate and surrounding skin, therefore, after use it is important to well nourish the nail plate and area with cuticle cream.

Nail hardeners

These are composed of formaldehyde resins and care must be taken to prevent the product coming into contact with the skin, otherwise excessive dryness will result. Many people are allergic to the resin and this may result in a swelling of the skin around the nail. It is a wise precaution to protect this area of skin and the cuticle with a smear of oil.

Note: The use of formaldehyde must be stated on the bottle. This is a statutory requirement by the Cosmetic Product (Safety) Regulations.

Nail polish (enamel or varnish)

Modern nail polish formulae are principally composed of a mixture of different resins, solvents and colour pigments, i.e.

1. a film-former and a resin, which carries the colour, are dissolved in a solvent, having drying properties;
2. a pigment for colour;
3. plasticisers, which are added to improve the flexibility of the film of polish and help to prevent chipping of the polish.

Nail polish is designed to enhance the appearance of the nail and should be smooth and easy to apply, have covering power and adhere to the nail. All polishes are drying to the nail, but cream polishes are very slightly less harmful to weak and splitting nails than the pearlised types.

Base coats usually have a thinner film as they contain a lower percentage of film-former and they dry more quickly than the high-gloss polish. However, their important role is to prevent the pigment in the polish from staining the nail plate, minimising nail irregularities and prolonging the life of the polish.

Some manufacturers put tiny stainless steel balls into the polish bottle as they maintain that these will promote colour uniformity and break down the thixotropic structure of the product to facilitate smooth application.

Nail polishes must be kept away from heat sources as they are flammable and should be stored away from sunlight to avoid fading of the colouring matter. The temperature in the salon may alter the flow of the polish, i.e. cold rooms will thicken the polish and warm rooms will make the polish more fluid.

Hand creams/lotions

These are in the main lubricants used for massage purposes and are normally high oil content creams, i.e. O/W emulsions. They may contain lanolin, mineral oil, acetyl alcohol, glycerol, stearic acid and water. Lotions may have the same ingredients but they will contain a higher proportion of water.

Preparation of the manicure table/trolley

Prepare your manicure table or tray with the following:

- towels
- 2 bowls – one containing liquid soap and water and the other with a weak solution of antiseptic (or manicure pill, which turns ordinary water into an effervescent softening solution)
- nail bleach
- nail polish remover
- cuticle knife and clippers
- nippers
- cuticle cream and remover
- small emery boards and orange-sticks
- cotton wool
- hand cream or lotion
- a small jar – padded at the bottom with cotton wool (to prevent blunting your tools) containing surgical spirit or strong antiseptic
- a small bottle of weak antiseptic
- base coat, nail polishes and a top coat or sealer

A quick-drying sealer is very helpful as the nails are touch-dry in seconds.

Wash your hands prior to the arrival of the client.

Manicure – plain

1. Seat the client comfortably in the chair and ensure sleeves (if worn) are placed above the elbow and that rings or bracelets are removed. Inspect the hands for skin or nail infections. Wash the client's hands well, rinse in the antiseptic solution and dry well.
2. Start with the right hand, working methodically from the thumb to the fourth finger, remove all traces of old polish with a nail-polish remover free of acetone and with a good oil base. Soak a piece of cotton wool with the remover and hold between the middle joints of your first two fingers and hold your thumb under the client's finger. Place the cotton wool on the nail plate for a second or two to soften the enamel and then wipe the nail plate with firm, downward strokes towards the free edge until all the polish has been removed. Finally a cotton bud soaked in remover should clean up the cuticle area and the free edge (see Fig. 29.1).
3. Look to see if the nails require shortening. The condition of the nail is important, varying from the very soft to the brittle type. It is advisable to shorten the length of the nail, in the first instance, with clippers/nippers. The reason is that filing tends to disturb the nail bed, apart from being a slower method, the exception being where there is no free edge and the nail plate is completely attached to the fingertip. This type of nail plate is very sensitive and should only be filed with the fine side of the emery board.

    The art of clipping for length should first be practised on a thick piece of paper, then on your own hands and finally on the hands of a friend. There is quite a difference between paper and a nail, as the former is flat and the nail is rounded. Hold the clippers loosely in the palm of your hand with the spring in the upright position holding the cutting edges apart. To prevent any movement of the nail plate bring down the top edge of the clippers/nippers to meet the

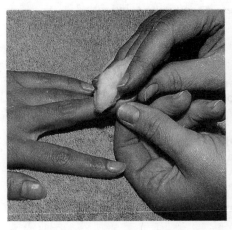 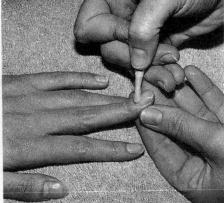

Fig. 29.1 Removing nail polish from the nail and cuticle area

underneath edge. If you are clipping for shape, slant the clippers on the right-hand side of the free edge and clip a small piece away, reverse the clippers and repeat on the left-hand side. You will then have the base for filing into shape. For a normal, healthy flexible nail, one clip is all that is required, but where the nails are thick or brittle, two or three clips are necessary taking very small pieces of nail each time. Very dry nails are brittle and are inclined to split. You will often find these on the hands of older people or on hands which are constantly immersed in very hot water or detergents. To lessen the brittleness, fill up the free edge of the nail with an emollient cream prior to clipping or filing.

4. For filing use a new emery board for each client and after use this can be given to the client or be thrown away. Hold the file lightly between the thumb and fingers and with short movements file from the sides to the centre. The top of the nail can be gently rounded. Never use see-saw movements as these disturb the nail bed and create friction. Which side of the emery board you use will depend on the type of nail and the amount to be filed, but always finish off with the fine side. The shape of the nail should relate to the nail and the finger. It can be made oval, almond or round. Be careful not to file into the corners of the nail plate as this will detach the nail from its bed. Complete all fingers and thumb on the right hand in this way. Run the pad of your thumb across the nail and check for any roughness or snags (see Fig. 29.2).

5. Fill the manicure bowl with clean, warm soapy water or use a manicure pill.

6. Take sufficient cuticle cream with an orange-stick to apply a small amount of cream to each finger and thumb of the right hand. Wipe the orange-stick with a tissue and place it in the jar of surgical spirit. With your thumbs, use the cuticle cream and massage all

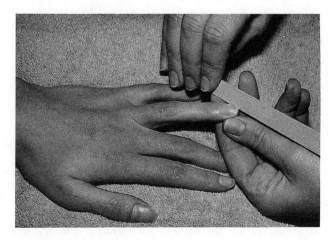

Fig. 29.2 Filing the nail

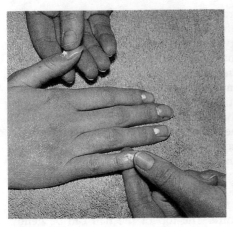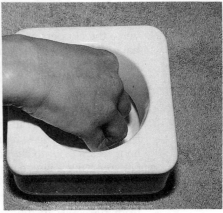

Fig. 29.3 Massage with cuticle cream, and placing right hand in bowl

round the cuticle and nail wall and place the right hand in the warm water (see Fig. 29.3).

7. Take the left hand, remove the nail polish, clip and/or file, use the cuticle cream and massage in well.

8. Take the right hand from the bowl and dry well. Place the bowl to the other side of the table/tray and place the left hand in the water. A word of caution here: do not let the fingers soak for too long in the water. Its purpose is just to soften the cuticle; if nails are soaked for any length of time they become spongy, lose their natural oils and the cuticles become so soft that there is a danger of their being trimmed and this is rarely necessary.

9. Pick up a tiny amount of cotton wool with an orange-stick and wind it around the hoof end. Dip this into the cuticle remover and lift the cuticles of the right hand. Some cuticle removers will have a brush for application – brush first and then use the orange-stick. If the cuticles have adhered to the nail plate it may be necessary to gently push them back first before lifting. Throw this cotton wool away and put the orange-stick back into the surgical spirit. Cuticle removers should not be applied to inflamed cuticles or irritated, damaged skin (see Fig. 29.4).

10. Take the manicure knife and from the centre of the cuticle (with the curved blunt end against the cuticle) gently lift the cuticle and work away at any dead tissue towards the right side of the nail. Reverse the knife, start again at the centre and work towards the left side of the nail. The knife must be held at right angles and at an almost horizontal level to ensure that no pressure is applied to the matrix. It is important to pay particular attention to the cuticles. They will often adhere to the nail and, as the nail grows, the cuticle is stretched until it reaches a certain point and then it will split. The result is a ragged cuticle which often causes hangnails and inflam-

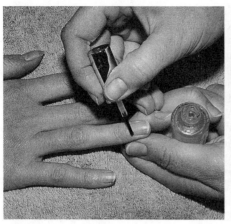
Fig. 29.4 Use of cuticle remover

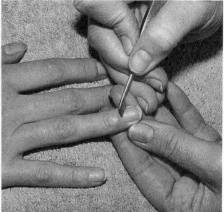
Fig. 29.5 Use of cuticle knife

mation. Dry cuticles are caused by excess acidity, easily recognised by a dry, white deposit underneath or near the cuticle, and is often found in the older client. Good knife work will minimise these problems. Advise the client to use cuticle cream every night to nourish the area (see Fig. 29.5).

11. Remember the left hand is still in water and this may be an opportune moment to dry this hand.
12. The use of cuticle clippers is very limited. They may be used to trim split or frayed cuticles or where a cuticle has been cut before and the condition is ragged (see Fig. 29.6). There is another exception

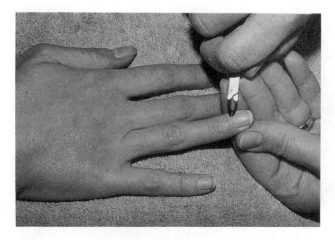
Fig. 29.6 Use of cuticle clippers

and this is when the cuticle is very thick and needs to be stretched and cut. Only an experienced manicurist should attempt to do this, as considerable harm can be done to the cuticles and matrix by careless or unskilled treatment. To cut the cuticle itself, it should be released from the nail with the knife and any deposits scraped away. Then the clippers should hold (but not cut) the cuticle and be pulled very gently towards the free edge. It will probably be about twice its original width. With the clippers trim only half the width of the cuticle. The trimming must be even and the edge smooth. If there is any need to cut the cuticle, dab the area immediately with cotton wool soaked in antiseptic. Advise the client to use cuticle cream nightly and ensure that she returns for treatment once a week until the cuticle has reached a narrow natural rim. Stretching the cuticle is very important as cutting without stretching can result in a thickening of the cuticle.

13. The free edge should now be cleaned of dirt or cream. Make a cotton bud and dip this into the antiseptic solution or nail bleach and clean under the free edge. Manufacturers sell this but it is extremely easy to make. Stir into 2 oz (57 gm) of 5 per cent peroxide, 2 oz (57 gm) of lemon juice and 0.25 oz (7 gm) ammonia. Pour this into an airtight bottle but leave a space at the top to allow for any expansion of the liquid. This bleach will also remove iodine or ink and some vegetable stains. You will probably have to use a damp pumice stone to remove nicotine stains. Be careful not to dig into the dividing line in an attempt to clear grime, as this will result in lifting the nail plate from the nail bed. Remember to throw away the cotton bud. The white pencil may now be used underneath the free edge (see Fig. 29.7).

14. Now check the filing and the cuticles and ensure a good, even base for polishing with a buffer or applying nail polish.

15. Return to the left hand and repeat from stage 9 to stage 14.

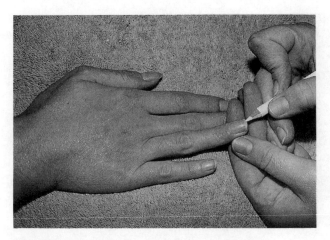

Fig. 29.7 Use of white pencil under the free edge

Massage of the arms and hands

This can be part of a body massage sequence or combined with a manicure.

If the latter, the client's sleeves should be above the elbow and the arms/hands resting comfortably on a clean towel or on the client's lap, or supported by a pillow or the arm rest of a chair.

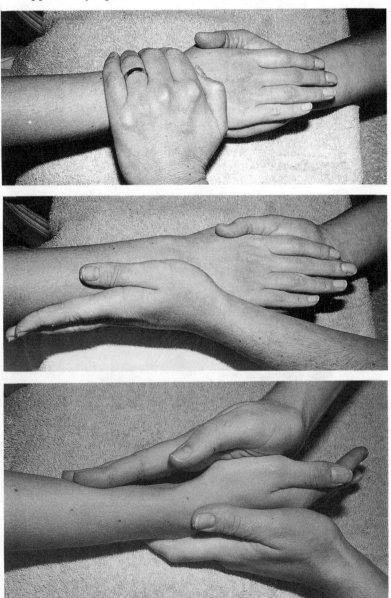

Fig. 29.8 (a) Effleurage over dorsal aspect (b) Effleurage over latera; aspect (c) Effleurage over posterior and medial aspects

Take sufficient massage cream/lotion between the palms of your hands.

1. Hold the client's right palm with your right hand and with your left hand held horizontally, give effleurage over the dorsal aspect of the right hand and arm (see Fig. 29.8(a)). Slide the hand over the elbow and down the lateral side of the arm to the hand and repeat three times.

   Using your hand in an upright position, effleurage the lateral side from the hand to the elbow and slide back (see Fig. 29.8(b)). Repeat three times.

2. Change you hands and repeat effleurage on the posterior and medial side of the arm (see Fig. 29.8(c)). The hands will be reversed when massaging the left arm.

3. Let the hand rest and slide your hands to the elbow and give thumb frictions around the elbow joint (see Fig. 29.9). Effleurage the area and slide hands back to the wrist.

4. Hold the client's hand and give thumb kneading movements from the extensor retinaculum over the extensor carpi ulnaris. With link effleurage, return to the retinaculum and repeat over digitorum, carpi radialis and other extensor muscles (see Fig. 29.10(a)). Turn the hand over and continue with the petrissage movements over the flexor muscles including the digitorum, brachioradialis and palmaris longus (see Fig. 29.10(b)). Give effleurage to the entire forearm.

5. Give thumb frictions over the extensor retinaculum with firm, circular movements, to alleviate any stiffness in the area (see Fig. 29.11).

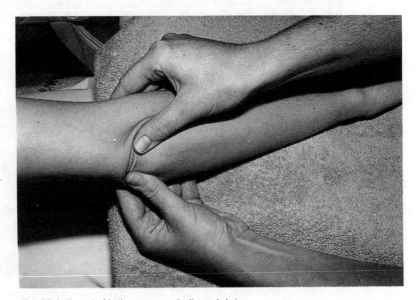

Fig. 29.9 Thumb frictions around elbow joint

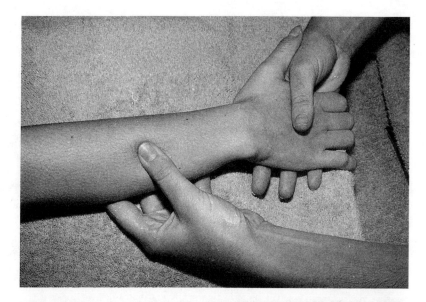

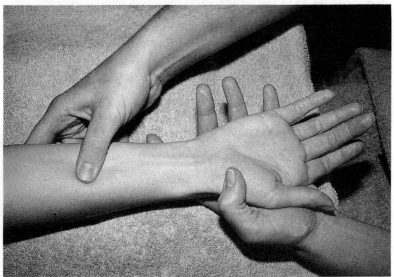

Fig. 29.10 (a) Kneading movements over the extensor muscles (b) Kneading movements over the flexor muscles

6. Take the client's hand, support the elbow and lift the arm/hand to an upright position. Slide the hand from the elbow to support the area just below the wrist. To stretch the muscle attachments and ligaments and improve joint mobility, the hand is rotated. Take the hand slowly forward, to the right, back, to the left – in a complete circle (see Fig. 29.12). Make three rotations to the left and to the right.

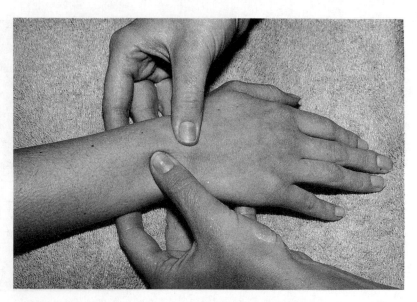

Fig. 29.11 Thumb frictions over the extensor retinaculum

7. With both hands place your thumb between the ring and little finger and the other thumb between the first finger and thumb of the client's hand. Make a brisk, rolling movement of the hand. This will help to stimulate circulation (see Fig. 29.13).

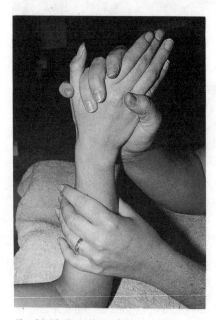

Fig. 29.12 Rotation of the hand

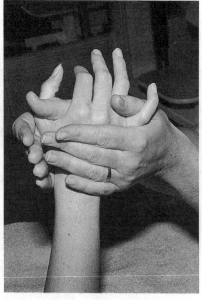

Fig. 29.13 Rolling movement of the hand

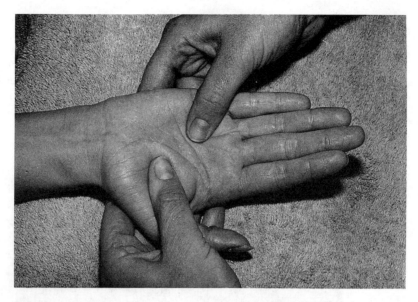

Fig. 29.14 Rotary kneading over palmar fascia and thenar eminence

8. Using both thumbs give rotary kneading over the palmar fascia (i.e. the sheet of fibrous tissue beneath the surface of the skin on the palm of the hand) and thenar eminence (see Fig. 29.14). Support either side of the hand.
9. Turn the hand over and give rotary kneading with your thumb between the metacarpals, effleurage back to the carpo-metacarpal

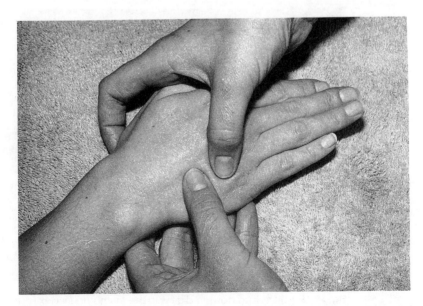

Fig. 29.15 Rotary kneading between the metacarpals

joint and repeat the movement on the remaining interosseus (see Fig. 29.15). Effleurage three times.

10. Hold the hand and take one digit at a time and give thumb rotary kneading over the joints, from the proximal to the distal end of the phalanx. Stroke down with your thumb and index finger (see Fig. 29.16(a)) and, in turning your hand, the third and index finger will be supporting either side of the digit. Very gently pull the phalanx

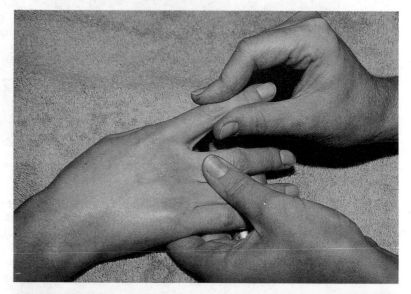

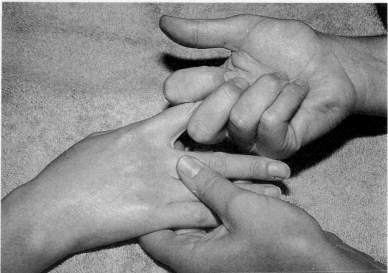

Fig. 29.16 (a) Stroking down a digit with the thumb and index finger
(b) Turning the hand, supporting the digit and stretching muscle fibres

as you slide your fingers to the distal end, so stretching the muscle fibres (see Fig. 29.16(b)). Repeat this movement for the remaining digits.

11. Repeat effleurage movements to cover the elbow, forearm, wrist and hand, the last movement terminating at the fingertips.
12. Repeat the massage for the other hand.
13. At this stage, wax baths or clay packs may be applied (see Chapter 30).

Application of nail cosmetics

For these to be applied, ensure that any grease on the arm or hand is removed by wiping the area with a toner or astringent. To make sure that the nails are completely free of grease, take a piece of cotton wool dampened with polish remover and wipe each nail carefully.

If the client does not wish for polish you can complete your manicure by polishing the nail plate with a buffer. This is an elongated pad over which a piece of chamois leather is clipped into place. You will need several pieces of leather as it should be washed after every client. The polishing medium is powder or cream which is either placed on the nail plate or on the leather itself. Always buff gently in one direction only, i.e. from the base to the free edge (see Fig. 29.17). This will not only stimulate circulation and encourage growth but will help to minimise ridges. However, you should remember that harsh buffing will cause friction which in turn creates heat, which is not good for the nail plate as it will become dry.

For both hands a nail strengthener can be applied (if required) together with a base coat which is left to dry.

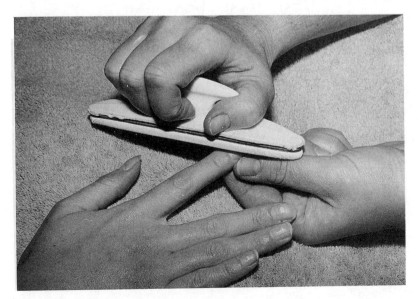

Fig. 29.17 Buffing the nail plate

Let the client choose the colour of the polish. Avoid shaking the bottle as this can create air bubbles which can be transferred to the nail plate, preventing an even smooth surface. It is better to roll the bottle upside down in your hands. The application of nail polish varies but as a guide, three or four strokes should be enough, e.g. one across the nail plate close to the cuticle and one each side from the centre of the nail plate to the free edge; or four strokes – one up from the centre to the free edge, one across the nail plate close to the cuticle and one each side of the nail plate (see Fig. 29.18). Practise various methods to find the one you prefer and perfect it.

Hold the bottle in the palm of the hand but low enough to leave your thumb and first finger free to hold the client's finger at the side of the nail. Usually two coats of nail polish are required and when these are dry, a colourless top coat or colourless fixator is applied. If possible then use a quick drying sealer. Make sure the polish is not only dry, but has had about twenty minutes to harden before the client leaves the salon. If a pearlised polish is used, apply three coats and leave out the top coat.

With regard to colours, show these to your client and let her choose. The lipstick she is wearing in the salon may not be the match she wants for her polish. Manufacturers do blend their colours for lipsticks and polishes and this often assists with choice. Where deep colours are concerned, these used to belong to the so-called sophisticated woman, but presently colours are chosen to match dresses or even eye shadows. For

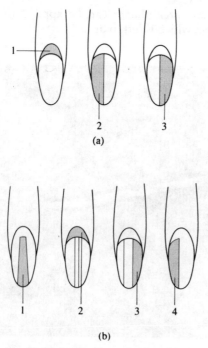

Fig. 29.18 Application of nail polish

the older woman, whose hair has turned grey or white and whose hands are ageing, do suggest a pale shade. Deep shades will make the hands appear much older.

With the wide selection of nail polishes available today, the necessity to mix a colour for that 'special occasion' is rare. However, should it occur, always use the same manufacturer's nail polishes and mix the colours with an orange-stick in a clean empty bottle.

Nail polish, whatever the quality, seals the nail and therefore dries it up. Advise your client to remove her polish after three or four days and explain that, with daily wear and tear, minute cracks will appear in the polish which in turn will result in corresponding fine lines in the nail plate. The end results will be flaky and brittle nails. If the polish is re-newed frequently these minute cracks will not appear and therefore no harm is done to the nail plate. The protective base coat will help by pre-venting the colouring pigments in the polish staining the nail plate. If the nails are already flaky and brittle do advise the client to leave off nail enamel for some time. Suggest polishing with a buffer. Cracks and flaky pieces can be filed down gently with the fine side of the emery board and a nail hardener applied. Nourishing nails nightly will help to improve the condition.

Wipe the top of the polish bottle with remover before screwing the top on tightly. Polish evaporates quickly when exposed to air and will become too thick to work with. A few drops of polish solvent will thin this out again.

Should the polish touch the skin or cuticles, dip an orange-stick with a cotton-wool tip into the nail-polish remover and touch very carefully to wipe away the excess of polish.

Contra-indications

- nail diseases or disorders
- bruised nails
- infections, cuts or abrasions of the cuticles or surrounding skin
- allergy to products.

Various nail shapes

Here are a few drawings of some of the shapes of nails that you will meet. When giving a manicure try to conform to the shape of the finger- or toe-tip as the sole purpose of a nail is to protect that area. Many women who work with their hands usually need short and rounded nails to avoid breakage and injury. This would indeed apply to a beauty therapist performing massage on the face or body and other treatments using the cushions of the fingertips. Long nails would in-hibit many movements and be uncomfortable for the client.

Nails should not be left to grow too long or filed to a point as this causes strain on the nail plate. Always discuss the shape of the nail with your client before filing. To make square and trapezoid nails appear narrower and longer, when applying nail polish, do not take the polish to the sides of the nail plate. Leave a small margin uncovered. For an-

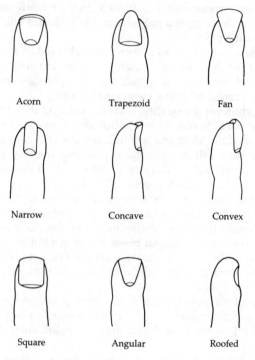

Fig. 29.19 Nail shapes

gular and fan-shaped nails, this small margin could be left at its widest point and perhaps the lunula could be left unpainted. For narrow nails, the reverse would apply. The polish would cover the entire nail. Convex and concave nails would perhaps benefit if a small margin was left unpainted at the accentuated curve.

Manicure – oil

This type of manicure is very good for ridged and brittle nails. The procedure is the same as for a plain manicure but with the following differences:

1. Use warm olive oil instead of soapy water. Always test the oil on yourself first to ensure that it is not too hot.
2. No cuticle cream is required.
3. Remove the oil from the arms and hands with a warm damp towel and apply a skin freshener.
4. Callouses can be rubbed gently with a damp pumice stone or the fine side of an emery board before immersing the fingers into the oil.

Remember, as you use your tools, that they must be returned to the jar with the surgical spirit. Clean paper tissues should be used to dry tools before using them on a client. If not using tools immediately, they should be cleaned and placed in a UV cabinet.

Emery boards and orange-sticks can be given to the client or broken and discarded after use. The manicure tray/table/trolley must be cleaned with surgical spirit. Used towels should be put in a laundry basket and fresh towels used for each client.

Hygiene and sterilisation

As mentioned in Chapter 1, good hygienic practices in a salon will prevent the transmission of infection. During a manicure or pedicure there is the possibility of the skin being accidentally cut. Use a prepacked spirit swab, leave it to dry and carefully discard the swab. The tool used, i.e. cuticle knife or nippers/clippers, should not be used again until they have been sterilised. If the cut continues to bleed use an aerosol form of styptic or shake styptic powder on to the cut and cover with a band-aid. Do not use a styptic stick directly on to the injury.

The best method for sterilising these implements is to place them under steam pressure, e.g. an autoclave (see Chapter 1, Fig. 1.1).

Self assessment

- what is the difference between a cuticle cream and cuticle remover and how are these used?
- explain the purpose of 'buffing' the nails
- explain how you would reduce the length of a nail
- explain how you would use a cuticle knife
- what is the purpose of an oil manicure?
- what are the contra-indications to a manicure?

30 Care of the hands

Groomed, well-cared-for hands are a pleasure to see and not difficult to achieve if a simple daily routine is advised. Hands are not only in continual use but take a lot of abuse and therefore age more quickly than other parts of the body. As with nail protection, you should advise the use of cotton gloves for dry work and rubber gloves for wet work but, after using gloves, wash the hands well in warm – not hot – water with a super-fatted soap and dry well. This will remove excess moisture and perspiration. Always advise that the gloves should be on the large side so that circulation is not impeded. For normal hands suggest a light hand-cream or lotion to keep them supple. If a client has hands where grimed-in dirt is apparent, massage olive oil into them first as it will help to loosen the dirt. Wipe the oil off with paper tissues before washing them.

Poor health and lack of exercise will often cause swelling, redness and numbness due to poor circulation.

These can be helped by showing the client exercises to do at home, and/or by use of clay packs, vibratory massage or paraffin-wax baths.

Exercises

There are several exercises to choose from or add a different exercise each week. In that way they can be remembered more easily.

1. Close the fingers and then open them and stretch the hand and fingers to their fullest extent (see Fig. 30.1). This can be repeated at least ten times.

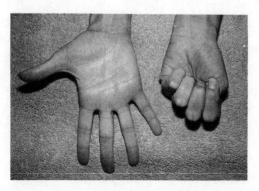

Fig. 30.1 Showing one hand fingers closed, the other hand at full stretch

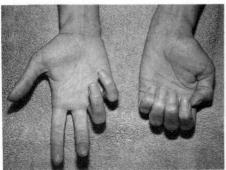 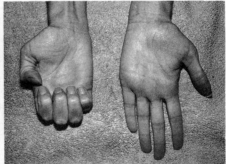

Fig. 30.2 Uncurling the fingers   **Fig. 30.3** Finger tips touching the base of the phalanges

2. Curl the fingers into a loose fist with the palms down. Turn the wrist inwards and upward and release the fingers one at a time as if they were petals of a flower (see Fig. 30.2). Do this slowly about eight times.
3. Bend all the knuckles and stretch the palm of the hand; all the fingertips should try to touch the base of the phalanges (see Fig. 30.3). This is followed by stretching the hand and fingers to their fullest extent. Repeat several times. This exercise will prove difficult for the person suffering from arthritis or simply swollen knuckles.
4. With very loose wrists the hands can be shaken. Start with the fingers left open and shake about six times. Shake again with the fingers closed about six times.
5. Hold the hands, palms facing as if in prayer and press them together. Turn the hands inwards towards the body and then outwards away from the body (see Fig. 30.4) six times. Still pressing the hands together, push the hands to the left and then to the right, i.e. pushing each hand towards the arm. This can be repeated six times.
6. Also for the wrist, stand up and place the palms and fingers of both hands on to a firm surface. Lean forward so that the arms move towards the backs of the hands. This can be repeated several times.

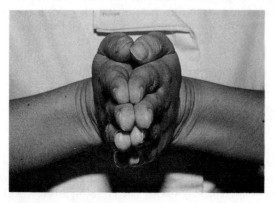

Fig. 30.4 Palms turned outward from the body

Here are only six exercises; there are many more which can be adapted from them. Also read magazines and books on exercises to widen your knowledge.

Contra-indications for exercises

There are none but exercises for clients suffering with rheumatism or arthritis in the hands or wrists should be carefully planned.

Clay packs

These are available at most chemists, but it is easy to make your own. Use kaolin and magnesia carbonate in equal parts, slowly mix water with them to form a thick creamy substance. You will need

- three hand bowls, one with warm water, one with the mixed clay and the other empty
- super-fatted soap
- a bottle of almond oil
- hand lotion
- two pieces of plastic or polythene film
- towels and tissues

Place one piece of plastic over the manicure table/tray and the other over the client to protect her clothing and the arms of the chair. Take the right hand and give a good deep massage but gently over the back of the hand if veins are evident. Wash off the massage cream with warm soapy water and dry the hand well (the clay will not adhere to a damp or greasy hand). Immerse the right hand in the bowl of clay and leave for about half a minute; remove the hand and put the wrist and arm on the arm-rest with the hand hanging over the edge. Place the empty bowl under the hand to catch the drips of surplus clay. Take the left hand and repeat the massage/wash/dry sequence. Immerse the left hand in the clay, remove it and put the wrist and arm on the arm-rest and remove the bowl to the other side to catch the surplus drips from the left hand. Wash the clay pack off the right hand and dry it well. The clay should remain on the hands for about ten minutes. When the left hand is ready, remove the clay. Massage both hands again, this time with the almond oil. Surplus oil can be removed with tissues. The piece of plastic should be removed.

Contra-indications for clay packs

- nail disorders or diseases
- infections, cuts or abrasions of the cuticles or surrounding skin
- allergy to the clay.

Vibratory massage

This deep massage can be used by itself, using talc or cream/oil or following a treatment, e.g. clay packs. The vibrator, an electrical appliance (see Fig. 34.3 using the same vibrator on the foot) penetrates deeply into the tissues, thereby increasing circulation, but should be used very gently on the back of the hand and not at all if veins are evident as bruising can occur.

Place the client's hand, palm down on the tray/table/trolley. Carefully avoiding nails and cuticles, lift each digit and vibrate down the centre and sides. As with manicure, start with the right hand, working methodically from the thumb to the fourth finger. Gently vibrate over the metacarpals to the wrist. Now place the client's elbow on a firm surface with the palm facing towards you and run the vibrator down each digit from the cushion pad at the tip to the base of the finger. Follow this with vibrations to the palm of the hand. Remove talc or cream/oil with a toner or simply use tissues.

Contra-indications to vibratory massage

- nail diseases or disorders
- infections, cuts or abrasions on the hand
- over the back of the hand if veins are evident.

Waxing, paraffin-wax baths

In the main there are two types of wax baths. The older type, which is still in use, has an outer casing (which is partially filled with water) and which accommodates an electric heater and thermostat control. The inner casing contains the wax. The more modern bath is usually made of stainless steel and has only one casing for the wax. When purchasing a wax heater read the manufacturer's instructions carefully. Some baths have a thermometer dial, others have an automatic high-temperature safety switch which prevents overheating.

When the heater is switched on, the small pilot light which is governed by a thermostat control will glow. The wax will then be heated to a temperature of 47–53 °C (116–27 °F). The whiteness will disappear and the melted wax will be clear.

Benefits from the wax are:

- a deep cleanse cause by sweating
- nerve endings are soothed
- due to increased circulation the skin texture and colour is improved
- deep heat eases aches and pains
- penetrates the tissues to relieve stiffness in joints
- relaxes muscles.

Apart from the wax therapy for the face described in Chapter 17 it can be used prior to massage, before or after manicure or pedicure.

For the hand or foot treatments, the limb can be immersed in the wax bath or a brush used to paint on the wax. If the hand is being treated all jewellery should be removed.

Method of application

Ensure that the wax in the paraffin-wax heater has melted to the required temperature and test this by applying a little to the inside of your wrist with a brush. Have ready:

- paper towels or tissues
- plastic sheets or foil, large enough to wrap around each hand
- a small heated blanket, two towels or two padded mitts.

For the brush method

1. Ensure that paper towels/tissues are placed under the area where the wax is to be applied in case of drips or spills.
2. Apply two coats of wax, on the palmar surface, from the wrist to the cushion tips of the fingers.
3. Turn the hand over and apply two coats of wax to the dorsal surface (see Fig. 30.5).

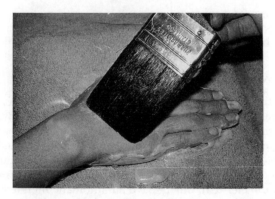

Fig. 30.5 Applying wax to dorsal area

4. Repeat this three times – six coats in all – to ensure that a thick film of wax covers the entire area.
5. Wrap in plastic or foil, cover with the towel or place the hand in the mitt. Repeat for the other hand. If you have a small electric blanket, plug this in and place over the towels/mitts to maintain the heat of the wax.
6. After twenty minutes remove blanket/towels/mitts and then take off the wax from the wrist down to the tips of the phalanges. The wax and plastic/foil must be thrown away.

For the immersion method

1. Test the temperature of the wax.
2. Have ready plastic sheets or foil, blanket/towels or mitts.
3. Dip one hand into and out of the wax at least six or seven times until a thick film is obtained (see Fig. 30.6).
4. Wrap the hand in plastic sheet/foil etc. (continue as for the brush method).
5. Repeat for the other hand.

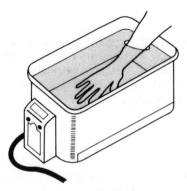

Fig.30.6 Immersion of hand in wax heater

For both methods

After twenty minutes, the blanket/towels/mitts and plastic or foil are removed. The wax is peeled off from the wrist down to the tips of the fingers and the plastic/foil and wax are *thrown away*. Check the hands carefully, as sometimes the wax becomes trapped in the cuticles or grooves or under the free edge of the nail. Massage of the hands may follow or the residue of the oil in the wax can be removed with paper towels, followed by the use of a skin toner.

Contra-indication to paraffin wax

- nail diseases or disorders
- infections, cuts or abrasions.

Dry hands

These are very common and require good nourishing creams to be rubbed in every night and covered with loose cotton gloves. Frequent washing of the gloves is important as creams do contain a percentage of moisture, which is detrimental to the skin. Most cosmetic houses have good nourishing creams for the hands but you can make your own quite simply. Mix with a wooden spoon equal parts of cold cream, lanolin, white petroleum and almond oil. Wash dry hands as little as possible and use a barrier cream after they have been dried. The constant use of soap and water will only increase the dryness.

It has already been mentioned that hands age quickly and in doing so, brown patches which look like freckles appear on the dorsal aspect. There is really no cure for these, one or two commercial products will help to fade the marks and a general bleaching will help. You can make a bleach pack using equal parts of almond meal and kaolin mixed with water to a thick, creamy substance. This can be placed on the hands and left for 10–15 minutes. Wash the hands well in warm water with a super-fatted soap. Dry the hands well and apply a hand cream or lotion.

Moist and clammy hands

These are often found in people suffering from a form of nervousness. You can only advise treatments of a temporary nature and suggest that the client see a doctor if it is a worry. Using an astringent several times a day will help; also the use of talcum powder two or three times a day will make the hands feel more comfortable.

Enlarged knuckles

Many older clients will suffer with enlarged knuckles which are caused by either an internal factor, such as rheumatism or osteoarthritis, or long immersion in water or damp substances, i.e. a gardener, handling damp soil or nurses who are continually using water and spirits. It can also be caused by tight rings impeding circulation. Before any treatment is given, the client's doctor should be consulted, as it may be better for the client to see a specialist or physiotherapist. Ascertain from the doctor that certain treatments may be carried out, such as radiant heat, massage, electrical vibrations, wax baths or clay packs and exercises. Advise the client to lift heavy articles with the palm and phalanges of both hands to relieve the weight on the knuckles and keep the latter out of water. There is one treatment with water which could help relieve the condition, i.e. salt water.

Mix equal parts of Epsom salt, kitchen salt and water and pour this into a bowl of hot water. If the client lives in a hard-water area, the water for the mixture should include a water softener. The hands should be immersed until the water is cool and this should be followed by a massage. Wipe the knuckles dry with soft tissues.

Warts

Warts on the client's hand must not be touched. It does not come within your jurisdiction and should be referred to a doctor.

Self assessment

- give three exercises for the hands to promote flexibility
- how would you use a vibrator on the hands?
- how would you make your own clay pack?
- what is the maximum temperature at which paraffin wax could be applied and how would you ensure that it is not too hot for the client?
- what advice would you give to a client with moist and clammy hands?

31 Nail repairs, artificial nails and sculptured nails

Nail repairs

Nail repairs are useful for nails which are damaged mainly by misuse, e.g. accidental breaks, incorrect filing during a manicure and excessive use of harsh detergents or other chemicals, which can dry out the nails causing them to split or flake. There are other contributory factors, e.g. ill health, poor circulation etc., which will also affect the condition of the nails.

Nail-patching kits are available which consist of special tissue or mending paper and strong fixatives or cement. Paper repairs can be made to:

1. nail tips which have started to split or the top layer has peeled off
2. attach a piece of nail which has started to break off
3. repair a split at the side of the nail plate
4. re-attach a broken nail.

Contra-indications

- nail diseases or disorders
- bruised nails
- infections, cuts or abrasions of the cuticles or surrounding skin.

Preparation

Your trolley should contain everything required for a manicure, plus:

- special tissue or mending paper
- nail fixative or nail cement
- nail enamel solvent
- cotton buds.

Method of use

1. *To repair the nail tip*
   (a) Clean the nail plate with nail enamel remover and very gently file if this is required to smooth the area.
   (b) Tear off a piece of mending paper (the ragged edge is easier to apply to the nail plate and disguise). Place the paper on the nail and trim the paper to the shape of the nail allowing about $\frac{1}{8}$ in (32 mm) to protrude over the free edge.

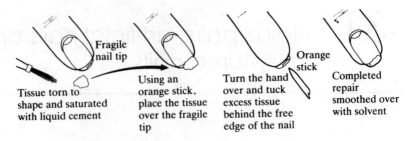

Tissue torn to shape and saturated with liquid cement — Using an orange stick, place the tissue over the fragile tip — Turn the hand over and tuck excess tissue behind the free edge of the nail — Completed repair smoothed over with solvent

Fig. 31.1 Repairing the nail tip

(c) Saturate the paper with the liquid fixative/cement and lay it flat on to the nail plate. Moisten your finger with cotton wool previously dampened with polish remover/solvent and lightly smooth out the patch.

(d) Turn the client's hand over and push the excess paper under the free edge with an orange-stick dipped in polish remover/solvent and press firmly (see Fig. 31.1).

(e) Any excess liquid can be wiped away with a cotton bud. Make sure the cap is completely dry as it can slip if the base coat and polish are applied too soon.

2. *To attach a piece of nail that has started to break off*
   (a) Ensure the nail plate is clean (as in 1(a)).
   (b) Take a double piece of mending paper and saturate with the liquid fixative/cement.
   (c) Place the tissue over the broken part of the nail and make sure it overlaps the free edge.
   (d) Again moisten your finger with cotton wool as in 1(c) and repeat 1(d) and (e).

3. *To repair a split at the side of the nail plate*
   (a) Make sure the nail plate is completely clean (as in 1(a)).
   (b) Take a narrow strip of mending paper, repeat the saturating process and apply diagonally across the split.
   (c) Again tuck the excess paper under the free edge and smooth as in 1(d).
   (d) If the split is quite deep a second patch may be needed for reinforcement. Make this patch slightly longer on the nail plate to cover the first patch to avoid a definite ridge caused by the paper. Again make sure that the patch is thoroughly dry before applying the base coat and polish.

4. *To re-attach a broken nail*
   This is not always successful and rarely will a client bring her piece of nail into the salon! However, it can happen, but the client should understand that it will be a very temporary repair, and can be mended to last for a few hours, i.e. an evening dance or party.
   (a) Again make sure the nail is clean.
   (b) Take a wisp of cotton wool, longer than the nail and the broken

piece and saturate it with the liquid fixative/cement. Then lay it flat on the nail leaving a little over the free edge.

(c) Apply the fixative/cement to the broken piece and place this on top of the cotton wool, matching the broken edge of the nail plate.

(d) Dip an orange-stick into the nail enamel solvent and turn the cotton wool over the break and very gently press.

(e) For reinforcement, take a piece of the mending paper, saturate with the liquid, lay it diagonally across the nail and fold the excess paper under the nail.

(f) As before, moisten the finger with the cotton wool dampened with polish remover, smooth down the free edge and allow to dry thoroughly before completing the manicure.

Semi-permanent nails

'Stick-on' type artificial nails

The nails usually come supplied with a special adhesive glue or liquid cement and glue solvent. These are very useful as they help to conceal broken or badly shaped nails and will also protect nails against breaking or splitting. However, they should not be worn for any length of time as the nail plate weakens and becomes spongy. They are often used for helping onychophagia, but should never be applied if the fingertip is bulbous or there is no nail plate for the artificial nail to completely adhere.

Where it may be advantageous for ten artificial nails to be worn by actresses or models, the majority of clients will find it impracticable as the extra length on all ten nails will feel strange and difficulties will be found in everyday use.

Contra-indications are the same as for nail repairs and also any allergy to the products.

Preparation

Again your trolley should contain everything required for a manicure, plus:

- adhesive glue or liquid cement
- shapes of artificial nails
- fine emery paper
- adhesive strips
- bowl of warm water.

Most of these items are usually supplied in a kit by the manufacturer/supplier.

Method of use

1. Complete a manicure up to but before the base coat stage and ensure the nails are absolutely clean and devoid of grease.
2. Judge the width of the client's nails. If the angle of the artificial nail is too shallow, soak the nail in warm water and curve it around a

pencil or pen; if the nail is too curved take it from the hot water and flatten it out.

3. Each nail should be tried in place and then clipped and filed to the right length. If you are using ten nails, these should all be prepared at the outset. The preparation of the artificial nails is very important and you should take care and time.

4. Roughen the underside of the artificial nails with the fine emery paper and leave the nails in the warm water to maintain pliability.

5. Dry the nails with tissues and place them on the adhesive tape with the inside uppermost; or you can take each nail separately from the warm water and dry one at a time. Apply the special adhesive to the sides of the nail plate and to the inside of the artificial nail.

6. Press the artificial nail firmly down on to the nail plate with the lower edge resting just beneath the tip of the loosened cuticle and hold in position for about half a minute. With modern day adhesives the nail will quickly adhere.

7. Clean away any excess glue with a cotton bud dampened with nail polish remover.

8. Repeat the process for the other nails and when completely dry and firm, any further shaping may be filed with the fine side of the emery board, but the artificial nail must not move.

9. Complete the manicure with the base coat, polish, top coat and sealer.

Removal of stick-on type artificial nails

Prior to removing the nails take off any polish with an acetone-free remover as some plastic resin nails may dissolve if acetone is used.

To remove these artificial nails put a drop of glue solvent into the sides of the nail plate and place the hands in hot water. The nails can be peeled off once the glue has softened. Clean the nail plate and the underside of the artificial nail with the glue solvent followed by warm water. The nails can be placed on the adhesive strip and used again at a later date.

Sculptured nails

This type of artificial nail is becoming increasingly popular and there are many companies distributing nail systems world-wide. It is wise to check out each type of system and to ensure that you have chosen a professional nail supplier, a company who is a member of a trade organisation, e.g. the International Nail Association.

This is important as this type of supplier will run training courses; promote the nail industry, e.g. help with the promotional material; keep up-to-date with current trends; provide you with backing, which in turn ensures peace of mind knowing that there is nearly always someone at the other end of the telephone should you ever require assistance.

Remember, you cannot give a professional service if you have simply read an instruction leaflet/book or watched a video. Training is paramount for whichever system you choose. Nail technology is advancing all the time with new or improved products and keeping in touch with the nail supplier you have selected will ensure that you are being kept up-to-date.

The system and where to train is always a difficult choice as so many companies have slightly different variations on the same theme. The three main systems use either gel, fibreglass or acrylic and these can be used for both a complete nail extension or to lengthen a tip. In general terms:

1. The gel system
   This is where the gel forms a direct bond to the nail and is non-porous. The application of gels is fairly straightforward and can be used with nail forms (e.g. 'horse-shoes'/metal shields) or with a tip. Some gels need to be cured, i.e. exposing the sculptured nails to ultra-violet light (some companies will provide a 'light box') or by the use of a special setting spray.

2. The fibreglass system
   The fibreglass nail is extremely thin and after application it is difficult to see the division between it and the nail plate. To give the nail strength a strip of mesh is applied before layers of sealant are added.

3. The acrylic system
   All liquid and powder systems are acrylic and these also look completely natural without nail polish and can withstand most of the pressures put on them by the client. This can be applied to any length of natural nail either by using a nail form or a pre-formed tip.
   Whichever system you choose, additional products are applied to the new growth area, therefore, maintenance is required every 2–4 weeks dependent upon on the rate of growth of the nails.

Contra-indications

Again these are the same as for a manicure but the client must be advised that some of the chemicals used are known sensitisers and allergies may result, e.g. inflammation of the surrounding tissues. Sculptured nails are not easily removed and, should this happen, extra care has to be taken over several months to avoid further infection at the site or at the new growth area if the sculptured nail or tip is allowed to grow out.

Self assessment

- what products would you need to repair a nail?
- why is it important for 'stick-on' nails to be removed after a short period of time?
- give a list of the contra-indications for artificial nails
- how would you remove artificial nails?
- give reasons why it is so important to use a reputable nail supplier when considering a sculptured nail service?

32 Anatomy of the lower leg and foot

Bones of the lower leg

1. The **tibia**, the larger bone below the knee, runs down the front and medial side of the leg. It is triangular in shape and has two extremities and a shaft. The upper extremity articulates with two condyles (i.e. a rounded eminence) of the femur (the thigh bone) to form the knee joint. Distally the tibia articulates with the fibula and with the talus (in the foot).
2. The **fibula** has a slender shaft and runs parallel with the tibia and articulates with it at both extremities, although it does not enter the knee joint itself. The projection at the upper extremity, the head of the fibula, articulates with the lateral condyle of the tibia. The lower extremity is prolonged downwards as the lateral process. The talus fits into a boxlike socket to form the ankle joint by the medial and lateral malleoli (i.e. projections of the tibia and fibula respectively) (see Fig. 32.1).

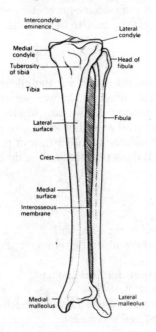

Fig. 32.1 The left tibia and fibula with the interosseous membrane

3. The **patella**, or knee cap, is the largest sesamoid bone in the body. It is located in the quadriceps femoris (a thigh muscle) as a projection to the underlying knee joint. It can be clearly seen through the skin when the knee is flexed.

Bones of the foot

There are 26 bones in the foot, 7 tarsus, 5 metatarsus and 14 phalanges.

The tarsus comprises the entire ankle and is made up of the following (see Fig. 32.2):

- calcaneum
- talus
- cuboid
- navicular
- cuneiforms (lateral, medial and intermedial).

The five tarsal bones in front of the calcaneus and talus articulate with the five metatarsal bones and these in turn articulate with the phalanges. Beneath the first metatarsal there are two sesamoid bones.

The longitudinal arches of the foot (see Fig. 32.3) are:

1. medial arch which is formed by the calcaneus, talus, navicular, cuneiforms and three metatarsals; and
2. lateral arch which is formed by calcaneus, cuboid and two lateral metatarsals.

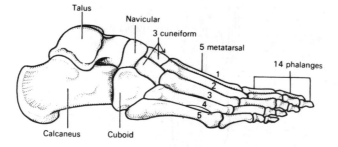

Fig. 32.2 The bones of the foot (Lateral view)

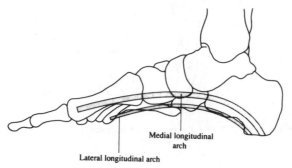

Fig. 32.3 Longitudinal arches

Muscles of the lower leg and foot

Muscles of the lower leg are detailed in Fig. 32.4 and Table 32.1; muscles of the ankle and foot are detailed in Fig. 32.5 and Table 32.2.

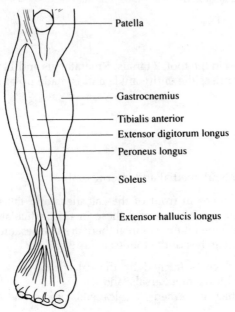

Fig. 32.4 Muscles of the lower right leg (anterior view)

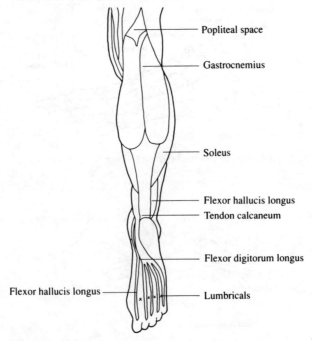

Fig. 32.5 Muscles of the lower right leg (posterior view)

Table 32.1 Muscles of the lower leg

Name	Location	Origin	Insertion	Action
Gastrocnemius	Back of lower leg (thick with two heads)	Medical and lateral condyles of femur	Calcaneum of the heel through the tendon calcaneum (or Achilles tendon)	Flexes foot at ankle and assists in raising leg
Soleus	Back of lower leg	Fibula and tibia	As above	Flexes foot at ankle
Tibialis anterior	Front of lower leg	Tibia	1st cuneiform, base of 1st metatarsal	Flexes and inverts foot
Peroneus longus	Down outer lower leg beneath foot	Fibula	Base of 1st metatarsal, 1st cuneiform	Supports arch
Extensor digitorum	Lower front leg to phalanges	Fibula	2nd and 3rd phalanges of lateral 4 toes	Extensor of the leg and foot
Extensor hallucis	Lower front leg to big toe	Fibula	Base of distal phalanx	Extensor of the leg and foot
Tendon calcaneum or Achilles tendon	Thick tendon at the heel	Fibula	Into the spur of the heel	Raises foot in walking

Table 32.2 Muscles of the ankle and foot

Name	Location	Origin	Insertion	Action
Lumbricals	Sole of the foot	Tendons of long flexor muscles of the toes	Medial side of base of proximal phalanges of 4 lateral toes	Aids in flexing proximal phalanges
Flexor digitorum longus	Sole of the foot	Calcaneum	2nd and 3rd phalanges of 4 lateral toes	Flexes foot
Flexor hallucis logus	Sole of the foot	Calcaneum	Base of big toe	Flexes foot

Circulatory system of the leg and foot

The main arteries of the lower leg and foot are shown in Fig. 32.6 and these are:

- popliteal
- glenicular
- anterior tibial
- posterior tibial
- peroneal
- dorsalis pedis
- arcuate
- dorsal metatarsal
- plantar arch
- plantar metatarsal.

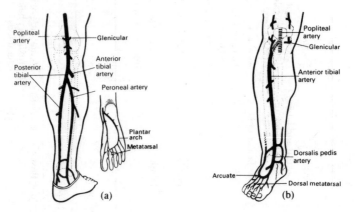

Fig. 32.6 Popliteal artery and its main branches (a) Posterior view (b) Anterior view

The main veins of the lower leg and foot are shown in Fig. 32.7 and these are:

- great saphenous
- anterior tibial
- posterior tibial
- small saphenous
- dorsal
- dorsal venous arch
- deep plantar venous arch.

The lymphatic nodes, seven in all, are embedded in fat in the popliteal space.

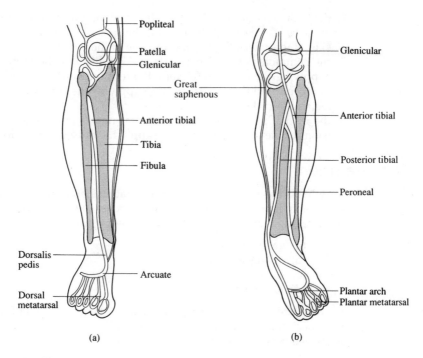

Fig. 32.7 Main veins of the leg

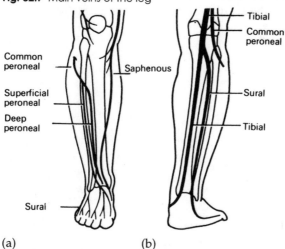

Fig. 32.8 The main nerves of the leg (a) Anterior view (b) Posterior view

Nerves of the lower leg and foot

The *principal* nerves of the leg are sensory-motor and these are (see Fig. 32.8):

1. sciatic nerve which passes through the thigh muscles and divides into:

2. the tibial nerve (medial popliteal) – the motor nerves, supplying the muscles of the calf of the leg and the sensory nerves supplying the skin of the calf of the leg and the sole of the foot;
3. the common peroneal nerve (lateral popliteal) – the motor nerves supplying the evertors (turning the foot outward) and dorsiflexors of the foot and the sensory nerves supplying the lateral surface of the leg and dorsal surface of the foot;
4. the medial plantar and lateral plantar nerves are the terminal divisions of the tibial nerve which supply the muscles of the foot.

Self assessment

- what is the difference between the patella and popliteal space?
- explain how the medial and lateral arches of the foot are formed
- give origin and insertion for the following muscles:

   (a) gastrocnemius
   (b) tibialis anterior
   (c) soleus
   (d) lumbricals

- what are the main arteries and veins of the lower leg and foot?
- where are the lymphatic nodes situated?
- which nerves supply the following areas?

   (a) the calf muscles
   (b) the evertors and dorsiflexors of the foot.

33 Pedicure and massage of the lower legs and feet

Pedicure

This is the care of toe-nails, feet and legs up to the knee and is quite similar in treatment to that of a manicure. However, it cannot replace the skills of qualified chiropodists. Many conditions should be referred to them, such as corns, bunions, verrucae, infection or inflammation of the feet, nail plate or cuticles. It is advisable to know the name, address and telephone number of your local chiropodist.

Before the client arrives ensure that you have everything to hand for the pedicure, i.e.

- three of four towels
- a bowl, large enough to take both feet
- a foot-rest for the client covered with a paper towel
- nail polish remover
- antiseptic solution
- antiseptic foot drops (these usually contain potassium undecylenoyl, hydrolysed benzalkonium chloride, an alcohol content and oils etc.)
- nail clippers and cuticle knife
- cuticle cream and cuticle remover
- steel diamond cut file and emery boards
- cotton wool
- massage medium (oil or cream etc.)
- a small jar – padded at the bottom with cotton wool (to prevent blunting your tools) containing surgical spirit or strong antiseptic
- pedi-pads (polystyrene pads for insertion between the toes)
- base coat, nail polishes and a top coat or sealer.

1. The client may have walked some distance before arriving at the salon, so after helping her to remove shoes and tights/stockings, put her feet into warm soapy water with a few drops of an antiseptic solution added, or use a foot spray to deodorise and disinfect the feet. The latter is often preferred as soaking the feet in water is inclined to soften the nails, making it difficult for the therapist to file well.
2. If you have used water, take out both feet and dry well with disposable paper and refill the bowl with warm water adding a suitable antiseptic solution.
3. Examine the feet for any contra-indications, i.e. infections.

4. Wrap the left foot in a towel. If you have used a foot spray ensure the water in the bowl is warm.
5. Remove any nail polish on the right foot. Apply the foot drops around the cuticle and in between the toes.
6. Look to see if the nails require shortening with nail clippers. If so, take very small pieces each time, clipping straight across (not shaped as fingernails) until the desired length is obtained (see Fig. 33.1). Never make a toenail shorter than the tip of the toe, the nail is there to protect this area and never clip or file into the corners of the nail plate, as this will encourage ingrowing toenails. The nail plate must adhere to the full length of the nail grooves and nail bed.
7. A sterilised diamond-cut steel file may be used if the nails are thick and hard, otherwise an emery board will suffice. The toe pad is very sensitive, so care must be taken to ensure that the file does not touch this area. File down the free edge and use a final sweep to round off sharp corners.
8. Take sufficient cuticle cream with an orange-stick and apply to each toe, rub this in well and place the right foot in the prepared water.
9. Unwrap the left foot and repeat steps 5 through to 8.
10. Dry the right foot. Pick up a little cotton wool, wind it around the end of an orange-stick and dip it into the cuticle remover, or use the brush provided to paint on the remover. Gently push back the cuticles with the orange-stick or rubber hoof stick (see Fig. 33.2). Throw away the cotton wool and orange-stick or put the rubber hoof stick in the surgical spirit.
11. The cuticle knife may now be used (as in manicure, see Fig. 29.5) to scrape away any debris and clear the cuticle from the nail plate.
12. The use of cuticle clipper again is limited, mainly for loose pieces or

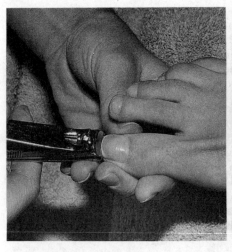

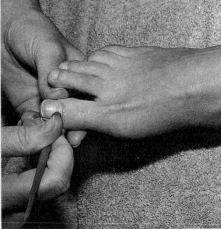

Fig. 33.1 Clipping the toenail   **Fig. 33.2** Pushing back the cuticles

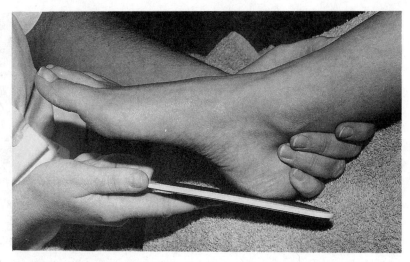

Fig. 33.3 Use of a foot scraper

trimming split or frayed cuticles (again in the same way as for the manicure shown in Fig. 29.6).
13. Make a cotton bud, dip this into the antiseptic solution and clean under the free edge and around the nail grooves. Nail bleach is rarely needed for toenails. Check your filing and cuticles.
14. Dip the right foot into the water and then use a pumice-stone, foot scraper or hard skin remover to remove dead skin and rough patches (see Fig. 33.3).
15. Rinse the right foot well to get rid of dead skin and cuticle cream and dry well.
16. For the left foot repeat steps 10 through to 15.

Massage of the legs and feet

This massage can be combined with a pedicure or used as part of a body massage sequence.

1. Commence effleurage at the phalanges with the hand in a horizontal position. Stroke over the dorsal aspect of the foot and tibialis anterior to the patella (see Fig. 33.4). Lightly slide the hand down the side of the leg to the phalanges and repeat three times.
2. Hold the foot and give effleurage from the tendocalcaneus to the popliteal space covering the calf muscles (i.e. soleus, gastrocnemius – see Fig. 33.5). Slide the hand down and repeat three times.
3. Change hands and give effleurage to the other side of the leg, covering peroneus longus and extensor digitorum longus to the popliteal space (see Fig. 33.6). Slide the hand down and repeat three times. Hold the foot and give single-handed effleurage, the strokes are firm and the leg does not move.
4. Support the foot and slide one hand towards the patella and, using kneading movements with the heel of the hand, circle down the

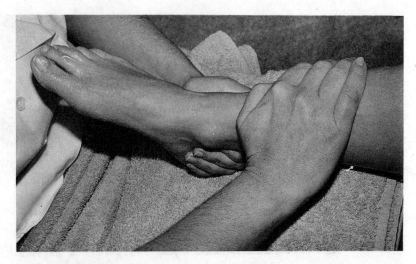

Fig. 33.4 Massaging the dorsal aspect of the leg

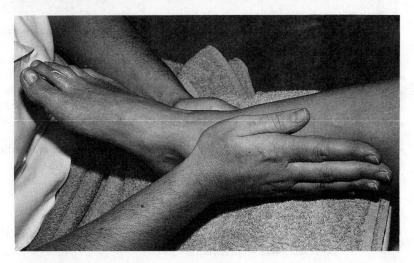

Fig. 33.5 Massaging the medial aspect of the leg

tibialis anterior to the ankle (see Fig. 33.7). Deep stroke back to the patella and repeat three times.

5. From the ankle, palmar knead the calf muscles. Support the heel with the left hand and with the right hand palmar knead, lifting the muscles medially, exert pressure and relax. Move upwards slowly with the hand in a new position each time, until the entire calf area has been covered. Pressure will depend on the condition and bulk of the muscles. Slide the hand back to the ankle, reverse the hands – holding the ankle with the right hand and palmar knead the muscles with the left hand (see Fig. 33.8). Repeat three times each side of the leg.

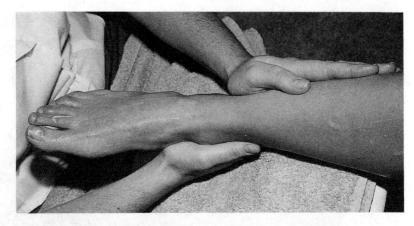

Fig. 33.6 Massaging the lateral aspect of the leg

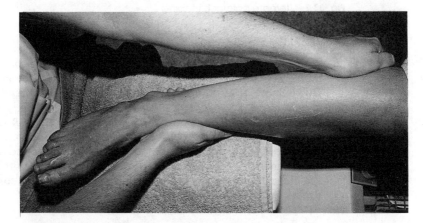

Fig. 33.7 Kneading the tibialis anterior

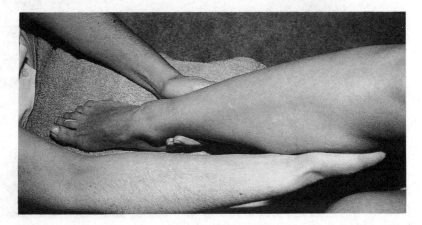

Fig. 33.8 Palmar kneading the calf muscles

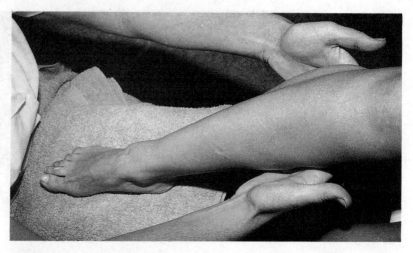

Fig. 33.9 Alternate palmar kneading

6. With link effleurage, alternate palmar kneading with both hands from the popliteal space to the ankle – three times (see Fig. 33.9). This is more of a rolling movement, stretching and strengthening muscle fibres.
7. Dependent upon the condition of the muscles, a brisk clapping movement may be given by cupping the hands and using the alternate palmar areas to lift the muscles laterally and medially for approximately 30 seconds (see Fig. 33.10). Follow this with effleurage from the ankle to the popliteal space and give superficial strokes down the dorsal aspect of the leg.

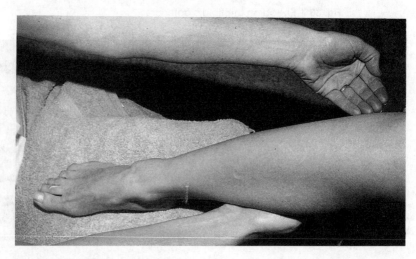

Fig. 33.10 Clapping movement

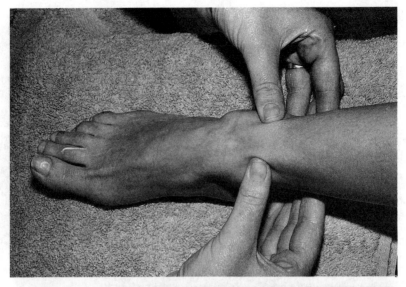

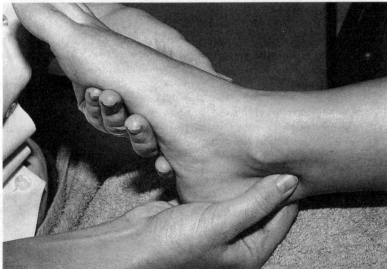

Fig. 33.11 (a) Kneading around the malleolus (b) Thumb kneading the Achilles tendon

8. Using both thumbs give kneading around the lateral and medial malleolus (the two rounded prominences either side of the ankle) (see Fig. 33.11(a)), then hold the foot and knead the Achilles tendon (see Fig. 33.11(b)). Effleurage the entire area.
9. Hold the foot and give thumb kneading between the metatarsals, i.e. between the first and second metatarsal to the proximal end of the toes (see Fig. 33.12). Effleurage with the thumb back to the base

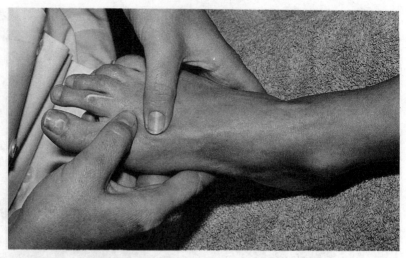

Fig. 33.12 Thumb kneading between the metatarsals

between the second and third metatarsals; then repeat the kneading until the four areas between the metatarsals have been covered.
10. Hold the foot and give thumb rotary kneading over the phalanges – especially over the joints to increase circulation. Stroke down the hallux (big toe) with the thumb and index finger, turn the hand and very gently pull the phalange to stretch the muscle fibres (same as the manicure step in Figs. 29.16(a) and (b). Repeat this movement on the remaining four toes.
11. Circle the toes. Hold the foot with the palm of one hand on the dorsal aspect (thumb on the posterior) and the other hand grasping all toes firmly (see Fig. 33.13). Circle the toes to the right and then to the left – six times each way.

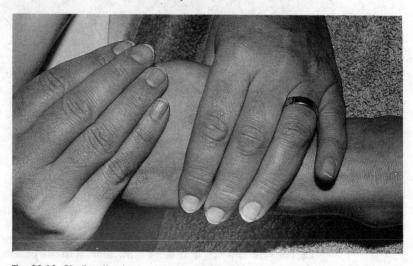

Fig. 33.13 Circling the toes

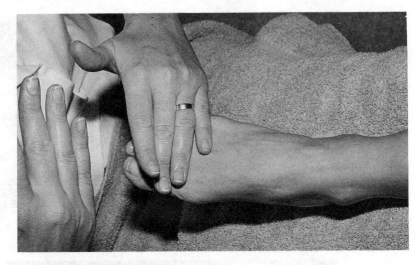

Fig. 33.14 Tapotement over the toes

12. To increase circulation of the toes use stimulating movements. Make light tapotement strokes with the fingers over the toes rapidly in an upward direction (see Fig. 33.14). To avoid any discomfort these movements should not be performed over inflamed areas or corns.
13. To give deep stroking on the sole of the foot and to extend the toes, hold the foot with the fingers resting on the dorsal aspect and the thumbs under the metatarsals. Criss-cross the thumbs with firm pressure from the base of the phalanges towards the calcaneum (see Fig. 33.15). Deep stroke with the thumbs up the sole of the foot extending the toes at the base of the phalanges. Repeat three times.

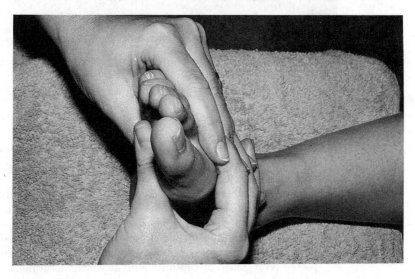

Fig. 33.15 Criss-cross movements on the sole of the foot

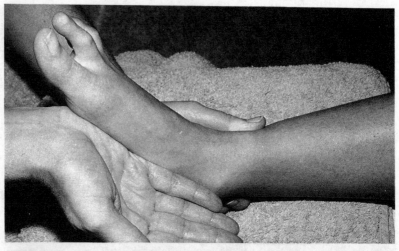

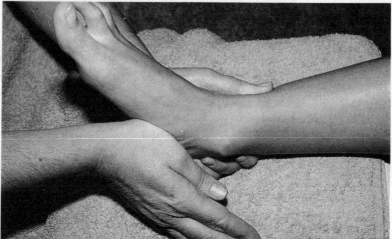

Fig. 33.16 (a) Using the ulnar border of the hand (b) Using the thenar eminence of the hand

14. To massage the arch of the foot, hold the heel and with the other hand perform deep strokes with the ulnar border (see Fig. 33.16(a)) and then turn the hand and use the thenar eminence – from the base of the hallux to the heel (see Fig. 33.16(b)). Repeat six times.
15. Make deep strokes around the lateral and medial malleolus and finally perform effleurage over the foot and leg.
16. Repeat the massage for the other leg. If required, the massage medium may be removed with a toner. The pedicure can be completed with polish or continue with any other treatment, i.e. paraffin wax.

Application of nail polish

This is applied in the same manner as for manicure. Ensure nail polish remover is wiped over the nails to remove any grease. Insert pedi-pads or cotton wool between the toes and apply base coat, nail polish and top coat or sealer.

Leave the feet on the footstool, wrapped in a towel but avoiding the nail polish.

When the nails are completely dry, remove the pedi-pads between the toes. Sprinkle medicated foot powder, especially between the toes, over and under both feet.

Give the client her shoes and tights/stockings and if necessary help with these.

Escort the client to the Reception Desk for payment.

As with manicure, discard all orange-sticks, emery boards and paper towels. Clean your instruments and steel file and place them in the steriliser. Put towels in a basket for washing and generally clean up.

It is suggested that dark towels, maybe brown, are used for the feet as this will ensure that these, even when washed, are never used for the face.

Contra-indications

- infections or diseases (i.e. onychomycosis or onychia)
- common warts and verrucae
- knife work or use of clippers/nippers, is a contra-indication for clients taking steroids, anti-coagulants or who suffer from diabetes.

Self assessment

- why is it important not to file into the corners of a toe-nail plate?
- what is the purpose of a cuticle knife?
- how would you remove hard skin on the foot?
- when would you not use a clapping massage movement on the calf muscles?
- list the contra-indications for a pedicure.

34 Care of the legs and feet

Conditions affecting the feet

Nearly everyone is born with perfect feet and during childhood most parents ensure that children's feet are measured and the right shoes purchased with growth in mind. However, as children grow up, fashion usually dictates the type of footwear worn, i.e. high heels or narrow, pointed shoes. You can advise your client, especially when you see cramped toes, corns, chilblains and bunions.

Before giving a pedicure, you will have examined the feet closely and will have decided whether there are any contra-indications, i.e. infections or disease of the nails. Athlete's foot already described in Chapter 28, can easily be picked up in saunas, communal bathrooms, shower and swimming-pool areas. Verrucae, occurring on the soles of the feet, are caused by a virus which may also be picked up in moist areas. They are easily recognised as 'foot warts' or 'corns' but, if not treated quickly, will grow bigger and multiply. Here medical treatment should be obtained as the condition can be quickly and effectively corrected. If you have touched the area at all observe the strictest hygiene and clean the hands with surgical spirit. Pressure by shoes will create numerous problems, as will heels higher than 1.5–2 in (3.8–5 cm).

Ill-fitting shoes can often lead to nail-bed infections, metatarsalgia, hammer toes, hallux-vulgus, bursitis, corns and flat-feet. High heels will distort the natural curve of the spine, posture will suffer as the body's weight is unevenly distributed.

The following are some common foot faults.

Nail-bed infections

These are often caused by pressure of the shoe, with very little air around the toes and sometimes through lack of cleanliness.

Metatarsalgia

This is pain in the metatarsus. The wearing of high heels will force the metatarsals to take the body's weight thereby stretching the ligaments of the feet. Joints can become inflamed, resulting in pain.

Hammer toes

These are recognised by a clawlike appearance, where the proximal phalange of the toe is extended and the second and distal phalanges are flexed and humped.

Hallus-vulgus

Hallus is the name given to the big toe and vulgus is the condition where the big toe is pushed either under or towards the other toes, generally known as a *bunion*. This is often caused by shoes being too tight and heels too high. There are conditions affecting the big toe which are easily recognised:

- *hallux varus* means that the big toe is moving away from the other toes;
- *hallus malleolus* is a hammer toe affecting the big toe;
- *hallus flexus* means that the big toe is bent.

Bursitis

This is the inflammation of a bursa which is a small connective tissue sac lined with synovial membrane and containing synovial fluid. It is always located where pressure is exerted over moving parts as its purpose is to facilitate the gliding of muscles or tendons over bony or ligamentous surfaces. This can occur if shoes are too tight or rubbing the heel, causing an inflammation of the bursae around the achilles tendon. This condition is often found around the patella and can be aggravated by wearing of high heels.

Corns

Hard corns found on the toes are a conical keratinous mass, always caused by friction or pressure, again by poorly fitting shoes. They are a nuisance and quite painful when the point of the conical mass causes pressure on the nerve endings in the corium. For older people they can be quite disabling. Soft corns are usually found, as a white mass, between the fourth and fifth toes. Again pressure will make this condition painful.

Callouses

These denote hard, dead skin. It is the thickening of the stratum corneum which can grow over any body prominence but is usually found on the ball of the foot. This is a condition you may be able to alleviate with a foot scraper, but it usually requires the expert attention of a chiropodist. A paraffin-wax foot bath will also help to soften hard skin and callouses.

Flat feet

This is recognised by the absence of the normal arch of the sole of the foot. It can be the result of constant standing, being overweight, lack of exercise or again ill-fitting shoes. Muscles lose their tone, the ligaments binding the bones of the feet together stretch and the arches flatten out.

Chilblains

The basic cause of these are sensitivity to cold or poor circulation which can also affect fingers and ears as well as feet. They appear as painful erythema accompanied by inflammation and swelling. Shoe pressure will aggravate this condition. Recommend direct high-frequency treatment around the area (but not on the chilblain centre) to help circulation.

Tired and aching feet

This can often be the cause of any of the above foot faults. A clay pack (see pp. 326–7) is most refreshing and helps to reduce swelling. However, swelling of the ankles often needs a more in-depth knowledge of the client. Females often experience a little swelling prior to menstruation but this is only caused by an increase in the production of progesterone. Pregnancy also increases this hormone. If your client experiences sudden severe swelling either around the entire ankle or even to one side suggest seeking medical advice. In serious circumstances it may suggest heart trouble or water retention but usually there is a simpler explanation – the consumption of too much coffee!

Excessive perspiration

For feet which perspire too much, giving off unpleasant odours, suggest the following daily treatment at home.

1. Wash the feet in lukewarm water and rinse them under a cold running tap. Dry the feet well and apply an astringent all over them.
2. If inflammation is present but not serious enough to consult a doctor, calamine cream or lotion can be applied to the area.
3. When feet are perfectly dry, especially between the toes, apply a medicated foot powder.
4. Changing stockings/tights and shoes every day is important.
5. If the changing of shoes every day is not possible, advise inner soles which can be washed frequently. There are also commercially available products which can be sprayed inside the shoes to keep them fresh.
6. Air to the feet is important, advise leaving off tights and wearing of sandals whenever possible.

Ingrowing toe-nails

These can be painful and are usually the result of the nail plate being cut or filed. As the nail tries to regain its original form it cuts into the nail groove and any pressure, by walking or wearing tight-fitting shoes or tights, will aggravate the condition. To allow the nail plate to return to its natural groove, saturate a wisp of lamb's wool in olive oil and, with an orange-stick, wedge this between the nail groove and the nail plate. Show the client how this is done so that the treatment can be continued at home.

Conditions affecting the legs

Varicose veins

These are mainly hereditary and do not come within the scope of the work of a beauty therapist. It must be stressed that faradic, vibratory or hand massage may not be given over varicose veins. Clients should be advised to rest their legs when possible, wear support hose and walk up to three miles a day.

Blemishes (i.e. 'thread' veins) or bruises

These may be slow to disappear or they may be embarrassing but they seldom have any serious effect and can be disguised with a suitable leg tint.

Treatment for the legs and feet

Foot exercises

Feet benefit from a basic exercise routine to strengthen the supporting structures around the ankle bone, arch of the foot and toes. Exercise will improve circulation, thereby bringing warmth to cold feet and help to alleviate chilblains.

1. In a sitting position, place the right ankle on top of the left knee. Stretch and bend the right foot from the ankle, i.e. turn the foot upward as far as it will go, then stretch the foot down and back to its fullest extent. Then circle the ankle clockwise and anti-clockwise. Change the left ankle to the right knee and repeat the plantar flex and inversion followed by the circular movement with the left foot.
2. Sitting in a chair with a broom handle on the floor, slowly curl the toes around the broom handle, release and repeat. This will stretch the metatarsophalangeal joint.
3. 'Pedalling' can be done by either sitting on a chair or on the floor. When sitting, raise one heel off the floor and as it is lowered, raise the other heel. The ball of the foot is not raised but left firmly on the floor. When sitting on the floor, one foot is dorsiflexed and the other plantarflexed and again you have a 'pedalling' movement, but the knees must be kept straight.
4. Sit on the floor, bend the knees outward so that the feet are turned inward. Hold the ankle of one foot with one hand and make a fist with the other. Working with the knuckles, perform slow, circular movements from the arch to the base of the toes, back to the heel and then to the arch. Repeat on the other foot. This can be done several times and will relax and stimulate the soles of the feet.
5. Standing, raise the heels slightly off the floor and hold for a count of five. Then raise the heels higher and again hold to the count of five. Finally raise the heels as high as possible, hold to the count of five and very slowly lower the heels to the floor to a count of six. This

also requires balance so initially advise the clients to support themselves using a chair or doorway.

6. Goose-stepping tones up the feet and legs. Simply raise one leg at a time with the feet turned upward. Then place the heel on the floor and repeat with the other leg.

Only six exercises are detailed but read articles in magazines and books to further your knowledge.

Intermittent compression massage

This is a treatment which helps to improve venous and lymphatic circulation of the legs by using inflatable leggings, known as 'boots'. It will not reduce the size of the legs or improve cellulite, but it will relieve the feeling of tired, heavy legs often caused by standing, especially in one position for any length of time, e.g. shop assistants, hairdressers, etc.

The machine itself has an electrically operated pump for inflation, indicator lights for the on/off switch and for the air pressure and an air-pressure gauge or controller. At the side of the machine are outlets into which are pushed the long plastic tubes from the boots. The boots themselves come in various sizes, i.e. large, medium and half leg, and are made of washable polyurethane material and all are fitted with zips to facilitate use. At the top of the boot there is a valve (outlet) with a ring which is pulled out to deflate the boots.

The benefits of intermittent compression massage

- Improves venous flow and can be used over varicose veins at low pressure
- Helps to eliminate waste toxins.
- Improves both peripheral and lymphatic oedema.
- Useful for sports injuries, where bruising or oedema is evident.
- Relieves feeling of tired, heavy swollen legs and ankles.

Contra-indications

- Acute thrombo-phlebitis.
- Any known or suspected recent deep vein thrombosis.
- Acute pulmonary oedema.
- Congestive heart failure.

Preparation

Ensure that the client's record card has been completed, especially any medical history – including any medication being taken, before commencing the treatment. Request the client to remove shoes, tights/stockings etc. and assist her/him on to a couch in a semi-reclining position. Place the machine on a stable surface and plug into a socket.

Note: For photographic purposes the machine has been placed at the end of the couch in Fig. 34.1.

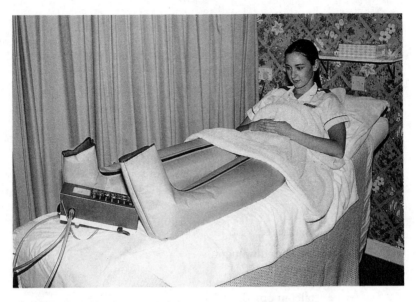

Fig. 34.1 Intermittent compression massage using the 'boots'

Method of use

1. Lightly massage the legs with a suitable gel/cream or leg balm (e.g. containing essential oils of camphor or peppermint for a cooling effect) and cover the legs with two sheets of plastic.
2. Place the client's legs on the boots which are then zipped up to the top. The long plastic tubes are fitted into the outlets at the side of the machine and the pull ring is inserted into the valve (outlet) at the top of the boot.
3. Switch on the machine and both indicator lights will illuminate. The air-pressure control, which will read from 20 to 120 mm Hg should be turned up to approximately 25 mm Hg. The machine will take approximately five minutes to achieve normal running pressure and then the client will feel inflation and decompression of the tissues on alternate legs. More modern machines inflate and deflate simultaneously on both legs. You should adjust the pressure accordingly to ensure that the compression is adequate, but on the other hand it should not be too strong.
4. When the treatment has been completed (usually after 30 minutes) the pull ring is released to allow for deflation before unzipping the boots. Use damp cotton wool to remove perspiration, gel/cream or balm from the legs and apply a skin toner.
5. The usual courtesies are extended to the client before leaving the salon.
6. The maintenance of the equipment is minimal. The plastic tubes must be kept clean and the boots washed (inside and outside) after use.

Faradic foot bath

A faradic foot bath can be given to re-educate the muscles of the foot. This treatment should not be attempted until you are totally familiar with the faradic current.

Contra-indications

- client wearing a pacemaker
- high blood pressure
- highly strung nervous clients
- cuts, abrasions or any areas of septic foci.

Preparation

You will need:

- faradic equipment
- electrodes
- a large plastic bowl
- talcum powder
- towels.

Method of use

1. Have sufficient warm water in the bowl to cover the toes. On this occasion you will not need salt.
2. Place both feet in the water and ensure that the client is sitting comfortably, thighs well supported and the knees at right angles to the feet when they are in the bowl.
3. Place an electrode under the heel and another under the meta-tarsophalangeal joint of each foot. (It may be that you have large electrodes which can cover both areas and therefore only two electrodes will be required.)
4. Switch on the current and turn it up until the usual prickly sensation in felt. The current can then be turned up very slowly until the muscles begin to contract. Between each contraction make sure that the toes straighten out.

   Your client may be apprehensive about the thought of water with electricity. Do not leave the client at any time and the first treatment should not last for more than ten minutes. It is an excellent treatment which can be given daily. This is not always possible in a salon but do suggest two or three treatments a week initially and once a week thereafter. The duration can be increased by three to five minutes as treatments progress but do not exceed the maximum of twenty minutes.

Clay packs

Make your own clay pack with equal parts of kaolin and magnesium carbonate mixed with water to a thick creamy consistency.

Contra-indications

These are few, mainly diseases or septic foci, cuts or abrasions.

Preparation

- a low stool for yourself
- a leg rest covered with a piece of plastic
- a larger sheet of plastic to spread on the floor
- two small plastic trays
- a paint brush $1\frac{1}{2}$–2 in (3.8–5 cm) wide
- large bowl
- massage cream
- almond oil
- astringent
- medicated foot powder
- super-fatted soap
- 2–3 towels
- paper tissues

1. Spread the large sheet of plastic over the floor. Wash the feet well in warm, soapy water with an antiseptic solution added and dry. Throw away this water and refill with warm water.
2. Place the left leg on the leg rest and the right foot on a plastic tray. With a brush apply the clay liberally all over the right foot and ankle and leave the foot in the tray.
3. Massage the left foot and leg and remove the cream with an astringent.
4. Dry the left leg and foot and place the left foot in the second plastic tray and apply the coating of clay (see Fig. 34.2). Leave both feet in the clay for ten minutes.
5. Take the right foot and wash off the clay, dry and massage the leg and foot. Remove the cream with an astringent.
6. Wash the clay off the left foot and dry well.
7. Massage both legs and feet with almond oil and remove any surplus oil with paper tissues.

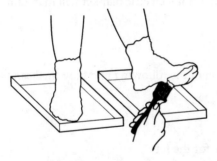

Fig. 34.2 Applying clay pack

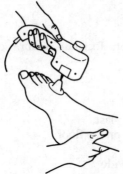

Fig. 34.3 Use of vibrator on the foot

8. With an astringent perform friction movements over the feet and ankles and dry well with paper tissues and apply medicated foot powder.
9. Remove trays, plastic sheeting, water and bowl of clay before assisting client to dress.

If you are giving a pedicure the clay pack would be applied prior to the application of the base coat.

Vibratory massage

Using an electric vibrator on the feet and legs will stimulate circulation (see Chapter 30 for contra-indications and use). On the legs, as with massage by hand, move the vibrator from origin to insertion on the muscles. Avoid any bony areas, i.e. the tibia. The balls of the feet and the heels may be vibrated, but avoid the arch of the foot as the veins are near the surface (see Fig. 34.3).

Paraffin-wax baths

Paraffin wax application for the hands has been explained in Chapter 30 and the benefits from the wax and method of use (either brush or immersion method) can be equally applied to the feet. Paraffin wax will also help to soften hard skin and callouses. Padded booties (instead of mitts) or towels are used after the feet have been waxed and placed in a plastic sheet/foil and a small electric blanket will maintain the heat of the wax.

Self assessment

- give an explanation of the following and how they can be avoided:

    (a) metatarsalgia
    (b) corns
    (c) callouses

- list three exercises for the feet
- give the benefits of:

(a) a clay pack
(b) a faradic foot bath
(c) a vibratory massage

- give the contra-indications for intermittent compression massage.

35 Bleaching, depilation and waxing

Superfluous hair is an excess of hair which is regarded as unattractive if it appears on areas of the body which women prefer to be hairless, e.g. face, underarms, abdomen, bikini line and legs. However, there are races and sects who regard hair in some of these areas to be acceptable and wish the hair to grow there naturally.

There are many reasons for superfluous hair, but hormonal influences are the most common. This is noted at the onset of puberty when underarm and pubic hairs appear. Often there is an increase during pregnancy and at the menopause. Other causes include glandular disturbances which, in the extreme, cause 'hirsutism', a condition of excessive hair growth often associated with a malfunction of the ovary or adrenal glands. Heredity factors, old age and certain drugs will also influence hair growth.

Temporary removal methods include shaving, using abrasive gloves, plucking, the use of chemical or waxing depilatories.

The first two are rarely used by the beauty therapist in the salon. During a shave the hairs are cut off at skin level and new growth appears bristly and uncomfortable. However, it is doubtful, if left to grow, that the hairs will be any thicker or stronger. Abrasive gloves are used in circular movements to 'rub' off the hairs. The regrowth is not impaired and appears less bristly.

Plucking is an obvious way to deal with isolated hairs, e.g. eyebrows (see Chapter 16, pp. 166–7).

Waxing is popular; it removes the hair from its follicle but rarely destroys the root. The regrowth of hair appears over a period of four to six weeks.

For these treatments the client's clothing should be removed or protected with towels or paper.

Bleaching

Bleaching is an effective way of disguising unwanted hairs. With age excess hair tends to become slightly darker and thicker and the use of bleach, especially on a large area, is useful. Bleaching affects the cortex of the hair (Chapter 7, p. 75), as the melanin (brown or black pigment) and the pheomelanin (yellow or red pigment) are oxidised to become colourless. The most common oxidising agent used is hydrogen peroxide as it is an oxide with more than the normal proportion of oxygen. The catalyst to break down the peroxide to release the oxygen is an alkaline substance, usually a diluted ammonia solution.

Contra-indications

- skin infections
- cuts, blisters or burns (e.g. sun-burn)
- sensitive skins
- dry, flaky skins
- moles, warts or cold sores (herpes).

Inevitably the bleach will come into contact with the skin and therefore a patch is advisable. This will ensure that the strength of the bleach has been assessed correctly and that any skin reaction will be seen.

When the bleach has been made, place a small amount of the bleach on a clean area and leave for five minutes. Wash off with warm water and dry with a tissue. Check the hairs to ensure that the bleach has removed the colour, and the skin for any immediate reaction. Request the client to return to the salon after 24–48 hours to inspect the area again before proceeding with the treatment.

A bleach for hair on arms and legs

Bleaches are available commercially, but you can make your own by mixing:

- 2 fluid oz (57 gm) of 6 per cent (20 vol) hydrogen peroxide
- 10 drops of 28 per cent ammonia water
- magnesium carbonate (known as white henna) or Fuller's earth.

You will also need for any type of bleaching:

- cleanser
- spatula or brush
- cotton wool
- tissues
- clean towels
- antiseptic moisturiser.

Application

1. Place a towel under the limb.
2. Cleanse the area and remove the cleanser with damp cotton wool.
3. Mix the peroxide, ammonia water and one of the powders to a thin paste (or have the purchased products ready).
4. Apply the paste/cream to the area with a spatula or brush and leave for five minutes.
5. Check the hairs in a small area to ensure the bleach has removed the colour (if required it can be left for another minute).
6. Use hot damp towels to remove the paste/cream and ensure that none is left in the folds of the skin.
7. Wipe the area with warm water and cotton-wool pads.
8. Tissue dry and moisturise well.

A bleach for fine hair

- use equal parts of lemon juice, 6 per cent (20 vol) hydrogen per-oxide and witch-hazel together.

Application

1. This bleach can be painted on the area and be left for approximately 15 minutes but it is advisable to check the hair and skin at intervals after five minutes have elapsed.
2. Wash the bleach off with warm water, pat dry with tissues and apply an antiseptic moisturiser.

A bleach for the skin

- The mixture is egg-white and peroxide. The strength of the latter is important and it can vary from 3 per cent (10 vol) to 6 per cent (20 vol) depending on the skin.

This may not be so effective as the strength of the bleach must be mild. However, it can help sallow or sluggish complexions, especially the neck area, faded tans and discolouration above the lips and fingers due to nicotine staining.

Application

1. Apply to the area with a brush and leave for 10–15 minutes.
2. Check the area at intervals after five minutes have elapsed.
3. Wash the area well with warm water and pat dry with tissues.
4. Apply a moisturiser.

Chemical depilation

Chemical depilatories are used mainly as an alternative to hot or cool waxing. There are creams or pastes commercially available which can be applied to the hairs with a spatula. Providing there are no lesions these depilatories can be used over varicose veins.

Contra-indications

- skin conditions, i.e. spots, bruises inflammation, infectious or con-tagious diseases, psoriasis, eczema
- any moles or warts present must be avoided and any hairs on these should be cut with scissors
- herpes (cold sores).

To avoid any allergic reaction, a simple test should be made by placing a small amount of depilatory (cream or paste) on to a clean area and left for five minutes before wiping off. If any redness or irritation appears this will preclude the treatment.

You will need for chemical depilation:

- the depilatory cream or paste
- cleanser

- spatula
- cotton wool
- tissues
- clean towels
- antiseptic lotion/cream.

Application

1. Cleanse the area and dry thoroughly.
2. The depilatory is smoothed on thickly with a spatula covering the hairs well.
3. Dependent upon the hair growth leave the cream/paste for 7–10 minutes.
4. Gently remove with a spatula (using tissues to clean this as you work) taking care not to scrape the skin.
5. Rinse the area with cold water ensuring that all the depilatory has been removed.
6. Pat the skin dry with tissues and apply antiseptic lotion/cream.
7. Advise the client to avoid the use of sun-beds, hot baths, soaps or detergents and not to apply perfumed lotions for at least eight hours.

Wax depilation

There is more than one method of removing hairs (i.e. with hot or warm wax explained below) or other procedures where the manufacturer's instructions must be closely followed. New clients should be advised of the methods available and the possible sensitivity of waxing.

Contra-indications to both hot and warm waxing

- skin conditions (i.e. spots, cuts, bruises, inflammation, infections or contagious diseases, psoriasis or eczema
- moles or warts
- impaired circulation, i.e. diabetic condition, leg ulcers, etc.
- varicose veins
- aged or very thin skin
- herpes (cold sores)
- sun-bed immediately before or after treatment
- the use of a swimming pool after the treatment (the water usually contains chemicals).

Hot waxing

Hot wax is made from beeswax and resin. Use of good quality wax is essential as cheap versions tend to be brittle. New wax requires heating several times to thicken before use or it should be mixed with used clean wax, otherwise it will be thin, become brittle and break off in small pieces.

This wax can be used for legs, arms, underarms, bikini line, upper lip and chin. Waxing should not be attempted over varicose veins or thin skin as the removal of the wax could result in bruising or even tear the skin. Results are better achieved if the hairs are of a minimum length, i.e. 0.2 in (0.5 cm) to ensure a secure grip.

Regrowth hair is generally very fine but occasionally hairs can ingrow and cause discomfort. Further waxing in this small area should not be attempted again until the hair/s have worked their way out. If the ingrowing hairs appear on the legs the client can be advised to use a friction mitt gently over the area when in the bath or shower.

You will need for hot wax depilation:

- a thermostatically controlled heater with a filtering system
- magnifying lamp
- surgical spirit
- talcum powder
- wooden spatula and small brush
- tweezers
- soothing antiseptic lotion or cream
- soap and water or a cleanser
- clean towels
- for waxing the legs and bikini line it is more comfortable for the client if the couch also has plastic sheeting.

Application

For waxing the legs and bikini line the couch should be prepared with plastic sheeting or foil rather than a paper roll. This will prevent any spilt drops of wax sticking to the paper and the client's skin. Ensure the heater is on a stable base, i.e. a trolley, which can be brought close to the couch. Assist the client into position and protect any clothing not removed with towels or paper.

The following is the general method for all applications:

1. Check the areas to be waxed, under an illuminated magnifying lamp, for contra-indications and to determine the patterns of hair growth.
2. To remove natural surface oils, cleanse or wash the area well and dry thoroughly or use surgical spirit.
3. Make sure the wax has melted to a syrup consistency with a temperature of 48 °C (118 °F). The wax should be tested on the inside of the therapist's wrist before application to ensure the correct temperature.
4. Use talcum powder to the area *against* the hair growth, the small brush can be used to uplift any hairs lying flat on the skin. Test the wax.
5. Apply the wax with a spatula, again *against the hair growth* then smooth the wax with the natural growth and finally against the growth, i.e. three applications. The wax can be applied quite quickly but keep the edges of the wax thick. Until you perfect the method it is wise to keep the length of the strip of wax quite short.
6. Curl or flick up the edge of the wax and knead or press down the centre. Leave it for a minute and while the wax is still firm but flexible, take the flicked-up edge and rip off with one stroke.

Always hold the area just below the wax to save the skin being pulled and immediately soothe the area with pressure of the hand or fingers to momentarily exclude the air and the stinging effect.
7. Check carefully to see that no particles of wax are left on the skin. A stray hair may be removed with tweezers or a small area may be re-waxed if the skin does not appear red or feel sensitive.
8. Apply an antiseptic lotion or cream to alleviate the tightness of the skin.

Although application of wax in each area may differ, the direction of the hair growth or contour of the area should be followed. Much emphasis is placed on this as hairs grow at various angles especially on the back of the legs and thighs.

Ankle to knee waxing

After preparation of the area, check the hair growth first. It may be necessary to follow the contour of the leg instead.

(a) Apply the wax with a spatula along the anterior surface of the leg and build up the wax evenly. Until you are proficient this can be done in two sections.
(b) Keep the edges thick, flick the lower edge and press the wax down with your knuckles. Hold the ankle and rip off the wax. Always remember to soothe each area waxed with the pressure of the hand.
(c) Repeat above this area (if necessary) making sure that the new strip meets the edge of the area waxed.
(d) Apply two strips to the lateral and medial parts of the tibia (in two sections either side if required).
(e) When the anterior aspect of the leg has been completed, bend the knee, apply wax and remove any hairs. Repeat for the other leg.
(f) Request the client to turn over. Wax the posterior of the legs, either in long strips from the Achilles tendon towards the popliteal space, or in oblique or flat curves depending on the direction of hair growth (again this can be done in sections).
(g) Massage the entire area – anterior and posterior – with an antiseptic lotion or cream.

As a guide to the method of ankle to knee waxing see Fig. 35.1

Full leg waxing

(a) Complete waxing the anterior aspect of the lower leg and knee and then divide the thigh into sections and wax the front of thigh (see Fig. 35.2). Repeat for the other leg.
(b) Request the client to turn over and, commencing at the ankle, wax the posterior aspect of the lower leg. Again divide the thigh into sections and wax the posterior aspect. Repeat for the other leg (see Fig. 35.2).

The above are general guidelines. Check the hair growth carefully as this will dictate the angle of wax applied. Massage antiseptic lotion or cream over entire areas.

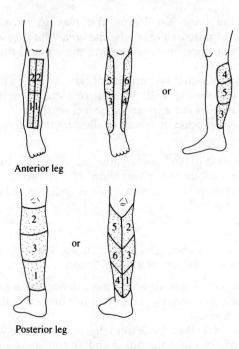

Fig. 35.1 Leg waxing – ankle to knee

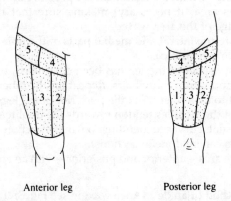

Fig. 35.2 Leg waxing – upper leg

Bikini waxing

(a) Request the client to wear plastic or disposable briefs as these will indicate the line of removal. If this is not possible, tuck into briefs, paper or tissues carefully for protection and for the line.

(b) Request the client to lie on the couch, open the leg and bend the knee to the side.

(c) Apply the wax in two small sections (see Fig. 35.3). Rip off and immediately soothe the area with antiseptic cream. Repeat for the other side.

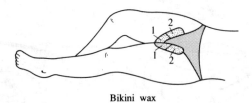

Bikini wax

Fig. 35.3 Bikini waxing

Remember to keep the wax and edges thick to ensure that all the hairs are removed in one attempt as it is not advisable to go over this area again. Blood spots or redness will require a dusting of anti-bacterial powder.

Abdomen waxing

Usually hairs only appear from the navel to the pubic line and these can be removed easily with one strip of wax.

Underarm waxing

This area should be treated with extreme caution as the skin in the axillae is delicate and any infection will cause the glands to swell.

(a) Check the skin carefully for contra-indications and cleanse well.
(b) Lift the arm and request the client to place her hand under her head. Apply talcum powder.
(c) Wax from the top outer edge towards the centre. Depending on hair growth this may require two strips of wax.
(d) Wax from the lower area to the centre for the complete removal of hair.
(e) Keep the skin taut to minimise discomfort and soothe immediately with an antiseptic lotion or cream.
(f) Repeat for the other underarm.
(g) Check both underarms. If blood spots or redness appears give a dusting of anti-bacterial powder.
(h) Advise the client to refrain from using anti-perspirants or deodorants for a minimum of twelve hours.

Lip waxing

(a) All make-up in the area should be removed and the area cleansed and dried thoroughly or use the surgical spirit. Use talcum powder and uplift the hairs.
(b) The spatula should not exceed 0.5 in (1.3 cm) in width and due to the sensitivity of the area the wax should be slightly cooler.
(c) Apply the wax in sections (see Fig. 35.4) against the hair growth, usually from the corners of the mouth towards the nostrils and across the area above the lips. Keep the skin taut by stretching it between your fingers as you pull off the wax. Immediately place your fingers over each area as it is de-waxed.

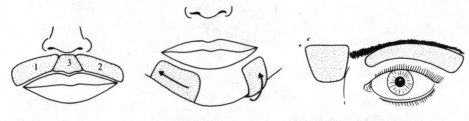

Fig. 35.4 Lip waxing   **Fig. 35.5** Chin waxing   **Fig. 35.6** Eyebrow waxing

(d) Redness in the area can be reduced by applying a small cold-compress. This can be made with an ice cube wrapped in a small towel – no fridge! – use thin cucumber slices. Always finish with the antiseptic lotion or cream and advise the client to avoid make-up in the area for a minimum of two hours. If this is not possible use a medicated foundation to avoid infection.

Chin waxing

Apply the wax against the hair growth, which may mean starting under the chin with small strips and/or applying the wax along the mandible. Use the same procedure as for lip waxing (see Fig. 35.5).

Eyebrow waxing

Another very delicate area and discussion with the client is very important for the required shape and thickness of the eyebrows.

(a) Smooth the eyebrows and with a small brush or orange-stick separate the unwanted hairs.
(b) Cover the eyes with damp cotton-wool pads (in case of an accident with the wax).
(c) Using a very small spatula, apply a very thin strip of wax under the brow (proceed as for lip waxing for both eyebrows).
(d) If necessary apply wax to the area between the eyebrows. There are occasions when the client will request waxing above the eyebrows. Be careful not to make the brows too thin or uneven (see Fig. 35.6).

Cleaning the wax and heater

While you are working with a client, lay aside the used wax. As soon as time permits, the wax may be put back in the container to be cleaned of all loose hairs and reused. It is important to clean the filter regularly, depending on the amount of usage.

For small areas it is more hygienic to throw away the used wax, e.g. bikini line, underarms etc.

Use an equipment cleaner to keep the rings of the heater free of wax and, when not in use, the lid should be kept on the heater.

Warm waxing

Warm waxing (also known as cool waxing) is popular because it is easy to apply and remove, equipment costs are low and it is hygienic.

You will need for warm wax depilation:

- a thermostatically controlled heater to melt the wax to approximately 43 °C (110 °F), when it will become warm and clear
- wax in a container which should fit into the heater
- surgical spirit
- tongue depressors or thin wooden spatulas
- cleansers or pre-wax lotions
- talcum powder
- tweezers
- cotton wool
- cut strips of calico (or strong fabric) to suit the area to be waxed
- antiseptic lotion or cream.

The following is the general method for all applications:

1. Use a strong light (magnifying lamp) to inspect the area to be waxed for any contra-indications etc., as for hot waxing.
2. Cleanse the area well with either cleanser or pre-wax lotion or surgical spirit.
3. Follow the manufacturer's instructions, which often includes a fine dusting of talcum powder.
4. The therapist must test the temperature of the wax on the inside of her wrist.
5. Place the spatula in the wax and drain this on the side of the heater. Spread a thin film of wax *in the direction of the hair growth*, using the edge of the spatula at an angle of approximately 90°.
6. Place the strip of calico over the area, leaving the lower edge free and press firmly.
7. Take the free edge, support the skin below the wax and remove the calico swiftly *against the hair growth*. When removing the strip it should almost fold back on itself (see Fig. 35.7).
8. Soothe the area waxed with the pressure of your hand or fingers (as with hot waxing) and apply the antiseptic lotion or cream with effleurage movements.

The strip of calico can be used until it cannot pick up any more hair efficiently, however, the used strip can also remove the residue of wax which may be left. It should then be folded and thrown away. The number of strips used will depend on the area being waxed but as a guide (dependent on the amount of hair present) two to four strips will be needed for an ankle to knee wax.

Wax may be re-applied over hairs left behind but this will depend

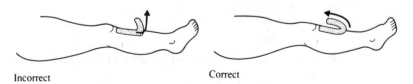

Incorrect   Correct

Fig. 35.7 Procedure for the removal of hair using a calico strip

entirely on the sensitivity of the skin and the client's tolerance. The odd hair may be removed by tweezers.

Apart from the application of the wax in the direction of the hair growth, the method is very similar to hot waxing. The same precautions must be taken and the same advice given to the client.

The following are possible reasons why hairs remain after depilatory waxing:

- the hairs were too short
- the skin was not stretched
- the wax was applied or removed in the wrong direction

Keeping the wax heater clean

'Collars', i.e. a circular band of white cardboard or thick paper, are commercially available and these are placed over the heater and cover the rims of the heater. These catch any drips of wax as the spatula is drained on the side of the heater. As these become messy they can be thrown away and replaced. When the heater is not in use replace the lid to avoid particles of dust entering the wax.

Cold waxing

There are manufacturers supplying jars with cellophane strips or wax-coated strips to smooth on. The same principle applies as with warm waxing but the manufacturer's instructions should be read carefully.

After any of the above treatments, assist the client with clothing and escort her to the reception desk. Return to the cubicle and dispose of spatulas, tissues, plastic sheeting (if used), paper, cotton wool etc. and ensure your equipment is clean and ready for the next client.

Self assessment

- when would you use bleach and how does it affect the hair?
- what are the contra-indications to bleaching?
- how would you make a bleach for fine hair?
- describe how you would make a patch test for chemical depilation
- give the temperatures for application of

    (a) hot wax
    (b) warm wax

- state the procedure, contra-indications and the advice given to the client for each of the following using the hot or warm wax method:

    (a) underarms
    (b) bikini line
    (c) lip
    (d) chin

- how would you clean your equipment for both hot or warm wax?

36 Heat and ultra-violet treatments

Heat

Heat is a form of energy and this is associated with the vibrations of the molecules.

Body heat is the by-product of the metabolic processes of the body and the temperature of the body is normally measured by a thermometer placed in the mouth. Normal body temperature varies from person to person and at different times of the day, but normally reads 98.6° on the Fahrenheit scale or 37° on the Celsius (formerly Centigrade) scale. To convert a temperature in Fahrenheit to Celsius, deduct 32 from the Fahrenheit figure, divide by 9 and multiply by 5, e.g.

$$100\,°F \text{ minus } 32 = 68 \div 9 = 7.5 \times 5 = 37.5\,°C.$$

To convert Celsius to Fahrenheit divide by 5, multiply by 9 then add 32, e.g.

$$20\,°C \div 5 = 4 \times 9 = 36 + 32 = 68\,°F$$

Heat can be transferred from one place to another by convection, conduction or radiation. During convection heat travels by the movement of heated molecules and this occurs in both liquids and gases. Conduction is where heat is passed from one molecule to the next or between solid objects which are in contact with each other. Radiation is where heat travels in the form of rays through gases or space.

Infra-red, visible, and ultra-violet rays are produced by heat and when an object is heated the increased vibration of the molecules displaces the electrons from their orbits, energy is released and electromagnetic waves are produced.

Electromagnetic waves

All electromagnetic waves are produced by movement of electrons. However, different electron movements will produce rays of different wavelengths. For example, a wavelength is the horizontal distance between corresponding points on adjacent waves. (Radio waves are quite long and expressed in metres.) Some electromagnetic waves are very short and a special measurement is used, i.e. a nanometer (nm) (being a thousand millionth of a metre). Wavelengths can also be measured in angstrom (Å) units and $10\,\text{Å} = 1\,\text{nm}$. The sequence of events that takes place between a point on one wave and the same point on the next wave is called a cycle. The number of cycles which occur in unit time is

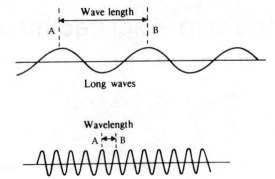

Fig. 36.1 Wavelength

known as the frequency. The distance travelled by a wave in the course of one cycle is a wavelength. The product of the wavelength and frequency gives the distance travelled by the wave in unit time which is called the velocity. Thus,

velocity = frequency × wavelength

The velocity is constant for all electromagnetic waves, but the frequency varies inversely with the wavelength.

Figure 36.1 shows two waves which take the same amount of time to travel from A to B, but the lower wave has a much shorter wavelength than the upper wave and therefore requires more cycles to reach the same distance, and therefore has a higher frequency.

The electromagnetic spectrum

This is an analysis of the electromagnetic waves as they vary considerably from radio waves to gamma waves. Figure 36.2 shows the complete spectrum.

There are rules which govern the radiation of infra-red, visible, and ultra-violet rays and these are refraction, reflection and absorption and also the law of inverse square.

Refraction

This is the deviation of a beam of light (or ray) in transversing obliquely a medium of differing intensity, i.e. if a ray passes from a less dense medium – e.g. air into a denser medium – e.g. glass – a change of direction occurs as shown in Fig. 36.3

Reflection

This can also change the direction of a ray, e.g. if a light is directed on to a mirror it will be reflected or thrown back. More rays are reflected from mirror or polished surfaces than from dark matt surfaces. When this occurs the angle of the incident ray to normal is exactly equal to the reflected ray to normal (see Fig. 36.4).

Type of wave	X-rays and gamma rays	Ultra-violet			Visible light	Infra-red		Radio
		UVC	UVB	UVA	V I B G Y O R	Short	Long	
Wave length	Short	100 nm	280 nm	315 nm	400 nm 700 nm	1400 nm		1 mm Long
Frequency	High							Low
Description		Cold invisible rays			Visible rays	Warm invisible rays		
Skin penetration		Superficial epidermis	Deep epid.	Blood vessels of dermis	Subcutaneous tissue	Superficial epidermis		
Sun's radiation at Earth's surface		⟷						

Fig. 36.2 The electromagnetic spectrum

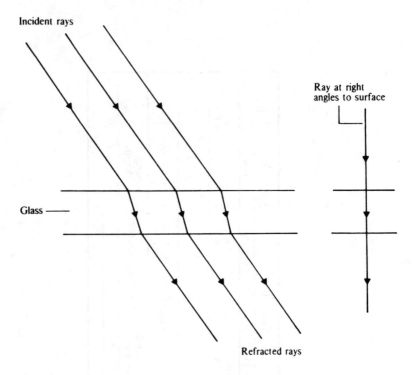

Fig. 36.3 Refraction

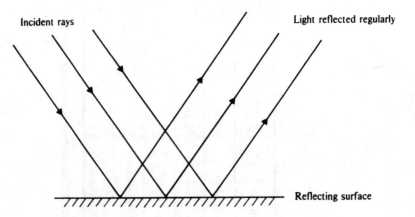

Fig. 36.4 Reflection

Absorption

When rays strike the surface of a new medium, the proportion of rays absorbed is dependent on the nature of the medium, the wavelength of the rays and the angle at which they strike the medium.

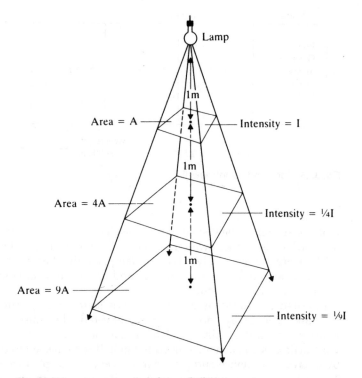

Fig. 36.5 Inverse square law for radiation

Inverse square law

The intensity of rays travelling from a lamp lessens as the rays spread out over a greater area when the distance from the lamp increases. For example, in Fig. 36.5 it will be seen that the intensity of the rays from the lamp varies inversely with the square of the distance from the lamp. Therefore the intensity of the radiation is 4 times greater at 1 m than at 2 m.

This law especially applies to infra-red, visible and ultra-violet lamps but is exact only if the lamp used is small compared with the distance from the lamp to the skin. To calculate times and distances, doubling the distance will reduce the intensity 4 times. Therefore if the lamp were positioned at

18 in (45 cm) from the body for 1 minute, or
36 in (90 cm) from the body for 4 minutes,

the same effect would be produced.

Infra-red rays

Infra-red rays are electromagnetic waves and extend from 400,000 to 779 nanometres and infra-red (IR) radiation can be divided into near IR

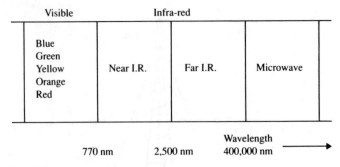

Fig. 36.6 Near and far infra-red

which is nearer to the visible part of the electromagnetic spectrum and far IR which is further away from the visible spectrum (see Fig. 36.6).

There are in the main two types of lamp, a radiant heat lamp radiating near IR from a luminous source and an IR lamp radiating far IR from a non-luminous source.

Infra-red produced by a non-luminous source rarely emits visible light and is generally known as 'pure' infra-red. There are several varieties of lamp but usually the filament is a core of black fire clay with a wire, acting as an element, embedded in it. It is connected to the circuit by a screw-cap device and placed in the centre of a spherical reflector. This is usually mounted on a stand and its position can be adjusted as required. Most lamps have a wire guard to prevent inadvertent contact with the element. All non-luminous elements need time to heat up to reach maximum intensity and this usually takes from five to ten minutes. These are the longest rays and are less penetrating than those of the luminous source, but have a soothing effect on the skin.

Radiant heat is produced by rays emitted from a luminous source, usually by an incandescent lamp which consists of an airless bulb inside which is a filament. The latter is usually made of tungsten as this material permits repeated heating and cooling. The element is visible and the lamp produces a few ultra-violet rays as well as infra-red rays. These rays are shorter and penetrate to the deeper parts of the dermis. As the skin absorbs the rays a chemical reaction takes place which may have an irritating effect. However, most lamps have a red glass filter which eliminates this. Light and heat are produced immediately they are switched on. The glass of the lamp becomes very hot and should not be touched as a burn could result. Care should be taken to ensure that the lamp is not knocked or splashed with water otherwise it may explode.

Method of use of lamps

1. If using 'pure' IR, turn the lamp to face the wall or away from the client and switch it on.
2. Touch the skin before the treatment to feel if it is hot or cold as this

will determine the distance of the lamp from the skin and the amount of time to be given.

3. Prepare the client as for a facial treatment and place dry cotton wool over the eyes. Alternatively cotton wool dampened with boracic lotion may be used.

4. If using radiant heat, switch on the lamp and explain to the client the effect of the lamp. A comfortable warmth only should be felt.

5. Direct the lamp on to the client so that the rays are at an angle of 90° to the skin at the distance required. This can range from 18 in to 30 in (45–75 cm) and is measured from the post protuberant part of the client, i.e. the tip of the nose. The distance should be recorded for reference at future treatments.

6. Set the timer or watch for five to ten minutes depending on skin type, i.e. no more than five minutes for a sensitive skin.

7. Never leave the client, and watch for any skin irritation.

8. When the treatment has been completed, switch off the lamp and move it away from the client.

9. It is preferable for keep the client warm for a few minutes after the treatment.

Safety precautions

1. Make sure that lamp reflectors are bright, clean, free of dust and that they are also free of dents. Dents in a reflector will cause over concentration at the point and results in 'hot-spots' which can cause burns.

2. Ensure that the client is not wearing jewellery.

3. Do not allow the client to touch the lamp.

4. Place the reflector at right-angles to the skin.

5. Ensure that there are no trailing flexes and the lamp is in a stable position.

6. Do not place the lamp directly over the client, it could shatter or fall and this could cause shock or injury.

Benefits of infra-red rays

- IR has a sedative effect on sensory nerve endings, relieves pain, stiff muscles and joints
- heats and relaxes the skin locally
- dilates blood vessels and increases lymph flow
- increases sweat and oil in the skin, thus aiding elimination of waste products and desquamation
- can be used to dry out face masks

Contra-indications

- infectious skin diseases or skin disorders
- inflamed areas
- cuts or wounds where bleeding can occur, e.g. varicose veins
- epileptics

- diabetics
- spastics
- respiratory diseases
- sunburn or hypersensitive skin
- loss of skin sensation
- metal plates or pins in the body

Ultra-violet rays

Ultra-violet rays are electromagnetic waves with wavelengths of between 100 nm and 400 nm and, just as IR is divided into near and far, the UV wavelength is divided into UVA, UVB and UVC (Fig. 36.7).

UVA (315–400 nm) waves are the longest wavelengths, closest to visible light and can penetrate the epidermis and the deeper layer of the skin, the dermis. They cause the skin to brown without burning.

UVB (280–315 nm) waves are considered the medium wavelengths, penetrating the epidermis and dermis, and stimulating the pigmentation of the skin. These are termed biotic rays being beneficial to life.

UVC (100–280 nm) waves are the shortest wavelengths and are absorbed in the superficial epidermis. These are termed abiotic rays as they are inimical to life. However, they do produce a germicidal effect.

The effect of ultra-violet rays

Erythema

All these rays can produce erythema but they are not all equally effective. Ultra-violet radiation, when absorbed in the skin, causes chemical actions which result in an irritation and destruction of cells. This in turn causes the release of a histamine-like substance called the 'H' substance which can dilate the blood vessels to the extent that reddening and swelling known as inflammation occurs. An excessive dose of UV exposure causes the skin to become very red, hot and sore, with exudation of fluid into the area resulting in swelling (or oedema) of the skin. The fluid then separates the stratum lucidum from the stratum granulosum and a blister is formed.

There are four degrees of erythema:

1st degree There is a mild reddening of the skin which should fade within twenty-four hours. There is no irritation or soreness.

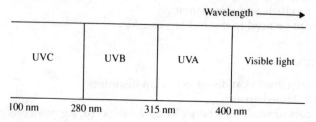

Fig. 36.7 Ultra-violet radiation

2nd degree   This is where a more marked reddening of the skin is seen with some slight irritation. It fades in two or three days but often this is followed by a fine, powdery peeling of the skin (desquamation).

3rd degree   There is a marked reddening of the skin which becomes hot, sore and oedematous with severe irritation. The erythema lasts for about a week, followed by considerable peeling of the skin.

4th degree   This is very similar to the third-degree reaction, except that blisters form.

Desquamation

Once erythema has subsided the superficial dead cells of the skin, which were destroyed by the ultra-violet rays, are shed. This is followed by an increase in the reproduction of the growth cells in the stratum germinativum which leads to a thickening of the epidermis.

Pigmentation

UVB rays penetrate the epidermis and the chemical reaction which results converts amino acid tyrosine into the pigment melanin. The degree of pigmentation varies in differing individuals (as outlined in Chapter 8).

Vitamin D formation

UVB rays also cause a chemical reaction with the ergosterol (a sterol or a chemical impurity found in the cholesterol contained in sebum) in the skin to form ergocalciferol, Vitamin D_2. Another constituent of sebum is 7-dehydrocholesterol and the chemical reaction of the UV rays converts this into Vitamin D_3. Vitamin D is necessary for the normal absorption of calcium and phosphorous into the bloodstream.

Increased blood supply to the skin

With the increased blood supply to the skin more oxygen and food-stuffs are made available and the condition of the tissue is improved. The body's resistance to infection is increased as the UV rays cause the reticulo-endothelial cells in the deep epidermis to be more efficient. The increased blood supply increases the number of white cells and antibodies which is beneficial when there is a presence of bacteria.

Tonic effect

It has been said the UV irradiation can produce a tonic effect whereby appetite and sleep are improved and nervousness, tiredness and irritability are decreased. This is certainly true of natural sunlight but there is no definite evidence of this effect by lamps or tubes.

Photosensitivity

This mainly concerns certain drugs or foods which increase the sensitivity of the skin where ultra-violet light is applied and which are included under 'Contra-indications' at the end of this chapter. It is important to obtain information from the client to avoid any adverse

---

SUN BED QUESTIONNAIRE

Client's Name: ....

Address: ....   Tel:...............................

....

Skin colour: .... Hair colour: ....

| Answer: Yes   or   No

1. Have you ever had any adverse reaction to sunlight
   other than normal sunburn?
2. In natural sunlight do you:-
   a). Always burn and never tan?
   b). Always burn and sometimes tan?
   c). Sometimes burn and always tan?
   d). Never burn and always tan?
3. Do you ever suffer from cold sores?
4. Have you ever had skin cancer?
5. Do you wear contact lenses?
6. Are you currently taking a contraceptive pill?
7. Have you any reason to believe you may be pregnant?
8. Have you recently undergone an operation?
9. Have you had an X-ray within the last 3 months?
10. Are you currently receiving any form of medical treatment?
    If YES, please give details ....

....

Please note:- If your answer to any question is YES you must see
your therapist before using the sun bed equipment.

I have understood the above questions and answered them to the best
of my belief and accept full responsibility for the sun bed treatment.

Signed: ....   Signed:...............................
                 Client   Therapist

Date:...

Fig. 36.8 Sun-bed questionnaire

reaction, i.e. excessive erythema, a rash, headaches or nausea. The use
of a form (Fig. 36.8) is helpful.

Use of UV lamps

UV lamps are supplied with elements either on a stand or suspended
from the ceiling, i.e. solariums. UV tanning should be given slowly,
otherwise blistering will occur. In giving a tanning be guided by Table
36.1.

Table 36.1 UV treatment times

Normal skin		Sensitive skin	
Session	Time	Session	Time
1st and 2nd	1 min.	1st and 2nd	30 secs.
3rd and 4th	1 min. 30 secs.	3rd, 4th, 5th	1 min.
5th and 6th	2 mins.	6th and 7th	1 min 30secs.
7th	2 mins. 30 secs.	8th	2 mins.
8th	3 mins.	9th	3 mins.
9th	4 mins.	10th	4 mins.
10th	5 mins.	11th	5 mins.
11th	6 mins.	12th	6 mins.
12th	7 mins.		

If you are in any doubt at all, give an actinic test, e.g. cut two strips of light cardboard – one 10 in × 5 in (25 cm × 12 cm) and another piece slightly smaller. Make four holes equidistant about 1 in (2.5 cm) in diameter in the larger piece. Sticky-tape this to the buttocks and slide the smaller piece of cardboard underneath the larger piece, exposing one hole. Expose this aperture to UV for 30 seconds, slide the cardboard to expose the second aperture for 30 seconds and likewise for the third and fourth holes. This will mean that

the 1st aperture has had UV for 2 mins
the 2nd aperture has had UV for 1.30 secs
the 3rd aperture has had UV for 1 min
the 4th aperture has had UV for 30 secs

Ask your client to return the following day to examine the skin.

Use of sun-beds

These are used extensively. Normally they are modified couches containing a series of low-pressure mercury vapour (LPMV) tubes. In modern equipment the short UVC and UVB rays have been cut out or cut down completely to produce mainly UVA with the possibility of a little UVB included. Sun-beds are considered the safest way to obtain an artificial tan but there are safety precautions to be observed.

1. Ensure that the client does not exceed the recommended time because erythema is possible, especially if your equipment has a minimal amount of UVB rays.
2. Advise the client to wear the same clothing each treatment time to avoid any erythema reaction on under-exposed areas.
3. Check that the area where the sun-bed is situated is well ventilated to prevent a build-up of heat.
4. Ensure that the client wears goggles and it is also advisable for the therapist to wear some form of eye protection. Some manufacturers state that this is not necessary but where light is reflected, ultra-violet is also likely to be reflected.
5. Regularly check all electrical safety precautions, i.e. wiring, plugs, overhead canopy, straps and the tubes. Some models have a digital

monitor for the number of hours the tubes have been used but if the sun-bed does not have this facility a daily record should be kept. This is important as waste deposits build up in the tubes, so lessening the intensity.

6. It is inadvisable to give a client a sun-bed immediately after a sauna, steam bath or any other form of heat treatment as ultra-violet exposure will mean that the reaction of the skin is increased.

General method of use

1. Take off all jewellery.
2. Preferably shower before use, but all make-up, perfume, colognes and pre- or after-shave lotions must be removed.
3. No suntan lotion or preparation to be applied unless recommended by the manufacturer of the sun-bed.
4. Ensure that contact lenses are removed.
5. Ensure that the skin is completely dry.
6. Check that the sun-bed is operating efficiently and ensure that it is hygienically cleaned after every client, i.e. use a diluted solution of disinfectant and wash thoroughly with clean water and dry. Surgical spirit will damage the acrylic surface. Constant client handling of the edge of the sun-bed will cause a build-up of oily matter. This should be cleaned well frequently.
7. Lay down disposable floor covering for each client.
8. Protective eye wear – goggles – to be worn for both client and operator.
9. The first session should not exceed fifteen minutes. Check at the next session to see if there are any adverse reactions before increasing the tanning time. Depending on the skin type, five minutes may be added each time with a maximum of thirty minutes per session.
10. Advise that sessions should be at least twenty-four hours apart. When the client has developed a satisfactory tan, sessions should be given once a month.
11. Use a timer or watch to ensure that the client is not given more than the prescribed exposure.
12. Advise the client not to get up quickly, otherwise fainting may result.
13. Moisturiser may be applied to the face and body.
14. All cleaning materials and waste paper to be placed in a bin with a close-fitting lid.

Keeping records
For the client:

    date of session
    period of time
    any adverse reactions
    progress

The therapist should keep records of the number of hours the sun-bed is used each day, i.e. potency life of the tubes.

Contra-indications

1. pregnancy
2. X-ray, radio therapy or chemotherapy within the last six months
3. cancerous skin conditions or operations (mastectomy or hysterectomy)
4. arteriosclorosis, elderly clients, kidney or liver disease, heart disease or high or low blood pressure (without doctor's consent)
5. recent scar tissue or open cuts or wounds to be covered with a towel or dressing
6. migraine (ultra-violet may cause headaches)
7. nervous disorders (i.e. shingles)
8. epilepsy (flickering light may cause fits)
9. cold sores (these will be aggravated)
10. eye conditions (glaucoma or cataracts)
11. thyroid condition or diabetes (this may cause irritating symptoms and itching)
12. pulmonary tuberculosis
13. dermabrasion or skin peeling
14. not before or after depilatory waxing, electrolysis, epilation, unless area is covered
15. certain drugs which are known to cause photosensitivity:

Antibiotics:

tetracyclines	e.g. Achromycin
sulphonamides	e.g. Bactrim, Septrim, Flagyl
naladixic	e.g. Negram
ozytetracycline	e.g. Bergmycen

Anti-depressants, sedatives and tranquillisers (only certain groups):

lithium	e.g. Camcolit
amitriptyline	e.g. Limbitrol, Lentizol
prochloroperazine	e.g. Stemetil, Vetigon
thioridazine	e.g. Mellerill
chlorpromazine	e.g. Largactil
trimpramine	e.g. Surmontil
promazine	e.g. Sparine
fluphenazine	e.g. Modecate, Moditen, Motipress, Motival
trifluoperazone	e.g. Stelazine

Diuretics:

cyclopenthiazide	e.g. Navidrex, Navidrex K
bendrofluazide	e.g. Neo-naclex
hydrochlorothiazide	e.g. Moduretic

Hypoglycaemics (for diabetes):

insulin and oral medication

Infections and infestations:

demeclocycline hydrochlor	e.g. Ledermycin

oxtetracycline   e.g. Terramycin
griseofulvin   e.g. Fulcin, Grisovin

16. drugs which may cause a reaction:

thyroid and antithyroid	e.g. Eltroxin, Tertroxin
antimalarials	e.g. Quinine and derivatives, Nivaquine, Daraprim

17. *photosensitisers* which may cause a reaction:

eosin	e.g. lipstick
hormone replacement pills	e.g. Premarim, Primolut N
contraceptive pills	e.g. Loestrin 20 or 30, Gynovlar 21 (these may cause chloasma)
aromatic oils	e.g. Bergamot (perfume) cedar oil citron oil clover fennel lavender oil sandalwood (perfume)
certain foods	e.g. angelica carrots celery eggs mustards parsley parsnips shellfish (i.e. lobster) strawberries

Self assessment

- what is normal body temperature in Fahrenheit and how would you convert this to Celsius?
- describe the meaning of velocity
- what is the difference between refraction and reflection of rays?
- explain the inverse square law and say why it is important to understand this when being used for either infra-red or ultra-violet treatments
- explain the difference between near and far infra-red rays
- give the method of using near infra-red and the precautions you would take when using this lamp
- what are the four degrees of erythema?
- what precautions would you take before giving a sun-bed treatment?
- state the general contra-indications to a sun-bed treatment

Appendix 1 Glossary of chemicals used in cosmetic products

acetates Esters formed by the reaction of an alcohol with acetic acid. They are often sweet and fruity smelling.

Amyl, butyl and ethyl acetates are all used as solvents in nail polish removers.

acetone A ketone; it is used in nail polish removers but it is very drying and highly inflammable.

AHA or **alpha hydroxy acids** The alpha hydroxy acids are lactic, citric, glycolic, tartaric and salicylic acid. They are found in fruit juices and are commonly called fruit acids.

alcohols Simple organic compounds containing an OH group. They are frequently used in cosmetics; ethyl alcohol, isopropyl alcohol are liquids used as solvents, cetyl alcohol and stearyl alcohol are waxy solids used to add viscosity and texture to skin-care products. Alcohol is a term commonly used for **ethanol**.

aldehydes Aldehydes are organic compounds; formaldehyde is a powerful biocide but no longer used in cosmetics. Some aldehydes find use in perfumery, benzaldehyde has a strong odour reminiscent of almonds.

almond oil, sweet Only the sweet almond oil is used in cosmetics, it is the oil obtained from the nut of the almond tree, *Prunus communis*. It is an excellent emollient oil and resistant to rancidity, hence its use as a carrier oil in aromatherapy.

aluminium silicate Silicates are natural minerals and many variations are obtained from around the world including **bentonite** and **kaolin**.

antimony sulphide Kohl which is used in eye-liner pencils.

astringent Describes compounds which have a tightening effect on the skin, e.g. ethanol and aluminium chlorhydrate.

avocado pear oil A rich, viscous oil obtained from the pear of the avocado tree, *Persea gratissima*. It is rich in vitamins A and B and highly prized in skin care and aromatherapy for its reputed cosmetic benefits.

beeswax The wax is obtained from the honeycomb, purified and bleached to make it suitable for cosmetic use. It was long used as an emulsifier in conjunction with borax, the original cold cream formulation, but is now more often used to add texture and body to cream and to stiffen lipsticks.

bentonite A mineral thickener used in face masks. True bentonite is only found as a mineral deposit in Wyoming in the USA.

benzalkonium A cationic surfactant with biocidal properties. It is used as a surface antiseptic and may be used as a preservative in eye products.

carbomer   A gelling agent and also used as an emulsion stabiliser.

ceteareth–20   A non-ionic emulsifier used in the preparation of cosmetic creams and lotions.

chitin   A generic term describing the shell material of various marine crustacea. It is a polysaccharide and the second most abundant material found in nature after cellulose. It has strong moisture retention properties but because of its insolubility it is chemically modified before use as a moisturiser and film former in cosmetics.

cocoamphocarboxyglycinate   A very mild surfactant sometimes used in eye make-up removers.

colours and **CI numbers**   The last items on a coloured cosmetic's list of ingredients are prefixed with the letters CI followed by a numerical code. These are the colours which may be dyestuffs or pigments. Dyestuffs are either water soluble or oil soluble and are mostly used in minute quantities to colour the product for aesthetic reasons. Many of these colours are also found in food. Pigments are insoluble materials, often synthetic derivatives of iron oxide or they may be organic colours absorbed on to insoluble substrates of aluminium hydroxide or a barium or zirconium salt; these colours are termed 'lakes'. Pigments and lakes are used in decorative make-up and their quality and usage is strictly controlled by legislation. CI refers to Colour Index and the actual colour being used may be found by reference to its CI number.

diatomaeous earth   A fine powder originating from ancient deposits of plankton shell and may be used as an **exfoliant**.

emollients   A term used to describe oils which have a skin softening effect.

emulsifiers   Binding agents which are used to combine the incompatible components of a cosmetic product together to form a stable and consistent product.

emulsions   A fine, stable dispersion of one liquid in another. Cosmetic emulsions are usually described as O/W or W/O. O/W emulsions tend to be light and cooling, such emulsions are commonly used as moisturisers. W/O emulsions are heavier and may frequently be found as night creams and water resistant sun protection products. Cleansing lotions may be either, often depending on skin type.

eosin dyes   Once used in lipsticks to stain the lips and give prolonged staying power, they tended to be sensitisers and are now seldom used.

esters   Compounds formed by reacting a fatty acid with an alcohol. They are normally oily liquids, insoluble in water and used to improve the spreading properties and reduce the greasiness of cosmetic oils.

ethanol   Also known as ethyl alcohol and often referred to as alcohol. It is the alcohol to be found in fermented vegetable material and is commonly used for its astringent properties in skin toners and as a solvent in perfumery.

exfoliants   Used to remove the outer, dead layers of the epidermis; they are usually mildly abrasive like ground nut shells and polystyrene beads.

fatty alcohols   Waxy solids used to add viscosity and texture to skin-care products.

gluceth–20 disterate   An O/W emulsifier derived from glucose. Glucose derived ingredients are increasingly popular because they come from renewable resources and are generally well tolerated by human skin.

glycerol or **glycerine**   Used as a **humectant** because of its moisture attracting properties.

grapeseed oil   A vegetable oil from the seeds of muscat raisins. It is lighter in feel and texture to many vegetable oils and relatively inexpensive. Beware of rancid notes if being used as an aromatherapy carrier oil or a massage oil.

gums, natural   Used as thickeners to build viscosity and improve the stability of cosmetic products and may also be used as hair fixatives. Once widely used, they were largely replaced by synthetic compounds but are now enjoying renewed interest in natural-based cosmetics. Commonly used ones include: Acacia, from the *Acacia* tree ('Gum Arabic'); Guar, obtained from *Cyanopsis tetragonalba*; Kuaraya, obtained from *Stericulis urens*; Tragacanth, obtained from *Astragus gummifer*.

humectants   Materials which have a strong affinity for water and are used to prevent cosmetic products and toothpaste from drying. They may also have skin moisturising properties.

isopropyl alcohol   Also called isopropanol; it is similar in nature to ethyl alcohol but has a more pungent odour. It may be used as a solvent in hair-setting lotions and as a biocide.

isopropyl mysristate   An **ester**. An oily liquid often used as a partial replacement for mineral oil to reduce greasiness. It has been implicated in comedone formation so is more often used in cleansers rather than moisturisers.

jojoba oil   Strictly speaking this is a wax, liquid at ambient temperatures, obtained from the seed of the desert plant, *Buxus chinensis*. It is remarkably resistant to oxidation and rancidity and is used as a replacement for spermaceti in cosmetics.

kaolin or **china clay**   A form of **aluminium silicate**. A fine off-white powder used in face masks for its drawing properties and ability to absorb oil-based grime.

ketones   Chemically similar to aldehydes and widely used in perfumery. Well known ketones are acetone and camphor.

lanolin   The sebum exuded from sheep and removed from the wool. Once highly regarded for its incomparable skin emollient properties, it fell into disfavour following reports of sensitisation caused by contaminants in the lanolin. Now purified forms are available it is rapidly regaining its popularity. Lanolin derivatives are perhaps the most widely used group of cosmetic materials and have not been implicated in any of the concerns attributed to lanolin itself.

liquid paraffin   Mineral-based oil from petroleum products.

magnesium aluminium silicate   Fine volcanic clay used as a thickening agent and for suspending pigments in cosmetic products. (See also **bentonite** and **kaolin**.)

magnesium stearate   Used in face and body powders to improve adhesion to the skin. It is a better fragrance carrier than talc and is often added for this purpose to powder products.

methyl glucose sesquistearate   A W/O emulsifier derived from glucose.

methyl cellulose   A cellulose-based thickener and film former used in decorative make-up to improve adherence of the pigments to the skin. It may also be used to impart viscosity and stability to cosmetic lotions. Many other cellulose derivatives are used, all for similar purposes under differing circumstances.

mineral oil   Chemically mineral oils are hydrocarbons and are by-products of the petroleum industry. They are odourless, colourless and chemically inert. Their cosmetic usefulness is largely confined to cleansing creams and massage creams; natural oils and esters being preferred in moisturising creams and lotions. Aka white oil, liquid paraffin.

orange flower water   When the blossom of the bitter orange tree is steam distilled to yield the essential oil, neroli, the aqueous distillate contains traces of the essential oil giving it a wonderful aroma. This orange flower water may be used as a mild skin toner and as a basis for preparing face masks.

PEG–20 methyl glucose distearate   An O/W emulsifier derived from glucose.

petrolatum   Also known as petroleum jelly or Vaseline. This is a pale unctuous mass used to impart an occlusive film in some skin-care products, or it may be used by itself to cover burns or to act as a skin protectant.

polymer   Formed when molecules of the same substance combine with themselves; plastics, most hair fixatives and resins are polymers.

polysorbate–20   A non-ionic emulsifier and solubilising agent.

potassium hydroxide   A strong alkali used to neutralise a fatty acid to form soap. Sodium hydroxide is similar in nature and use.

propylene glycol   A humectant and moisturiser.

polyvinyprrolidone (or **PVP**) A synthetic polymer used as a film former and hair fixative, it also has some moisturising properties when used in skin care.

potassium undecylenoyl   An antiseptic often used in foot drops.

rose water   When rose petals are steam-distilled to yield rose oil the aqueous distillate contains traces of the essential oil. This rose water may be used as a mild skin toner and as a basis for preparing face masks.

sodium lactate   Used in conjunction with lactic acid to buffer skin toners to match the natural pH of the skin's acid mantle, it also has moisturising properties.

solvent   A liquid in which another material may be dissolved. Thus acetone is a solvent for nail polish, ethanol is a solvent for perfume oils.

sorbitol   A humectant and moisturiser which may be obtained from sugar although it is usually prepared synthetically.

surfactant   Also known as surface active agents. These are materials which have the capacity to decrease the surface tension of liquids. The term embraces emulsifiers and detergents.

talc A naturally mined clay consisting of magnesium silicate and much used in body powders and face powders because of its slip and lubricity.

titanium dioxide Synthetic pigment of intense whiteness. It is used in decorative make-up for producing the correct shades and adding opacity to the product.

tocopherol acetate Vitamin E; a naturally occurring antioxidant.

triclosan An active ingredient which acts as an anti-bacterial agent.

triethanolamine A mild alkali often used in combination with stearic acid to form a soap type emulsifier, especially useful in cleansing lotions.

waxes Many natural and hydrocarbon waxes are used in cosmetic emulsions to impart body and texture to the product. They are also used in lipsticks and other make-up products. Examples:

beeswax: see separate entry.

candelilla wax: obtained from *Euphorbiaceae*, it is used in lipstick and other wax-based products.

carnauba wax: occurs as an exudate on the leaves of the carnauba palm *Copernica cerifera*. It is used to harden lipsticks and in anhydrous make-up.

ceresin wax: a purified ozokerite wax used to reduce greasiness in emulsions, also used in foundations, lipsticks and eyeshadows.

Japan wax: a fat expressed from the mesocarp of the fruit of *Rhus succedanea*, used in emulsions to add body and texture.

microcrystalin wax: a hydrocarbon wax with a fine crystalline structure used as an emulsion stabiliser and viscosity increasing agent.

ozokerite wax: a hydrocarbon wax used to give body and texture to emulsions, less greasy than paraffin wax and mineral oils.

paraffin wax or synthetic wax: a hydrocarbon wax with a fine crystalline structure used as an emulsion stabiliser and viscosity increasing agent. This is also used in paraffin-wax baths.

wheat-germ oil A natural oil obtained by expression from wheat germ, *Triticum vulgare*, and popular in cosmetics because of its high content of natural tocopherols.

witch-hazel Frequently used in skin toners because of its natural mild astringency, it is extracted from the leaves and bark of *Hamamelis virginiana*. It has a long history of use in the treatment of bruises and sprains.

zinc oxide A white powder used as a pigment and as a soothing agent. It is also mildly antiseptic so is used in pigment products that are used on irritated skins such as acne cover creams, post depilatory lotions and in the traditional Zinc and Castor Oil cream.

Appendix 2 Glossary of terms

abrasive silica grains   Abrasive grains consisting of a crystalline mineral compound.

agnails or **hang nails**   Where the cuticle or nail plate is split along the nail groove.

AIDS   Acquired immuno-deficiency syndrome; a virus infection

albumnoid protein   A simple water-soluble protein coagulable by heat.

allergen   A substance capable of inducing hypersensitivity.

amino-acids   The structural units from which proteins are built.

alopecia   Partial or total loss of hair.

ampere   Unit of electricity; size or intensity of current.

anaemia   Deficiency in the oxygen-carrying pigment haemoglobin in the blood.

anaphase   Stages of mitosis, duplicate chromosomes move to poles of dividing cell.

appendages   Attachments such as hair and nails are appendages to the skin.

aster   A cluster of filaments extending from each daughter centriole at the beginning of division of the nucleus of a cell.

atom   The smallest part of an element.

audio-sonic treatment   A vibrator is used to produce vibrations in soft tissue of a frequency in the range 50–100 Hz.

bacilli   Rod-shaped bacteria.

bacteria   A type of micro-organism that can be seen through a microscope.

Beau's lines   Transverse ridges across the nail plate due to a temporary interference of the formation of nail keratin.

bleaching   A method of disguising unwanted hair and fading skin discoloration.

bunion   Deformity of the bone at the side of the big toe.

burn   Damage to the skin caused by heat or strong chemicals.

bursa   A fluid containing sac or pouch, especially one located between joints or at points of friction between moving structures.

bursistis   Inflammation of a bursa.

callouses   Hard, dead skin, usually found on the ball of the foot.

cellular oxidation   A chemical reaction in the cells.

chilblains   Irritant red swellings which affect fingers, ears and feet.

chloasma   Hyperpigmentation of the skin usually on the nose and cheeks, often occurs during pregnancy.

cocci   Dot-shaped bacteria.

collagen   Principal organic fibrous constituent of connective tissue.

collagen fibres   Composed of an albumnoid protein present in the dermis.

comedo or **blackhead**   Waxy plug of sebum in the dilated orifice of a hair follicle.

compounds   Have fixed compositions; different compounds such as sugar, common salt and water can all be produced from around 100 existing elements.

conductors   Allow a free flow of electrons (i.e. an electric current) to pass through them.

conjunctivitis   Inflammation of the eyeball.

cubic   Like a cube.

cutaneous musculature   Muscles of the skin.

dehydrate   To lose moisture; become dry.

depilation   Removal of unwanted hair, by one of two methods:

   Chemical: using chemical depilatories (creams or pastes) to remove hair.
   Hot or cool wax: using types of heated wax to remove hair.

dermatitis   Inflammation of the skin caused by an external agent.

dermatosis   Any disorder of the skin.

desquamate   To shed, peel or come off in scales.

diffusion through the 'pores'   To pass through to the surface of the skin.

diplococci   Bacteria formed in pairs.

direct high frequency   HF current applied to the skin through a glass electrode.

DNA   Deoxyribonucleic acid; genetically inherited information required for the maintenance of cells and their reproduction.

earth wire   Safety device in electrical appliances and cables designed to prevent electric shock.

ectoparasite   Animal parasite living outside the body or just beneath the surface of the skin.

eczema   Inflammation of the skin with itching.

effleurage   Stroking massage movement.

electrolyte   A compound which exists as ions in water and able to conduct an electric current.

electrodes   Metal conductors.

electromagnetic waves   Produced by the movement and change of speed of electrons.

elements   In electro-physics they are the simplest substances; there are around 100 different commonly occurring elements.

EMF   Electrical pressure produced by battery or generator.

emphysema   Abnormal condition of the lungs causing laboured breathing.

endomysium   Sheath of delicate reticular fibrils surrounding each muscle fibre.

endoparasite   Animal parasite living inside the body.

enzyme   A substance, usually a protein, that can initiate or accelerate a chemical reaction.

ephelis   A freckle.

epilepsy   Characterised by sudden attacks of motor or sensory nerve malfunction with or without unconsciousness or convulsive movements.

erythma   A redness of the skin due to dilation of the blood capillaries.

erythrocytes   Red blood cells.

faradic current   An interrupted direct current used to cause muscle contraction.

fascia   A band or sheet of tissue, e.g. muscle sheath.

fibre   Thread-like structure.

flat feet   Absence of the normal arch of the sole of the foot.

fragilitas unguium   Brittle nails.

friction   Circular or to-and-fro massage movement.

fungi   A group of plant organisms which contain no chlorophyll, e.g. ringworm fungus.

fuses, circuit   Main fuses in the house/salon.

fuses, plug   Designed to protect the flex and its appliance.

galvanic current   Constant uninterrupted direct current used to produce chemical changes in the skin by a process called electrolysis.

galvanic iontophoresis   Introduction of ions into the body by a galvanic current.

genitals   External sex organs.

glycogen   A carbohydrate, stored or found in muscle tissue.

haem   An iron-containing compound which combines with the protein globin to form haemoglobin.

haemorrhage   Bleeding.

hallus-vulgus   A bunion.

hammer toes   Clawlike appearance of the toes.

hazard   A source of potential danger.

herpes simplex   Cold sores.

herpes zoster   Shingles.

high-frequency current A rapidly alternating current at a frequency in excess of 500,000 Hz.

hormones Glandular secretions from endocrine glands.

HPMV High-pressure mercury vapour.

hydric balance Balance of moisture in the skin.

indirect high frequency HF treatment where the client holds saturator and the therapist's hands are used for massage.

infra-red ray An electromagnetic wave with wavelength extending from 400,000 to 779 nanometres.

insensible Unnoticeable perspiration.

insulators Do not provide free electrons and so do not conduct electricity.

keratin A protein of which hair, nails and skin are composed.

keratinisation Formation of keratin.

lacunae Space or cavity, e.g. lacunae in bone contain bone cells.

lamellae Thin layers, as of bone tissue.

lentigo Pigment spot caused by increased deposition of melanin.

leucocytes White blood cells.

leukemia Proliferation of leucocytes suppressing the production of normal blood cells.

leukonychia White spots appearing on the nail plate.

melanin Dark pigment of hair and skin.

melanocyte Cell which produces melanin.

membrane Thin layer of tissue that covers a surface or divides an organ, e.g. mucous membrane.

menopause The period when menstruation ceases, usually between 45 and 50 years of age.

menstruation Monthly discharge of blood from the uterus.

metabolism The sum total of the physical and chemical processes and reactions taking place in the body.

metaphase A stage of mitosis, where chromatin is more definite in shape and forms dark rod-shaped structures.

metatarsalgia Pain in the metatarsal area.

migraine Severe headache.

milia or **whiteheads** Small, hard, pearly white raised spots in the skin caused by retention of sebum.

milliampere One thousandth of an ampere.

mitosis Reproduction or division of cells.

mixed nerves Having both sensory and motor fibres carrying impulses to and from the brain.

motor nerves Efferent nerves carrying impulses from the brain.

mycoses   Diseases caused by fungi.

naevi   Skin blemishes either cellular or vascular.

nail   The following items all relate to the nail:

Bed: lies under nail plate.
Cuticle: natural fold of overlapping epidermis.
Eponychium: extention of the cuticle at the base of the nail plate.
Free edge: part of the nail plate extending over finger/toe tip.
Grooves: furrows at the sides of the nail plate.
Hyponychium: part of the epidermis upon which the nail plate rests.
Lunula: the half-moon; the intermediate stage between the matrix and
   the nail plate.
Matrix: nail bed which extends beneath the nail root.
Perionychium: part of cuticle surrounding base of nail plate.
Plate: main body of the nail – rests on the nail bed.
Root: base of the nail.
Walls: folds of skin overlapping the sides of the nail plate.

nanometer   One thousand-millionth of a metre.

oedema   Swelling due to retention of fluid in the tissues.

oestrogen   Hormone produced chiefly by the ovaries intensified during ovulation, pregnancy and menstruation.

onychauxis   Hypertrophy (overgrowth) of the nail.

onychia   Extension of paronchyia causing inflammation of the nail bed.

onychitis   Inflammation of the matrix of the nail.

onychocryptosis   Ingrowing nails.

onychogryposis   Clawlike appearance of the nail.

onycholysis   Separation of the nail from the nail bed.

onychomycosis   Ringworm of the nail.

onychophagia   Nail biting.

onychopyma   Swelling of the nails.

onychorrhexis   Split or brittle nails.

onychosis   Term applied to any nail disease.

onychotrophia   Atrophy or wasting of the nail.

oxyhaemoglobin   Haemoglobin combined with oxygen.

parasite   A living creature that lives in or on another causing harm.

parasitic   Characteristic of a parasite.

paraffin wax   A white or colourless waxy solid mixture of hydrocarbons obtained from petroleum.

paronchyia   Infection originating in the folds of tissue surrounding the nails.

pernicious anaemia   A severe anaemia associated with the failure to absorb vitamin B12.

petrissage   Type of pressure massage.

pH A measure of acidity or alkalinity.

phenol Caustic, white crystalline compound in disinfectants.

progesterone Female hormone secreted by the ovaries prior to ovulation.

prophase First stage of mitosis, chromosomes become visible.

psoriasis Non-infectious skin condition which could result in severe scaling.

pterygium Forward growth of the cuticle on to the nail plate.

puberty Maturation in early adolescence when the individual becomes physiologically capable of sexual reproduction.

radiant heat Heat produced by infra-red rays emitted from a luminous source.

reflection Change in direction of a ray of light as it meets a surface.

refraction The deviation of a beam of light or ray as it passes from one medium to another, e.g. from air into glass.

RNA Ribonucleic acids.

saturator An electrode used during indirect high-frequency treatments.

sebum Oily secretion of the sebaceous gland.

sensory nerves Afferent nerves, carrying impulses from all parts of the body to the brain.

sphincter A circular muscle that constricts or closes a natural orifice such as the bladder.

spindle An elongated structure, wider in the middle and tapering at each end, e.g. centrosomes.

spirilla Spiral shaped bacteria.

squamous Scale-like.

squamous cell carcinoma Skin cancer.

staphylococci Bacteria formed in bunches.

sterols Unsaturated solid alcohols in the steroid group; have the properties of fat.

strata Plural of stratum, meaning layers.

streptococci Bacteria formed like string of beads.

stye Inflammation of one or more sebaceous glands of an eyelid.

synapse A point at which an impulse is transmitted from one nerve cell to another.

tapotement Percussion massage movement.

tinea Ringworm, a fungal infection of the skin.

tinea pedis Athlete's foot; ringworm of the foot.

tumours Three types of tumour are:

Viral: verrucae or warts.
Chemical: skin tags.

Naevi: epidermal and/or dermal including seborrhoeic warts and cellular naevus.

urticaria or **hives**   Raised patches or wheals on the skin caused by a temporary escape of fluid into the dermis.

UVA   Ultra-violet rays; they have wavelengths of 315–400 nm.

vacuum massage   Suction massage.

ventouses   Small vacuum cups used for facial vacuum massage.

venules   Minute veins.

verruca   A wart; a viral infection of the skin.

vertebrae   Bony segments of the spine.

virus   A minute infectious agent, smaller than bacterium, that requires susceptible host cells for multiplication and activity.

Wood's light   Light used for skin analysis and producing fluorescence of the epidermis.

Index